Thoracic Multidetector CT Comes of Age

Guest Editor

SANJEEV BHALLA, MD

RADIOLOGIC CLINICS OF NORTH AMERICA

www.radiologic.theclinics.com

Consulting Editor
FRANK H. MILLER, MD

January 2010 • Volume 48 • Number 1

SAUNDERS an imprint of ELSEVIER, Inc.

W.B. SAUNDERS COMPANY
A Division of Elsevier Inc.

1600 John F. Kennedy Boulevard • Suite 1800 • Philadelphia, Pennsylvania 19103-2899

http://www.theclinics.com

RADIOLOGIC CLINICS OF NORTH AMERICA Volume 48, Number 1
January 2010 ISSN 0033-8389, ISBN 13: 978-1-4377-1514-9

Editor: Barton Dudlick
Developmental Editor: Donald Mumford

Radiologic Clinics of North America (ISSN 0033-8389) is published bimonthly by Elsevier Inc., 360 Park Avenue South, New York, NY 10010-1710. Months of issue are January, March, May, July, September, and November. Periodicals postage paid at New York, NY and additional mailing offices. Subscription prices are USD 361 per year for US individuals, USD 545 per year for US institutions, USD 176 per year for US students and residents, USD 421 per year for Canadian individuals, USD 684 per year for Canadian institutions, USD 520 per year for international individuals, USD 684 per year for international institutions, and USD 253 per year for Canadian and foreign students/residents. To receive student and resident rate, orders must be accompanied by name of affiliated institution, date of term and the signature of program/residency coordinatior on institution letterhead. Orders will be billed at individual rate until proof of status is received. Foreign air speed delivery is included in all Clinics subscription prices. All prices are subject to change without notice. **POSTMASTER:** Send address changes to Radiologic Clinics of North America, Elsevier Health Sciences Division, Subscription Customer Service, 3251 Riverport Lane, Maryland Heights,MO63043. **Customer Service: Telephone: 1-800-654-2452** (U.S. and Canada); **1-314-447-8871** (outside U.S. and Canada). **Fax: 1-314-447-8029. E-mail: journalscustomerservice-usa@ elsevier.com** (for print support); **journalsonlinesupport-usa@elsevier.com** (for online support).

Reprints. For copies of 100 or more of articles in this publication, please contact the Commercial Reprints Department, Elsevier Inc., 360 Park Avenue South, New York, New York 10010-1710. Tel.: (+1) 212-633-3812; Fax: (+1) 212-462-1935; E-mail: reprints@elsevier.com.

Radiologic Clinics of North America also published in Greek Paschalidis Medical Publications, Athens, Greece.

Radiologic Clinics of North America is covered in *MEDLINE/PubMed (Index Medicus), EMBASE/Excerpta Medica, Current Contents/Life Sciences, Current Contents/Clinical Medicine, RSNA Index to Imaging Literature, BIOSIS, Science Citation Index,* and *ISI/BIOMED.*

Printed and bound in the United Kingdom
Transferred to Digital Print 2011

Contributors

CONSULTING EDITOR

FRANK H. MILLER, MD
Professor of Radiology; Chief, Body Imaging
Section and Fellowship Program and GI
Radiology; and Medical Director MRI, Department
of Radiology, Northwestern University Feinberg
School of Medicine, Chicago, Illinois

GUEST EDITOR

SANJEEV BHALLA, MD
Associate Professor of Radiology; Chief,
Cardiothoracic Imaging Section, Mallinckrodt
Institute of Radiology, Washington University
School of Medicine, Barnes-Jewish Hospital,
St Louis, Missouri

AUTHORS

NILA J. AKHTAR, MD
Radiology Fellow, Department of Radiology,
University Hospitals, Case Medical Center,
Cleveland, Ohio

KYONGTAE T. BAE, MD, PhD
Professor and Vice Chair, Department of
Radiology, University of Pittsburgh, Pittsburgh,
Pennsylvania

SANJEEV BHALLA, MD
Associate Professor of Radiology; Chief,
Cardiothoracic Imaging Section, Mallinckrodt
Institute of Radiology, Washington University
School of Medicine, Barnes-Jewish Hospital,
St Louis, Missouri

KRISTOPHER W. CUMMINGS, MD
Instructor, Cardiothoracic Imaging, Mallinckrodt
Institute of Radiology, Barnes-Jewish Hospital,
St Louis, Missouri

JEAN-BAPTISTE FAIVRE, MD
Department of Thoracic Imaging, Hospital
Calmette; University Lille Nord de France, Lille,
France

ROBERT C. GILKESON, MD
Professor of Radiology, Director of Cardiothoracic
Imaging, Department of Radiology, University
Hospitals, Case Medical Center, Cleveland,
Ohio

LAWRENCE R. GOODMAN, MD
Professor, Diagnostic Radiology & Pulmonary
Medicine, Department of Radiology,
Medical College of Wisconsin; Director, Section
of Thoracic Imaging, Department of Radiology,
Froedtert Memorial Lutheran Hospital, Milwaukee,
Wisconsin

FERNANDO R. GUTIÉRREZ, MD
Professor of Radiology, Cardiothoracic
Section, Mallinckrodt Institute of Radiology,
Washington University, St Louis, Missouri

ANNE-LISE HACHULLA, MD
Department of Thoracic Imaging, Hospital
Calmette; University Lille Nord de France, Lille,
France

HIROTO HATABU, MD, PhD
Clinical Director, MRI Program, Medical
Director, Center for Pulmonary Functional
Imaging, Brigham and Women's Hospital;
Department of Radiology, Center for Pulmonary
Functional Imaging, Brigham and Women's
Hospital, Associate Professor of Radiology,
Harvard Medical School, Boston,
Massachusetts

TRAVIS HENRY, MD
Mallinckrodt Institute of Radiology,
Washington University School of Medicine,
St Louis, Missouri

TRAVIS J. HILLEN, MD, MS
Clinical Fellow, Division of Diagnostic Radiology,
Section of Musculoskeletal Radiology,
Mallinckrodt Institute of Radiology, Washington
University School of Medicine, St Louis,
Missouri

CYLEN JAVIDAN-NEJAD, MD
Assistant Professor, Section of Cardiothoracic
Imaging, Mallinckrodt Institute of Radiology,
Washington University School of Medicine, St
Louis, Missouri

JANE P. KO, MD
Department of Radiology, New York University
Langone Medical Center, New York, New York

JEAN KURIAKOSE, MBBS, MRCP, FRCR
Division of Cardiothoracic Radiology,
Department of Radiology, University of Michigan
Health System, Ann Arbor, Michigan

HWA YEON LEE, MD, PhD
Associate Professor, Department of Diagnostic
Radiology, Chung-Ang University College of
Medicine, Seoul, Korea

JOSÉ A. MALDONADO, MD
Assistant Professor of Radiology, Chief,
Cardiothoracic Imaging Section, Department of
Diagnostic Radiology, University of Puerto Rico
School of Medicine, San Juan, Puerto Rico

ALAN H. MARKOWITZ, MD
Director, Heart Valve Center, Harrington-
McLaughlin Heart & Vascular Institute,
University Hospitals, Case Medical Center,
Cleveland, Ohio

MIZUKI NISHINO, MD
Staff Radiologist, Department of Radiology,
Dana-Farber Cancer Institute, Assistant
Professor of Radiology, Harvard Medical School,
Boston, Massachusetts

SMITA PATEL, MBBS, MRCP, FRCR
Department of Radiology, University of Michigan
Health System, Cardiovascular Center, Ann Arbor,
Michigan

FRANCOIS PONTANA, MD
Department of Thoracic Imaging, Hospital
Calmette; University Lille Nord de France, Lille,
France

JACQUES REMY, MD
Department of Thoracic Imaging, Hospital
Calmette; University Lille Nord de France, Lille,
France

MARTINE REMY-JARDIN, MD, PhD
Department of Thoracic Imaging, Hospital
Calmette; University Lille Nord de France, Lille,
France

BRADLEY S. SABLOFF, MD
Department of Radiology, University of Texas MD
Anderson Cancer Center, Holcombe Boulevard,
Houston, Texas

TERESA SANTANGELO, MD
Department of Thoracic Imaging, Hospital
Calmette; University Lille Nord de France, Lille,
France

NUNZIA TACELLI, MD
Department of Thoracic Imaging, Hospital
Calmette; University Lille Nord de France, Lille,
France

MYLENE T. TRUONG, MD
Department of Radiology, University of
Texas MD Anderson Cancer Center,
Holcombe Boulevard, Houston, Texas

GEORGE R. WASHKO, MD
Division of Pulmonary and Critical
Care Medicine, Brigham and Women's
Hospital; Instructor in Medicine,
Harvard Medical School, Boston,
Massachusetts

DANIEL E. WESSELL, MD, PhD
Assistant Professor, Division
of Diagnostic Radiology, Section
of Musculoskeletal Radiology,
Mallinckrodt Institute
of Radiology, Washington University
School of Medicine, St Louis,
Missouri

CHARLES S. WHITE, MD
Professor, Department of Diagnostic Radiology,
University of Maryland, Baltimore, Maryland

SEUNG MIN YOO, MD, PhD
Assistant Professor, Department of Diagnostic
Radiology, CHA Medical University Hospital,
Bundang, Korea

Contents

advances in technology have allowed for its application in realms that were previously exclusive to conventional pulmonary angiography. In this article, the authors address the use of MDCT in the evaluation of chronic thromboembolic pulmonary hypertension and pulmonary arteriovenous malformations. These examples demonstrate the potential for MDCT to expand the use of computed tomographic angiography in the evaluation of the pulmonary arteries. Technical parameters, diagnostic findings at MDCT, and therapeutic implications of such findings are discussed for each condition.

This article provides a summary of acute aortic syndrome (AAS), focusing especially on the multidetector CT technique and findings of AAS, as well as recent concepts regarding the subtypes of AAS, consisting of aortic dissection, intramural hematoma, penetrating atherosclerotic ulcer, and unstable aortic aneurysm.

Congenital vascular anomalies of the thorax represent an important group of entities that can occur either in isolation or in association with different forms of congenital heart disease. It is extremely important that radiologists have a clear understanding of these entities, their imaging characteristics, and their clinical relevance. The imaging armamentarium available to diagnose these diverse conditions is ample, and has evolved from such traditional methods as chest radiography, barium esophagography, and angiography to new modalities that include echocardiography, multidetector row CT (MDCT), and MR imaging. These imaging modalities have added safety, speed, and superb resolution in diagnosis and, as in the case of MDCT, provide additional information about the airway and lung parenchyma, resulting in a more comprehensive examination with greater anatomic coverage. This article reviews the most important congenital thoracic vascular anomalies, their embryologic foundation, clinical presentation, and imaging characteristics, especially those of MDCT.

The expanding imaging capabilities of multidetector computed tomography (MDCT) have made it an important part of the preoperative assessment of the cardiac surgery patient. Ever decreasing imaging times, superior spatial resolution, and the 3-dimensional capabilities of MDCT improve diagnosis and enhance surgical planning. Understanding the imaging advantages of MDCT enable improved outcomes in this important patient population.

With the increasing use of multidetector CT, small nodules are being detected more often. Although most incidentally discovered nodules are benign, usually the sequelae of pulmonary infection and malignancy, either primary or secondary, remains an important consideration in the differential diagnosis of solitary pulmonary nodules. This article reviews the role of imaging in the detection and characterization of solitary pulmonary nodules. Strategies for evaluating and managing solitary pulmonary nodules are also discussed.

Tracheobronchial imaging has undergone a major revolution. The improved spatial and temporal resolution has introduced newer techniques such as dynamic expiratory imaging to evaluate for tracheomalacia. This article describes these techniques and a practical approach to diagnosis of diseases of the central airways.

Expiratory high-resolution CT (HRCT) of the chest offers a powerful adjunct to inspiratory HRCT in the detection of lung diseases involving the small airways. In 2003 a clinical HRCT scan protocol was developed. It has since been used for evaluation of diffuse lung disease with suspected airway abnormalities. It provides volumetric assessment of the entire thorax at end-inspiration and at end-expiration, and allows for detailed analysis of the airway and parenchyma. It offers a powerful adjunct to inspiratory HRCT in the detection of lung diseases involving the small airways. This article explores its clinical applications for chronic obstructive pulmonary disease, bronchiectasis, and sarcoidosis. It concludes that standardization of image acquisition and post-processing in CT examinations will be necessary for the real application of quantitative data derived from volumetric expiratory HRCT to daily clinical medical practice.

Acute nontraumatic chest pain is a common presenting symptom to the emergency department. Often, it is evaluated by thin-collimation multidetector computed tomography scan (MDCT) using pulmonary embolism, aortic dissection, or coronary artery protocols. The parameters used for these protocols are very similar to those used in protocols for dedicated imaging of the musculoskeletal system. In essence, every MDCT of the chest is also a musculoskeletal examination of the chest. Familiarity with the MDCT-imaging appearance of common musculoskeletal causes of acute nontraumatic chest pain aids in interpretation of the images. This article discusses the MDCT appearance of a number of musculoskeletal causes of chest pain, including those of infectious, rheumatologic, and systemic causes.

Recent technological advances in multidetector computed tomography (CT) have led to the introduction of dual-source CT, which allows acquisition of CT data at the same energy or at 2 distinct tube voltage settings during a single acquisition.

The advantage of the former is improvement of temporal resolution, whereas the latter offers new options for CT imaging, allowing tissue characterization and functional analysis with morphologic evaluation. The most investigated application has been iodine mapping at pulmonary CT angiography. The material decomposition achievable opens up new options for recognizing substances poorly characterized by single-energy CT. Although it is too early to draw definitive conclusions on dual-energy CT applications, this article reviews the results already reported with the first generation of dual-source CT systems.

GOAL STATEMENT

The goal of the *Radiologic Clinics of North America* is to keep practicing radiologists and radiology residents up to date with current clinical practice in radiology by providing timely articles reviewing the state of the art in patient care.

ACCREDITATION

The *Radiologic Clinics of North America* is planned and implemented in accordance with the Essential Areas and Policies of the Accreditation Council for Continuing Medical Education (ACCME) through the joint sponsorship of the University of Virginia School of Medicine and Elsevier. The University of Virginia School of Medicine is accredited by the ACCME to provide continuing medical education for physicians.

The University of Virginia School of Medicine designates this educational activity for a maximum of 15 *AMA PRA Category 1 Credits*™ for each issue, 90 credits per year. Physicians should only claim credit commensurate with the extent of their participation in the activity.

The American Medical Association has determined that physicians not licensed in the US who participate in this CME activity are eligible for a maximum of *15 AMA PRA Category 1 Credits*™ for each issue, 90 credits per year.

Credit can be earned by reading the text material, taking the CME examination online at http://www.theclinics.com/home/cme, and completing the evaluation. After taking the test, you will be required to review any and all incorrect answers. Following completion of the test and evaluation, your credit will be awarded and you may print your certificate.

FACULTY DISCLOSURE/CONFLICT OF INTEREST

The University of Virginia School of Medicine, as an ACCME accredited provider, endorses and strives to comply with the Accreditation Council for Continuing Medical Education (ACCME) Standards of Commercial Support, Commonwealth of Virginia statutes, University of Virginia policies and procedures, and associated federal and private regulations and guidelines on the need for disclosure and monitoring of proprietary and financial interests that may affect the scientific integrity and balance of content delivered in continuing medical education activities under our auspices.

The University of Virginia School of Medicine requires that all CME activities accredited through this institution be developed independently and be scientifically rigorous, balanced and objective in the presentation/discussion of its content, theories and practices.

All authors/editors participating in an accredited CME activity are expected to disclose to the readers relevant financial relationships with commercial entities occurring within the past 12 months (such as grants or research support, employee, consultant, stock holder, member of speakers bureau, etc.). The University of Virginia School of Medicine will employ appropriate mechanisms to resolve potential conflicts of interest to maintain the standards of fair and balanced education to the reader. Questions about specific strategies can be directed to the Office of Continuing Medical Education, University of Virginia School of Medicine, Charlottesville, Virginia.

The faculty and staff of the University of Virginia Office of Continuing Medical Education have no financial affiliations to disclose.

The authors/editors listed below have identified no financial or professional relationships for themselves or their spouse/partner:

Nila J. Akhtar, MD; Kristopher W. Cummings, MD; Barton Dudlick (Acquisitions Editor); Jean-Baptiste Faivre, MD; Lawrence R. Goodman, MD; Fernando Gutierrez, MD; Anne-Lise Hachulla, MD; Travis J. Hillen, MD, MS; Cylen Javidan-Nejad, MD; Theodore E. Keats, MD (Test Author); Jane P. Ko, MD; Jean Kuriakose, MBBS, MRCP, FRCR; Hwa Yeon Lee, MD, PhD; José Maldonado, MD; Alan H. Markowitz, MD; Mizuki Nishino, MD; Smita Patel, MBBS, MRCP, FRCR; François Pontana, MD; Bradley S. Sabloff, MD; Teresa Santangelo, MD; Nunzia Tacelli, MD; Mylene T. Truong, MD; George R. Washko, MD; Charles S. White, MD; and Seung Min Yoo, MD, PhD.

The authors/editors listed below have identified the following financial or professional relationships for themselves or their spouse/partner:

Kyongtae T. Bae, MD, PhD is a patent holder with Covidien, AG, and Medrad, Inc.
Sanjeev Bhalla, MD (Guest Editor) is an industry funded research investigator for Medtronic.
Robert C. Gilkeson, MD is an industry funded research/investigator for Siemens Medical Systems.
Hiroto Hatabu, MD, PhD is an industry funded research/investigator for Toshiba Medical Inc.
Travis Henry's, MD spouse is employed by Genentech.
Jaques Remy, MD is a consultant for Siemens Health Care.
Martine Remy-Jardin, MD, PhD is an industry funded research/investigator for Siemens Health Care.
Daniel E. Wessell, MD, PhD is a consultant for Biomedical Systems and CareFusion.

Disclosure of Discussion of Non-FDA Approved Uses for Pharmaceutical Products and/or Medical Devices.
The University of Virginia School of Medicine, as an ACCME provider, requires that all faculty presenters identify and disclose any off-label uses for pharmaceutical and medical device products. The University of Virginia School of Medicine recommends that each physician fully review all the available data on new products or procedures prior to clinical use.

TO ENROLL

To enroll in the Radiologic Clinics of North America Continuing Medical Education program, call customer service at 1-800-654-2452 or sign up online at http://www.theclinics.com/home/cme. The CME program is available to subscribers for an additional annual fee USD 205.

Radiologic Clinics of North America

THE CLINICS ARE NOW AVAILABLE ONLINE!

Access your subscription at:
www.theclinics.com

Preface

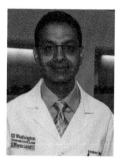

Sanjeev Bhalla, MD
Guest Editor

Over the past 2 decades, the role of computed tomography (CT) has expanded its role in the diagnosis of cardiothoracic conditions. The true potential of CT in the thorax has begun to be realized with multidetector CT (MDCT). With increasing number of detector rows, increasing number of x-ray sources, and decreasing slice thickness, we can now do clinically what was once only theoretically possible. Over the past decade, we have seen improvements in single-row, helical MDCT techniques and the emergence of new applications in cardiothoracic imaging. In the initial article, Dr Goodman beautifully provides a historical perspective on the advent of CT and its evolution over the years.

This issue of *Radiologic Clinics of North America* explores some of the ways in which MDCT has had a major impact in applications involving thorax. The authors were selected because of their passion in their chosen areas and because of their expertise. Their articles highlight applications of MDCT that allow the technology to become more than just a faster helical scanner. Some of the articles represent areas that have been improved by MDCT techniques while others discuss protocols that were never wholly realized in prior decades.

The article by Dr Bae offers a detailed discussion on contrast kinetics. As MDCT acquisition times get faster and injection rates increase, optimal contrast enhancement can be elusive. This article provides a background that should enable the practicing radiologist to tailor their protocols for their own practice.

Drs Kuriakose and Patel discuss the impact of MDCT on the pulmonary embolism (PE) protocol CT. They very nicely show how MDCT has transformed CT for PE from a novel technique to the workhorse of embolism imaging. Dr Cummings builds on the angiographic capabilities of MDCT by discussing how two additional applications of the PE protocol have helped push diagnostic angiography to more of a problem-solving technique.

Dr Yoo and colleagues truly convey the evolution in practice brought on by the use of MDCT. In their article on acute aortic syndrome, they show how MDCT has gained dominance as the diagnostic modality of choice and has challenged us by opening up possibilities for new protocols, such as the triple rule-out protocol. Dr Maldonado and colleagues also nicely show how CT has evolved from a technique to clarify vascular anomalies to the diagnostic method of choice when these entities are suspected. Postprocessing in this arena rivals surgical exposures for laying out the vascular anatomy. The anatomic detail is highlighted by Dr Akhtar and colleagues, who highlight the use of MDCT before sternotomy. At our institution, the Mallinckrodt Institute of Radiology, MDCT has almost become a prerequisite before redo median sternotomy.

Dr Truong and colleagues remind us of the approach to the solitary pulmonary nodule and provide us tips in the management of this entity in the MDCT and combination positron emission tomography–CT era. They also highlight one of the clinical problems that has plagued all of us who do routine, thin-section imaging: imaging the 4-mm ground-glass nodule. In her article, Dr Javidan-Nejad shows how MDCT has helped better understand and diagnose disease of the trachea.

Dr Nishino and colleagues highlight the role of expiratory imaging as part of the CT evaluation of

Radiol Clin N Am 48 (2010) xiii–xiv
doi:10.1016/j.rcl.2009.10.004

diffuse lung disease. With its expanded, multiplanar capability, volumetric expiratory high-resolution CT may help us better understand the physiologic insult of obstructive lung diseases.

With its isotropic and nearly isotropic data, MDCT of the thorax has blurred the line between the chest CT and a dedicated thoracic skeletal CT. Drs Hillen and Wessell remind us of this additional challenge and highlight tips useful for radiologists of all specialties.

Dr Remy-Jardin and colleagues bring into focus the frontier of dual-energy imaging and its use in the thorax. Knowledge of the potential of dual-energy imaging will enable practicing radiologists to improve their own equipment and make for more informed decision-making in the purchase of additional scanners.

As we enter the second decade of the twenty-first century and reflect on the first decade of

MDCT in clinical practice, these authors remind us that MDCT has gone from being fast CT to a whole lot more. I am indebted to their efforts in showing us the power of the modality and sharing their experience. As these protocols and articles remind us, MDCT of the thorax has come of age.

Sanjeev Bhalla, MD
Section of Cardiothoracic Imaging
Mallinckrodt Institute of Radiology
Washington University School of Medicine
Barnes-Jewish Hospital
510 South Kingshighway Boulevard
Campus Box 8131
St Louis, MO 63110, USA

E-mail address:
bhallas@mir.wustl.edu

The Beatles, the Nobel Prize, and CT Scanning of the Chest

Lawrence R. Goodman, MD[a,b,*]

KEYWORDS

- Tomography • Radiograph computed • Radiography
- Thorax • Diagnostic imaging • Imaging history

On June 6, 1962, the Beatles (Fig. 1A) had their first recording session with Electrical Musical Industries, Ltd (EMI). Their meteoric success changed the history of modern radiology and medicine forever. The money generated by record sales enabled the EMI basic science researchers to thrive in a cash-rich environment,[1–3] including the research of Dr. Godfrey Hounsfield, an electrical and computer engineer. He had spent years exploring whether back projection methods of producing an image could use differential X-ray attenuation values.

"YESTERDAY … SEEMED SO FAR AWAY"

In 1967, the first experimental computer axial tomography (CAT) scan was constructed on an old lathe, using americium as a gamma ray source.[2] The scan of a mouse took 9 days to complete. It required 2.5 hours of main frame computer time to reconstruct, but produced a recognizable image.[4] Four years later, in October of 1971, the first head scan of a living patient was performed using an EMI "Mark I" scanner.[2,4–6] The equipment used a translate-rotate gantry (step and shoot), an 80 × 80 matrix yielding a spatial resolution of 0.5 cm, and required a water bag for stabilization and normalization of the head. Reconstruction took all night but produced a recognizable image of a brain tumor. "My God, it does work!" exclaimed Hounsfield. The first EMI production model required 4 minutes per slice and 7 minutes per reconstruction. The first

description of a CAT scan in the radiology literature by Hounsfield and colleagues[4–7] was in the British Journal of Medicine in 1973.

Hounsfield apparently was unaware of prior work. In the 1960s, Dr Allan Cormack of South Africa, and later Tufts' University, a particle physicist, and Dr William Oldendorf, a Colorado neurologist, independently showed that multiple measures of radiograph attenuation around a target enabled one to compute an image of that target.[8,9] Unfortunately, without more powerful computers, there was little practical application of this concept.

Although Cormack (PhD) and Hounsfield (no formal degree) never met, and neither had a medical background or interest in medicine, both received the Nobel Prize in Physics and Medicine, in 1979, for the CAT scan, the "greatest advance in radiologic medicine since the discovery of the X-ray."[2] Cormack was cited for his math analysis that led to the CAT scan and Hounsfield for its practical development (Figs.1B and 2).[10] As CAT scans became more sophisticated, new areas of investigation opened up in radiology. Many opened up new approaches to surgery, and new understandings of medical conditions emerged.

"WITH A LITTLE HELP FROM (OUR) FRIENDS"

EMI estimated it needed to sell 25 CAT scanners worldwide to make it a commercially viable product. Others were more optimistic. Over the next few years, 18 companies, large and small,

[a] Department of Radiology, Medical College of Wisconsin, 9200 West Wisconsin Avenue, Milwaukee, WI 53226-3596, USA
[b] Section of Thoracic Imaging, Department of Radiology, Froedtert Memorial Lutheran Hospital, 9200 West Wisconsin Avenue, Milwaukee, WI 53226-3596, USA
* Department of Radiology, Medical College of Wisconsin, 9200 West Wisconsin Avenue, Milwaukee, WI 53226-3596.
E-mail address: lgoodman@mcw.edu

Radiol Clin N Am 48 (2010) 1–7
doi:10.1016/j.rcl.2009.09.008

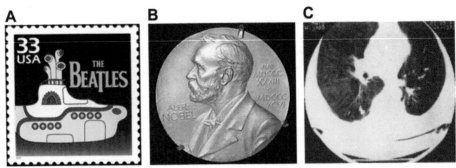

Fig. 1. (*A*) The Beatles. (*B*) The Nobel Prize Medallier. (*C*) Early chest CT scan from 1973. (Fig. 1C. *From* Sheedy PF 2nd, Stephens DH, Hattery RR, et al. Computed tomography of the body: initial clinical trial with the EMI prototype. AJR Am J Roentgenol 1976;127:23–51; with permission.)

competed for the growing scanner market. Over the first decade, many companies disappeared, leaving several major manufacturers as survivors.[9]

Gradually, computed axial tomography (CAT scanning) morphed into computed tomography (CT scanning). The first body CT scanner, which required no water bag, was developed at Georgetown Hospital by Dr Robert Ledley, a dentist (**Fig. 3**).[11] The automatic computerized transverse axial (ACTA) scanner was commercialized by Pfizer, with 30 photomultiplier tubes and a 256 × 256 matrix. The race to perform faster and better CT scans was on! Improvements in the translate-rotate scans by several manufacturers brought scan time down to 2 minutes per image (**Fig. 4**). By 1974, second-generation scanners from EMI, Ohio Nuclear, and Siemens brought scan time down to 1 minute, and then to 18 seconds (**Figs. 5** and **6**).[9,12] A 320 × 320 matrix replaced an 80 × 80 matrix.

In 1974, General Electric (GE) abandoned the translate-rotate approach and proposed a fan beam, which rotated around the patient (rotate-rotate) in synchronicity with a small curvilinear detector (300–700 elements) (see **Fig. 4**). This

was a small scanner prototype large enough to image the breast and, eventually, the head. By 1976, they produced a third-generation body scanner capable of producing 10 mm axial images with 9.5-second gantry rotation per image. Within a few years, GE and Siemens were the dominant producers of third-generation scanners.

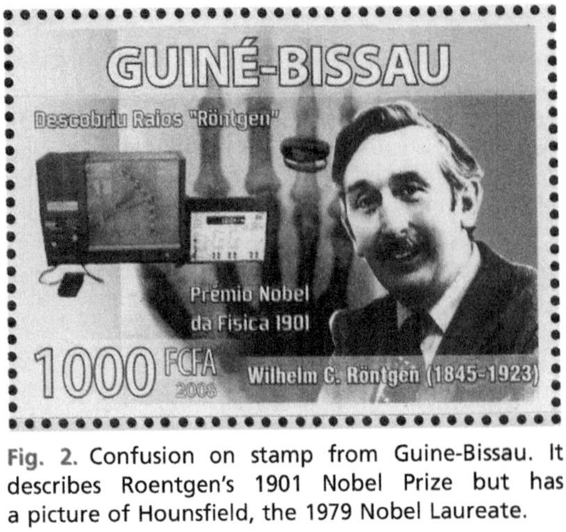

Fourth generation scanners, produced by Technicare (Johnson & Johnson), mounted a thousand stationary detectors around the gantry with a rotating radiograph tube. Technical problems eventually defeated this technique.[9,12] Imaging changed dramatically in 1989, when the first helical or spiral scanners were produced by Siemens. The tube rotated continuously as the patient moved through the gantry. Elscint produced a two-detector scanner and the multidetector race was on.

"YOU REALLY GOT A HOLD OF ME"

The life of the radiologist, and every physician, hospital, and patient, was never the same again. Although the original images were quite crude, the machinery was expensive, and validating studies were lacking, the CT scans were an instantaneous success.[1] It required only a brief look to realize that the CT scans were special and would replace many conventional techniques. By 1979, 6 years after its clinical introduction, 1,300 CT scanners were in use in the United States. By 1980, 3 million CT scans were performed and, by the year 2000, 62 million CT scans were performed annually.[1,13] With each generation of scanner, new applications arose, much of it made possible by the rapid increase in computer power and the markedly decreasing cost of memory.

The first published images of chest CT scans were in February of 1975, using the ACTA scanner.[14] Images were 7.5 mm thick and used a raster of 160 × 160. Images were displayed on a 19-in color monitor, photographed directly with a Polaroid camera, and the snapshots were archived. Later,

Fig. 2. Confusion on stamp from Guine-Bissau. It describes Roentgen's 1901 Nobel Prize but has a picture of Hounsfield, the 1979 Nobel Laureate.

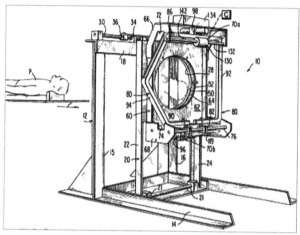

Fig. 3. Patent diagram of Ledley's 1974 ACTA scanner provided for "do it yourselfers." (U.S. patent #3,922,552; Nov 25, 1975.)

in 1976, others showed similar images obtained with EMI equipment (**Figs.** 1C, **5** and 6).[15,16] Predictions about the value of chest CT scans were mixed, "Considering that the scanning cycle takes about five minutes, one would expect that scanning of body parts containing moving organs, such as the chest and abdomen, would present a problem. However, we have been favorably impressed in particular by the quality of chest films obtained. Clear visualization of the lungs, heart, and mediastinal formations was possible."[16] Others expressed some doubt, "In the thorax, CT scans rarely surpass the diagnostic accuracy of conventional radiologic studies."[15]

"NOW MY LIFE HAS CHANGED IN OH SO MANY WAYS"

As this new expensive equipment spread, governments and insurers attempted to limit purchases. Certificates of Need were required in many states before a CT scanner could be purchased. However, the undeniable value of CT scanning—for both diagnosis and patient management—eventually overwhelmed attempts to control dissemination.[1] In the United States, in 2000, it is estimated that over 62 million CT scans were performed annually.[13] Today, approximately 30% of CT scans are of the thorax. Initially, most scanning was done

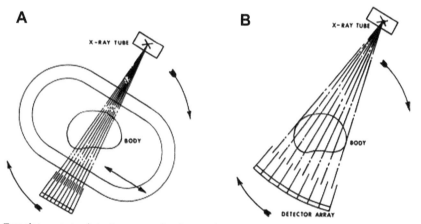

Fig. 4. (*A, B*) Translate-rotate detector versus fan beam detector. Original legends: "(A) Moving fan beam with rotation system. Fan beam produced from X-ray tube falls on X-ray detector and scans backward and forward, linearly, across the patient. At each scanning stroke, angle of scanning traverse changed by an amount equal to the angle of the fan beam. In this rotational method, all possible angles of scan across entire body will have been recorded after a 180 degree rotation. (B) Rotating fan beam system. X-ray tube produces fan beam as wide as large patient to be scanned. This was on wide array of 300 detectors. To obtain picture, assembly rotated around patient 360 degrees." (*From* Hounsfield GN. Picture quality of computed tomography. AJR Am J Roentgenol 1976;127:3–6; with permission.)[28]

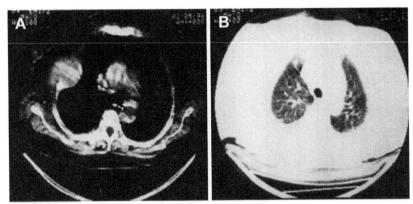

Fig. 5. Original legend: "CT scan of a 79-year-old woman who had subtotal thyroidectomy, three years earlier, for papillary adenocarcinoma. Destructive lesion had recently developed in the right third rib and in the right side of the pelvis. (A) Tomographic section through the chest revealing large destructive lesion in rib on right. Large potion of the mass projects into the chest, and tumor extends considerably into chest wall. (B) Lung parenchyma revealed after adjusting window height and width. Note tiny nodule in apex of right lung anteriorly, which was not appreciated on chest film." (EMI Body Scanner) (From Sheedy PF 2nd, Stephens DH, Hattery RR, et al. Computed tomography of the body: initial clinical trial with the EMI prototype. AJR Am J Roentgenol 1976; 127:23–51; with permission.)

for lung and mediastinal disease. With the advent of helical scanning, vascular and cardiac imaging has become a major focus. With each technical advance, new CT scan applications arose.

Lung

Initial scanning concentrated on parenchymal consolidation and tumor, as the peripheral anatomy of the lung was not well demonstrated on 10 mm slices with long breath holds (Figs. 1C, 5 and 7). With improved equipment, thinner and thinner scans became available. The first English language report of high-resolution CT (HRCT) scanning (1 mm slice every 10 mm, high-resolution algorithm) was in 1985.[17] HRCT became the hot new area in the late 1980s and 1990s. Multislice CT scanning now permits one to obtain

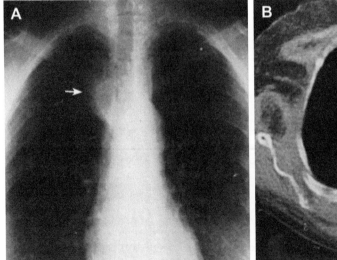
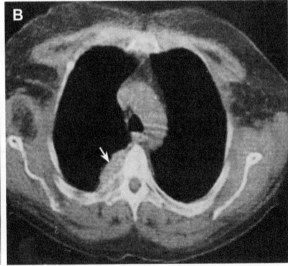

Fig. 6. Original legend. "(A) Currently asymptomatic 57-year-old with known multiple myeloma. A chest radiograph demonstrating 4 cm mass (arrow) in right posterior mediastinum. (B) CT scan showing the posterior mediastinal mass arises from contiguously destroyed posterior aspect of the right fourth rib (arrow), a manifestation of her known multiple myeloma." (EMI Body Scanner) (From Stanley RJ, Sagel SS, Levitt RG, et al. Computed tomography of the body: early trends in application and accuracy of the method. AJR Am J Roentgenol 1976; 127:53–67; with permission.)

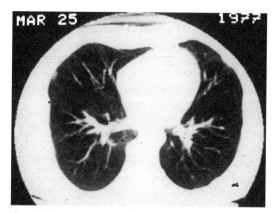

Fig. 7. CT scan on early fan beam scanner. Scan rotation time was 9.5 seconds and the slice thickness was 10 mm. (GE 5000 Scanner.)

sub-millimeter images using isotropic voxels and to perform high-quality multiplanar reconstructions. Now, lung detail and distribution of disease can be assessed at the sub-millimeter level in any plane. HRCT scanning has led to new understanding, classification, and reclassification of various forms of interstitial lung diseases and bronchial diseases. HRCT scanning has dramatically changed the way radiologists, pathologists, and clinicians diagnose and understand interstitial lung disease. As with most advances, as some areas become better elucidated, new questions arise.

Mediastinum

CT scanning was immediately embraced as the method for evaluating the mediastinum. Conventional radiographs and conventional tomography often failed to detect or adequately characterize mediastinal pathology because of lack of contrast between the normal structures and the pathologic structures (Figs. 5 and 6).[18] Because the mediastinum is less prone to respiratory motion, and intravenous contrast (administered by drip) provided sharp contrast boundaries, CT scanning rapidly became the modality of choice. It was soon touted as both sensitive and specific for staging lung cancer metastasis. With time, it was realized that CT scanning was an improvement, but fallible, for cancer staging. The recent fusion of CT and positron emission tomography scanning has overcome many of those problems.

Fast-drip intravenous contrast infusion was a valuable asset in distinguishing the major vessels from other structures, but little thought was given to using CT scans for evaluating the vessels beyond the superior vena cava and aorta. As axial imaging became faster, more detailed vascular

evaluation became possible.[19–21] Early studies of the aorta for trauma, dissection, or aneurysm were limited by motion and had limited acceptance in the radiologic and the surgical community. Aided by power injection of contrast, single-detector helical and then multidetector helical scanning, CT scanning is now the procedure of choice in the majority of patients with suspected aortic disease.

The first CT scan report on pulmonary embolism, in 1977, looked at parenchymal changes but did not even mention the visualization of intravascular clot.[22] The first mention of prospective evaluation for pulmonary embolus involved three cases using "rapid sequence of up to twelve 2.4-second scans, with a one-second delay between scans" (Fig. 8).[23] Although large pulmonary emboli could be visualized with axial CT scanning it was not until the advent of helical CT scan that large and midsized pulmonary vessels could be imaged routinely.[24] Single-detector helical scanning allowed one to scan only 12 cm of the chest in a 24-second breath hold at 5 mm intervals. Multidetector scanners shortened the breath hold to a few seconds, provided subsecond rotation time and submillimeter resolution. Helical CT scanning rapidly replaced perfusion scanning and angiography as the clinical procedure of choice and is now the gold standard.[25]

The same improvements, with 16-detector scanning and above, have made cardiac imaging and coronary artery imaging possible. Elegant 2- and 3-dimensional (D) reconstructions add a new

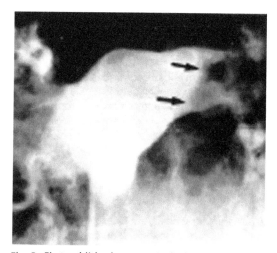

Fig. 8. First published prospectively diagnosed pulmonary embolism. 1977 Axial image using a fan beam/rotating detector with 9.5 second gantry rotation. (*From* Godwin JD, Webb WR, Gamsu G, et al. Computed tomography of pulmonary embolism. AJR Am J Roentgenol 1980;135:691–5; with permission.)

dimension. CT scanning's role is yet to be defined, as there are many competing modalities.

Lung Cancer Screening

CT scan screening for lung cancer is another recent addition to the diagnostic armamentarium. High-end scanners provide relatively low-dose images, capable of detecting even the smallest cancers.[26] Unfortunately, other clinically irrelevant nodules are seen with great frequency. The eventual role of lung cancer screening is still being debated.[27]

Other Developments

Many of the high-end applications discussed above are possible because of high quality 2D and 3D reconstruction. The development of the isotropic voxel has provided high-quality volumetric scanning and reconstruction in any two-dimensional plane or as three-dimensional images. Lung applications are numerous, including bronchiectasis and interstitial lung disease. Mediastinal and vascular applications include the trachea, the aorta, the great vessels, the pulmonary vessels, and cardiac applications—especially when gating is applied—include cardiac and coronary evaluation.

Early CT scans of the chest were 10 mm each. A chest CT scan consisted of 15 to 20 mediastinal and 15 to 20 lung images displayed on film. Now, with multidetector CT scans and routine reconstructions, such as coronal, sagittal, or maximum intensity projection pressure images, the chest CT scan is often well over 1,000 images. Picture archiving and communications systems have made it practical to view the staggering amount of data that each case presents. Computer-assisted diagnosis (CAD) offers a possibility of reducing the information overload confronting the radiologist on a daily basis. Sophisticated nodule detention and nodule quantization software promises to make these two tasks less burdensome. In addition, CAD programs, now in testing, can also detect pulmonary emboli to the subsegmental level and quantify emphysema.

"WILL YOU STILL NEED ME . . . WHEN I'M 64?"

As this article is written, the 64-slice multidetector scanner is the dominant CT scanner. Although it is a current workhorse, the industry is rapidly moving forward.

Phillips now has a functional 256-slice multidetector scanner that can provide images of the entire thorax within seconds and of the heart, in less than 2 beats. Toshiba (320 slice) can image the entire heart in one rotation. These newer scanners show the most promise for cardiac and coronary imaging and other small organ imaging. Technical limitations currently limit more general use.

Dual-energy scanning also has multiple potential applications in the lung. With dual energy, calcification can be more easily assessed and perfusion scanning of the lung is possible. This has potential applications for evaluation of pulmonary emboli and other clinical scenarios where perfusion information is helpful. Unlike nuclear studies, it provides both anatomic and functional information in the same scan. Myocardial infarct imaging, and perhaps coronary calcium removal, may be in the future. Dynamic respiratory imaging for airflow obstruction, tracheobronchial mechanics, and diaphragm motion are also possible with faster scanners.

SUMMARY

Chest CT scanning has come a long way since 1975. Anatomic images are now superb and functional imaging is in its early stages.

ACKNOWLEDGMENTS

Thanks to Dr Stanley Fox, PhD, for his historical insights, and to Mrs Sylvia Bartz, for her help in preparing this manuscript.

REFERENCES

1. Berland LL. Commentary on "Computed tomography of the body: initial Clinical Trial with the EMI Prototype" and "Computed tomography of the body: early trends in application and accuracy of the method". AJR Am J Roentgenol 2008;191:16–8.
2. Ambrose J. CT scanning: a backward look. Semin Roentgenol 1977;12:7–11.
3. The beatles. Available at: http://Wikipedia/org/wiki/beatles. Accessed August 1, 2009.
4. Ambrose J. Computerized transverse axial scanning (tomography): part 2. Clinical application. Br J Radiol 1973;46:1023–47.
5. Hounsfield GN. Computerized transverse axial scanning (tomography): part 1. Description of system. Br J Radiol 1973;46:1016–22.
6. Richmond C. Obituary. Geoffrey Newbold Hounsfield, engineer (b 1919, CBE, FRS), d 12 August 2004. BMJ 2004;329:687.
7. Perry BJ, Bridges C. Computerized transverse axial scanning (tomography): part 3. Radiation dose considerations. Br J Radiol 1973;46:1048–51.
8. Bui-Mansfield LT, Sutcliffe JB. Nobel prize laureates who have made significant contributions to radiology. J Comput Assist Tomogr 2009;33:483–8.

9. Robb WL. Perspective on the first 10 years of the CT scanner industry. Acad Radiol 2003;10:756–60.
10. Montgomery BJ. CT scanning recognized with Nobel Prize. Medical news. JAMA 1979;242:2380–1.
11. U.S. Patent #3,922,552 applied for Nov 25, 1975. Information for patent available at http://patft. uspto.gov.
12. Eisenberg RL. Computed tomography. In: Eisenberg RL, editor. Radiology, an illustrated history. St. Louis (MO): Mosby-Year Book; 1992. p. 467–77.
13. Brenner DJ, Hall EJ. Computed tomography – an increasing source of radiation exposure. N Engl J Med 2007;357:2277–84.
14. Schellinger D, Di Chiro G, Axelbaumn SP, et al. Early clinical experience with the ACTA scanner. Radiology 1975;114:257–61.
15. Stanley RJ, Sagel SS, Levitt RG, et al. Computed tomography of the body: early trends in application and accuracy of the method. AJR Am J Roentgenol 1976;127:53–67.
16. Sheedy PF 2nd, Stephens DH, Hattery RR, et al. Computed tomography of the body: initial clinical trial with the EMI prototype. AJR Am J Roentgenol 1976;127:23–51.
17. Nakata H, Kimoto T, Nakayama T, et al. Diffuse peripheral lung disease: evaluation by high-resolution computed tomography. Radiology 1985;157:181–5.
18. Mink JH, Bein ME, Sukov R, et al. Computer tomography of the anterior mediastinum in patients with myasthenia gravis and suspected thymoma. AJR Am J Roentgenol 1978;130:239–46.
19. Heiberg E, Wolverson M, Sundaram M, et al. CT findings in thoracic aortic dissection. AJR Am J Roentgenol 1981;136:13–7.
20. Heiberg E, Wolverson MK, Sundaram M, et al. CT in aortic trauma. AJR Am J Roentgenol 1983;140:1119–24.
21. Moncada R, Salinas M, Churchill R, et al. Diagnosis of dissecting aortic aneurysm by computed tomography. Lancet 1981;1:238–41.
22. Sinner WN. U.S. Patent #3, 922,552; 11/25/75. J Comput Assist Tomogr 1978;2(4):395–9.
23. Godwin JD, Webb WR, Gamsu G, et al. Computed tomography of pulmonary embolism. AJR Am J Roentgenol 1980;135:691–5.
24. Remy-Jardin M, Remy J, Wattinne L, et al. Central pulmonary thromboembolism: diagnosis with spiral volumetric CT with the single-breath-hold technique–comparison with pulmonary angiography. Radiology 1992;185:381–7.
25. Stein PD, Fowler SE, Goodman LR, et al. Multidetector computed tomography for acute pulmonary embolism. [PIOPED II]. N Engl J Med 2006;354(22):2317–27.
26. Henschke CI, McCauley DI, Yankelevitz DF, et al. Early lung cancer action project: overall design and findings from baseline screening. Lancet 1999;354:99–105.
27. Unger M. A pause, progress, and reassessment in lung cancer screening [comment]. N Engl J Med 2006;355:1822–4.
28. Hounsfield GN. Picture quality of computed tomography. AJR Am J Roentgenol 1976;127:3–6.

Optimization of Contrast Enhancement in Thoracic MDCT

Kyongtae T. Bae, MD, PhD

KEYWORDS

- Contrast agents • Intravenous • CT technology
- Optimization • MDCT • Thorax

Many clinical applications of thoracic computed tomography (CT) require contrast medium to enhance and delineate vascular, mediastinal, hilar, and cardiac structures, and differentiate normal and pathologic vascular or tumoral conditions. Multidetector row computed tomography (MDCT) is superior to single-detector row CT (SDCT) because MDCT permits more efficient and flexible use of intravenous contrast medium to achieve enhancement. However, to fully reap the benefits of MDCT contrast enhancement, the technical challenges associated with optimizing enhancement and scan timing in MDCT need to be solved. This article reviews the basic principles of CT contrast enhancement and discusses common clinical considerations and the protocol design modifications that are necessary to achieve optimal contrast enhancement in thoracic MDCT.

IODINE AND CT ATTENUATION

Iodine in blood vessels and organs will increase the absorption and scattering of x-rays within these structures and present stronger x-ray attenuation (CT contrast medium enhancement) on the CT images. The degree of CT contrast enhancement is directly related to the amount of iodine within the system and the level of x-ray energy (tube voltage). For a given voltage, the proportionality of contrast enhancement to iodine concentration is near constant,[1] typically in the range of 25 to 30 HU per 1 mg I/mL at 100 to 120 kVp. At a lower peak voltage, the proportionality is higher, yielding stronger contrast enhancement per iodine concentration (40 HU per 1 mg I/mL at 80 kVp).

Therefore, to achieve the same degree of contrast enhancement, substantially less contrast medium is required with a tube voltage of 80 kVp than with 120 kVp.[2] However, to keep the image noise constant, the tube current should be increased using a low tube-voltage protocol rather than a high tube-voltage protocol.

CT CONTRAST MEDIUM PHARMACOKINETICS

As contrast medium circulates throughout the body, it is diluted by the blood and the bolus disperses as it moves downstream through the circulatory system. The effect of dilution is greater in organs more distal from the injection site (typically antecubital vein). The contrast enhancement profile broadens with a flattened peak in the downstream circulation. The circulation of contrast medium throughout the body is mainly governed by hemodynamic physiology, but the injected contrast medium may affect and disturb the hemodynamics of the cardiovascular system.[3] In particular, a slow intrinsic peripheral venous blood flow would be perturbed and accelerated by a fast, large bolus of contrast medium injected with a power injector. As a result, contrast enhancement peaks higher and narrower with shortened contrast arrival and peak contrast enhancement times (Fig. 1). Peak aortic enhancement occurs earlier than the temporal sum of the injection duration plus T_{arr} (contrast arrival time). When contrast medium is considered as a pharmaceutical injected intravenously, its in vivo concentration can be predicted by using a physiologically based computer model developed from the

Department of Radiology, University of Pittsburgh, 3362 5th Avenue, Pittsburgh, PA 15213, USA
E-mail address: baek@upmc.edu

Radiol Clin N Am 48 (2010) 9–29
doi:10.1016/j.rcl.2009.08.012
0033-8389/09/$ – see front matter

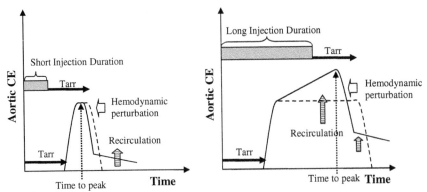

Fig. 1. Time-enhancement curve diagrams illustrating the effect of the injection duration and hemodynamic perturbation on peak contrast enhancement. In a theoretic physiologic model without recirculation or hemodynamic perturbation, aortic contrast enhancement would show a rapid increase and then a uniform steady-state plateau (a flat broad peak). The time to the end of the plateau enhancement corresponds to the sum of the injection duration plus T_{arr} (contrast arrival time). In reality, however, a fast large bolus of contrast medium affects and perturbs the hemodynamics of the cardiovascular system, particularly the slow peripheral venous blood flow. This will result in hastening the contrast arrival as the contrast bolus increases. Because of this effect and recirculation, the steady-state plateau contrast enhancement cannot be sustained and becomes elevated and compressed, resulting in a higher and narrower peak contrast enhancement. The time to peak aortic enhancement becomes shorter than the sum of the injection duration plus T_{arr}.

pharmacokinetics.[1] This model was used to simulate the time-enhancement curves presented in this article.

FACTORS AFFECTING CONTRAST ENHANCEMENT

The principal factors affecting contrast medium enhancement in CT imaging can be grouped into 3 categories: the patient, the contrast medium, and the CT scan. Contrast pharmacokinetics and contrast enhancement are solely determined by the patient and contrast medium factors and are independent of the CT scanning technique. CT scanning factors, however, play a critical role by permitting the acquisition of enhanced images at a specific time point of contrast enhancement. Many patient and contrast medium factors are interconnected and contribute to the final distribution of contrast medium and ultimately, the enhancement. Some of these factors are more influential on the *magnitude*; others are more prominent on the *temporal pattern* of contrast enhancement.

Patient Factors

The key patient-related factors affecting contrast enhancement are body size (weight and height) and cardiac output (cardiovascular circulation time). Other less influential factors include age, gender, venous access, renal function, hepatic cirrhosis, portal hypertension, and various other pathologic conditions.

Body weight, mass, and surface area

The most important patient-related factor affecting the magnitude of vascular and parenchymal contrast enhancement is body weight.[4–8] For a given dose of contrast medium, the magnitude of contrast enhancement decreases proportionally with increase in the patient's weight (**Fig. 2**). Thus,

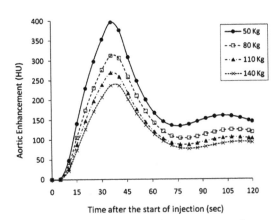

Fig. 2. Simulated thoracic aortic contrast enhancement curves with 4 different body weights. Simulated enhancement curves were based on a hypothetical adult male (60 years old, height 170 cm) with 4 different body weights (50, 80, 110, and 140 kg), subjected to the same injection of 120 mL of 370 mg I/mL contrast medium at 4 mL/s. The magnitudes of contrast enhancements are inversely proportional to the body weight. To achieve a consistent degree of enhancement, larger amounts of contrast medium are required in heavier patients.

when a consistent contrast enhancement is desired, the amount of iodine should be adjusted for the body weight; a large patient will require more iodine load than a small patient to achieve the same magnitude of enhancement.

One simple method for calculating the amount of iodine mass for the body weight uses a 1:1 linear scale (doubling the iodine mass when the patient's body weight doubles).[5] This direct body weight–based linearity may not, however, provide an accurate adjustment of the required contrast medium dose for body size, particularly in obese patients. Patients with a lot of body fat that is not metabolically active contribute little to dispersing/diluting the contrast medium in the blood. Thus, the 1:1 linear weight-based dosing may overestimate the amount of contrast medium required. To overcome this limitation of 1:1 linear weight-based iodine dosing, other body size parameters such as lean body weight (LBW)[9–11] and body surface area (BSA)[12] were proposed. Three recent studies[9–11] reported a consensus that LBW is a better body size adjustment index than total body weight and that iodine dose calculated from LBW resulted in more consistent contrast enhancement with less inter-patient variations. Another recent study[12] reported that the BSA provides a better adjustment of iodine dose for a wide range of body sizes than body weight. Because the BSA is directly related to weight $(kg)^{0.65}$,[13] this nonlinear weight-scaling can be used as a proportionality to adjust the contrast medium dose for body size, instead of the traditional linear 1:1 proportionality.

Cardiac output and cardiovascular circulation

The most important patient-related factors affecting the timing of contrast enhancement are cardiac output and cardiovascular circulation.[14] When cardiac output decreases, the circulation of the contrast medium slows. This results in a delayed contrast bolus arrival and peak enhancement and a slow clearance of contrast medium from the circulation (**Fig. 3**). The time of contrast bolus arrival and the time to peak enhancement in all organs are highly correlated with, and linearly proportional to, the reduction in cardiac output.[14,15] Thus, when scan timing is critical for CT imaging, scan delay should be individualized for each organ using a test-bolus or bolus-tracking technique. A slower clearance of contrast medium caused by a reduced cardiac output or circulation results in a stronger, prolonged contrast enhancement.

Contrast Medium Factors

The key contrast medium factors related to contrast enhancement include injection duration,

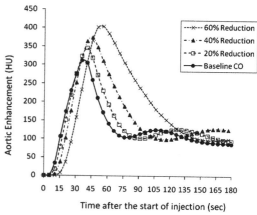

Fig. 3. Simulated thoracic aortic contrast enhancement curves at baseline and reduced cardiac outputs. Simulated enhancement curves were based on a hypothetical adult male (60 years old, weight 80 kg, height 170 cm) subjected to injection of 120 mL of 370 mg I/mL contrast agent at 4 mL/s. A set of aortic contrast enhancement curves was generated by reducing the baseline cardiac output by 20%, 40%, and 60%. With a reduced cardiac output, contrast bolus arrives slowly and clears slowly, resulting in a delayed contrast bolus arrival, and delayed and elevated peak arterial enhancement.

injection rate, injection bolus shape, contrast medium volume (= injection duration × rate), concentration, and the use of a saline flush.

Injection duration

Injection duration, defined as the time from the beginning to the completion of injection or alternatively defined by the contrast medium volume divided by the injection rate, critically affects the magnitude and timing of contrast enhancement.[3,16–24] A longer injection (without lowering the injection rate) results in the administration of a larger contrast volume into the body and thus proportionally increases the magnitude of contrast enhancement (**Fig. 4**).

The appropriate injection duration is determined by the scanning conditions and the clinical objectives of the examination. The injection duration should be prolonged for a long CT scan to maintain good enhancement throughout image acquisition. When a large dose of iodine is needed for CT but the injection rate and contrast concentration cannot be increased (eg, a large patient with a limited vascular access), a longer injection dispenses more iodine into the body. However, sometimes, the injection duration may be intentionally shortened to increase the injection rate for a fixed amount of contrast volume. The increased injection rate helps to achieve high arterial enhancement but has a reduced influence on

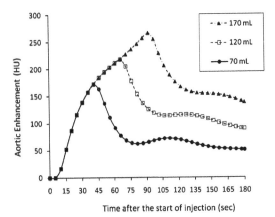

Fig. 4. Simulated thoracic aortic contrast enhancement curves with 3 different contrast medium volumes (durations). Simulated enhancement curves were based on a hypothetical adult male (60 years old, weight 80 kg, height 170 cm) subjected to 3 different volumes (70, 120, and 170 mL) of 370 mg I/mL contrast medium injected at the same rate of 2 mL/s. A larger volume requires a longer duration to inject. Both the time to and the magnitude of the peaks of enhancement increase with the contrast medium volume (injection duration).

parenchymal or venous enhancement because the parenchymal and venous enhancement are primarily determined by the total iodine dose administered into the body and less by the injection rate.[3,7,17–19,21,25–29]

Injection duration is the most important injection factor to be considered for determining CT scan timing, because it directly affects the time to peak

contrast enhancement in an organ or vessel as shown in several contrast enhancement studies on aorta.[3,21,30–32] When the injection duration increases, the time for the maximum deposit of contrast medium (the completion of the injection) is delayed and subsequently the time to peak contrast enhancement increases (see **Fig. 4**). A short injection duration (ie, low volume or high injection rate) protocol results in an earlier arterial peak and parenchymal enhancement, and requires a short scan delay to maximize contrast enhancement during the scanning. Conversely, a longer injection duration (ie, high volume or low injection rate) protocol results in a later peak enhancement and necessitates a longer scan delay. Therefore, when determining CT scan timing, it is more appropriate to use the completion of injection (the injection duration) as opposed to the start of injection, as the reference time variable.

Injection rate
When the duration of injection is fixed, a faster injection rate increases the delivery rate and the total delivered amount of contrast medium. It also results in a higher magnitude of vascular and parenchymal enhancement. On the other hand, when the total amount of contrast medium is fixed, a faster injection increases the delivery rate but shortens the injection duration and the time to peak enhancement (**Fig. 5**). This faster delivery of a fixed volume increases the magnitude of the aortic enhancement and, to a lesser degree, the magnitude of the visceral parenchyma (hepatic) or venous enhancement.[24,30,33,34] An

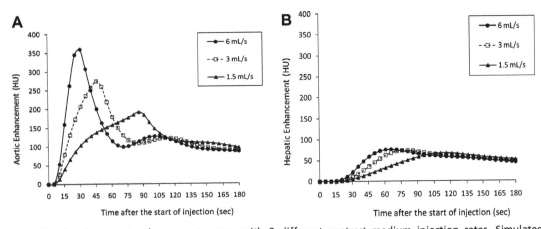

Fig. 5. Simulated contrast enhancement curves with 3 different contrast medium injection rates. Simulated enhancement curves of the (*A*) abdominal aorta and (*B*) liver based on a hypothetical adult male (60 years old, weight 80 kg, height 170 cm) subjected to a fixed volume 120 mL of 370 mg I/mL contrast medium injected at 1.5, 3, and 6 mL/s. As the rate of injection increases, the magnitude of contrast enhancement increases but the duration of high-magnitude contrast enhancement decreases. This trend is far more pronounced in the aortic than the hepatic enhancement.

increase in injection rate (up to <10 mL/s) steeply increases the magnitude of peak aortic enhancement. Conversely, the peak visceral parenchyma (hepatic) enhancement increases much more gradually and is apparent only at low injection rates (<3 mL/s).[30]

An increase in injection rate for a fixed volume of contrast medium results in a higher arterial enhancement, which is beneficial for arterial CT applications such as MDCT CT angiography (CTA) (see Fig. 5). However, this protocol may result in a reduced temporal window for CT scanning. Because of the shortened injection duration, more precise scan timing is required to achieve a high degree of enhancement. Although a fast injection is appropriate for procedures with short scan durations, a slower injection generating a prolonged vascular enhancement may be more suitable for procedures requiring long scan durations.

Injection rates of 2 to 5 mL/s via an antecubital vein are commonly used in clinical CT imaging. Although contrast administration at higher rates of 3 to 5 mL/s are reported to be feasible and safe using certain central venous catheters,[35–37] low injection rates of 1.5 to 2.0 mL/s are typically used with central venous catheters, peripherally inserted central catheters, and small-caliber catheters placed in forearm or hand veins because of safety concerns[38] and the pressure performance envelope of power injectors.[39] High injection rates of 5 to 10 mL/s are often used for CT perfusion imaging to generate a high peak enhancement with a short peak time. An increase of the injection rate greater than 8 to 10 mL/s is not likely to improve the enhancement. This is because of the inherent mixing or dispersion of contrast medium in the central blood compartment, which dampens the effect of fast injections propagating to a target organ.[40–43] Furthermore, a fast injection may result in a high retrograde reflux of contrast medium into the inferior vena cava and hepatic veins, even with the absence of right-sided heart disease.[44]

Injection bolus shaping

The shape of injected contrast bolus can be tailored to achieve a desired enhancement pattern. Contrast medium is commonly administered at a constant injection rate (uniphasic-rate) injection protocol. The second most commonly used injection bolus shape is a biphasic-rate injection: a fast constant-rate injection followed by a slow constant-rate injection. The biphasic-rate injection protocol is useful to prolong injection duration and maintain contrast enhancement for a long CT scan duration without increasing the amount of contrast medium.[17,45–49] Thus, the biphasic-rate injection was widely practiced with

slow CT scans, particularly during the prespiral CT era, and continues to be used in some MDCT applications that require long acquisition times, such as whole-body scans[48] and peripheral CTA.[49]

A recent variation of the biphasic injection is the injection of 2 different concentrations: the injection of higher concentration (undiluted) contrast medium followed by a lower concentration (diluted) contrast medium. The lower concentration is typically achieved by simultaneously injecting the undiluted contrast and saline loaded separately in syringes of a dual-head injector. The biphasic-concentration injection technique has been reported to be useful in improving right ventricular chamber enhancement and reducing the artifact resulting from the dense, undiluted contrast medium in the superior vena cava.[50–52]

The shape of the contrast bolus injection can be further tailored to achieve a desired enhancement pattern. With uniphasic-rate injection, the time-enhancement response progressively increases and peaks shortly after the completion of the injection, followed by a rapid decline in enhancement. This enhancement pattern is referred as a hump or peaked enhancement, which lacks a true plateau peak enhancement. A biphasic-rate injection typically results in a double-peaked arterial contrast enhancement pattern. To improve uniformity in the arterial enhancement while reducing double-peaking, the injection rates at the biphasic-rate injection can be customized algorithmically for each patient using the information extracted from a test-bolus injection acquired before the biphasic-rate injection.[36,53,54] Another more sophisticated injection bolus shaping technique used to achieve uniform vascular enhancement is the multiphasic, exponentially decelerated injection.[55,56]

Contrast medium concentration

Intravenous contrast media are available commercially in a wide range of concentrations, 240 to 370 mg I/mL. Contrast media with high iodine concentration ($\geq$350 mg I/mL) were widely used and reported with MDCT.[23,29,57–77] This trend reflects the fact that a high rate of iodine delivery is desired with a fast MDCT scan to maximize the arterial enhancement for CTA and improve the depiction of hypervascular tumors. When the volume, injection rate, and duration of the contrast medium are fixed, a higher concentration contrast medium will deliver a larger dose of iodine faster. This results in a higher magnitude of peak contrast enhancement and a wider temporal window for CT imaging at a given level of enhancement (Fig. 6). The time to peak enhancement is unaffected because the

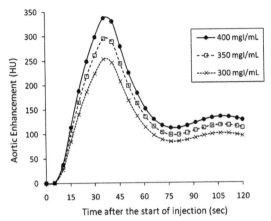

Fig. 6. Simulated thoracic aortic contrast enhancement curves with contrast media of a fixed volume but 3 different concentrations injected at a fixed rate. Simulated enhancement curves were based on a hypothetical adult male (60 years old, weight 80 kg, height 170 cm) subjected to injection of 120 mL of contrast medium with 3 different concentrations (300, 350, and 400 mg I/mL) at 4 mL/s. Contrast medium with a higher concentration delivers a larger dose of iodine faster and results in a higher magnitude of peak contrast enhancement and a wider temporal window for CT imaging at a given level of enhancement.

duration and rate of the injection remain unchanged. On the other hand, when the total iodine mass and injection rate are fixed, the injection volume and duration vary depending on the concentration; the bolus volume using a higher concentration contrast medium is smaller than that of a lower iodine concentration. Contrast medium of a higher concentration (but a fixed iodine mass and a smaller volume) injected at a fixed injection rate would result in arterial enhancement with earlier peak and greater peak enhancement. This is a result of faster delivery of iodine mass per unit time but a shorter duration of enhancement caused by a smaller volume of contrast medium (Fig. 7).[72] This trend in enhancement is the same as that for injecting contrast medium of a fixed total volume at a higher injection rate (see Fig. 5) because both procedures lead to a faster rate of iodine delivery per unit time with a reduced duration of injection.

Some clinical applications of thoracic CT may favor the use of contrast media with low concentration, particularly when saline flush is not used. One study[78] reported that diluted contrast medium (150 mg I/mL) injected faster in thoracic CT examinations resulted in less perivenous artifacts and higher aortic enhancement than undiluted contrast medium (300 mg I/mL). An additional benefit of a contrast medium with low concentration is low viscosity. High viscosity leads to the elevation of the injector pressure and thus may prohibit fast delivery of iodine when a rapid peripheral intravenous injection is desired.[39,79,80]

Saline flush

A saline flush pushes the tail of the injected contrast medium bolus into the central blood volume and makes use of contrast medium that would otherwise remain unused in the injection

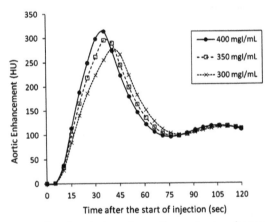

Fig. 7. Simulated thoracic aortic contrast enhancement curves with contrast media of a fixed iodine mass but 3 different concentrations injected at a fixed rate. Simulated enhancement curves were based on a hypothetical adult male (60 years old, weight 80 kg, height 170 cm) subjected to 4 mL/s injection of a fixed of iodine mass (42 g) but at 3 different concentrations and volumes: (300 mg I/mL, 140 mL), (350 mg I/mL, 120 mL) and (400 mg I/mL, 105 mL). The time-enhancement curves demonstrate that the use of high-concentration contrast material is associated with earlier and greater peak aortic enhancement.

tubing and peripheral veins. A saline flush therefore increases the efficiency of contrast medium utilization and the level of contrast enhancement.[40,81–90] Additional advantages of a saline flush include (1) improved bolus geometry as a result of reduced intravascular contrast medium dispersion, (2) reduced streak artifact from dense contrast medium in the brachiocephalic vein and superior vena cava on thoracic CT studies,[81,83] and (3) increased hydration to reduce contrast-induced nephrotoxicity.

With the increasing clinical applications of CTA and double-barrel CT contrast injectors, saline flush is widely accepted in CT imaging to improve the efficiency of contrast medium utilization and may reduce the iodine dose without negatively affecting the level of contrast enhancement. The maximum amount of contrast medium saved by use of a saline flush is equal to the volume of contrast medium retained in the injection tubing plus the contrast medium that remains in the peripheral venous space between the brachial vein and the superior vena cava. The peripheral venous space volume is related to patient size. Based on the results of recently published data and factoring in the patient's peripheral venous size, it is estimated that 12 to 20 mL of contrast medium could be replaced by a saline flush in the venous space. Therefore, with approximately 10 mL of contrast medium remaining in the tubing between the injector and venous access, an injection of more than 20 to 30 mL of saline flush would not save contrast medium nor would it contribute to further improvement of contrast enhancement. This amount of saving was supported by a recent phantom experimental study.[91] On the other hand, when a saline flush is applied with no reduction in the amount of contrast medium, there is a slight increase (5%–10%) in the magnitude of the peak arterial enhancement and the time to peak arterial enhancement is prolonged.[84,89–93]

CT Scan Factors

CT scanning factors play a significant role by determining the acquisition of contrast-enhanced images at a specific time point of contrast enhancement. Scanning parameters that critically affect contrast enhancement include the scan duration, scan direction, multiphasic acquisitions during different phases of contrast enhancement, and scan delay from the start (or completion) of contrast medium injection to the initiation of scan.

Scan duration and scan direction
To achieve diagnostically adequate contrast enhancement during CT scanning, it is vital to know the duration of the scan acquisition. Scan

duration information is crucial for the calculation of the injection duration and scan timing. For a long scan, an extended injection is likely required.

Although clinical contrast-enhanced CT scans are usually performed with the scan direction commensurate with the direction of contrast bolus propagation, 1 notable exception is a caudocranial scan of pulmonary CTA for the detection of pulmonary emboli. Scanning the lower lobes first is beneficial because if the patient breathes while scanning the lower lobes (which more frequently have emboli than the upper lobes), there is more excursion of the lower lobes compared with the upper lobes.[94]

Determination of contrast arrival time: test-bolus versus bolus-tracking method
When CT scan timing is individualized the contrast bolus transit time (which is closely associated with an individual patient's circulation time) can be measured before the diagnostic CT scan and factored into the calculation of scan timing for the diagnostic CT scan. Two methods, test-bolus and bolus-tracking, are commonly used to measure the transit time, or contrast arrival time (T_{arr}) (**Fig. 8**). For both methods, the contrast arrival time is measured by repeatedly scanning a target organ following the injection of contrast medium, placing a region of interest (ROI), and measuring the contrast enhancement over the target organ. Because contrast medium disperses during the transit, the profile of contrast enhancement broadens when it reaches the organ of interest. Therefore, the T_{arr} is determined from the time to peak enhancement (for the test-bolus) or time to reach a certain threshold (for the bolus-tracking). Contrast arrival time (T_{arr}) measured using the bolus-track with a 50-HU threshold of the aortic enhancement is likely equivalent to the time to peak test-bolus aortic enhancement measured from sequential CT scanning after an injection of a small amount of contrast medium.

The time determined by the test-bolus or bolus-tracking techniques simply represents the time of contrast arrival or contrast bolus transit.[3,95] This time should not be simply assumed to serve as the scan delay, but rather as a means of individualizing the scan delay relative to it, by including an adequate post-trigger delay (or diagnostic delay).[3,60] The post-trigger delay or diagnostic delay is defined as a delay from the T_{arr} (test-bolus peak time or bolus-tracking trigger time) to the initiation of the diagnostic scan, that is, the scan delay is determined to be the sum of T_{arr} plus the post-trigger delay. The requirement of post-trigger

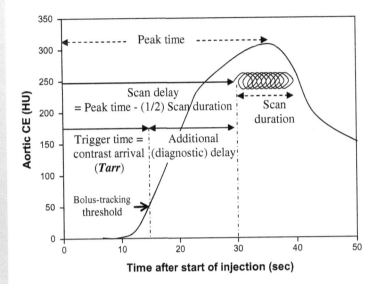

Fig. 8. Contrast medium injection, enhancement, and scan time variables illustrating the determination of scan delay from measured contrast arrival time and additional diagnostic delay. Scan delay should be determined by considering contrast medium injection duration, contrast arrival time, and scan duration. Contrast arrival time (T_{arr}) can be measured with a test-bolus or bolus-tracking method. In the figure, when bolus-tracking is used, T_{arr} corresponds to the time for the aortic enhancement to reach a 50-HU threshold. The scan delay is determined as the sum of T_{arr} plus an additional (diagnostic) delay. The additional diagnostic delay should be formulated considering the injection duration and scan duration such that the peak enhancement is centered in the middle of the CT scan (scan delay = peak time − (1/2) scan duration).

delay for optimizing the scan delay is particularly critical for fast MDCT. The post-trigger delay depends on several factors including the injection duration, scan duration, hemodynamics, and location of the target organ.

Although the bolus-tracking method is preferred because of its efficiency and practicality, some radiologists continue to use the test-bolus method, particularly for cardiac CTA examinations. The test-bolus injection provides an additional opportunity to test the integrity of the venous access site and to get the patient accustomed to the injection of contrast medium before the full injection of the contrast medium bolus. Another example of when the test-bolus is more appropriate than bolus-tracking is when performing a very short injection (an injection duration <10 seconds). A short injection results in narrowly peaked vascular enhancement. In this setting, there may not be sufficient time for the bolus-tracking to trigger and scan during the peak enhancement. A test-bolus injection also allows for mathematical modeling of each patient's cardiovascular and contrast pharmacokinetic response, which can then be used to optimally adjust the diagnostic contrast bolus shape in CTA.[53,96,97]

CLINICAL CONSIDERATIONS IN THORACIC MDCT PROTOCOLS

The key anatomic structures to be considered for thoracic CT contrast enhancement are pulmonary artery, aorta (including cardiac), and upper abdomen (Fig. 9). Clinical considerations associated with the contrast enhancement of these structures are addressed in 3 common thoracic CT protocols: aortic/cardiac CTA, pulmonary CTA, and routine chest CT. Key contrast

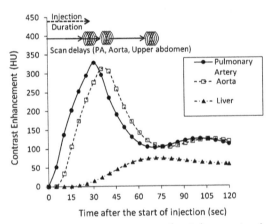

Fig. 9. Tim-enhancement curves for 3 key anatomic structures to be considered for contrast enhancement in thoracic CT. Simulated enhancement curves were based on a hypothetical adult male (60 years old, weight 80 kg, height 170 cm), subjected to injection of 120 mL of 370 mg I/mL contrast medium at 4 mL/s. To image each target organ at its specific peak contrast enhancement (CTPA, aortic or cardiac CTA, and routine chest including upper abdominal viscera), the CT scan should be delayed appropriately from the start or completion of contrast injection with consideration of the injection duration and circulation time.

enhancement variables for these protocols are summarized in **Table 1**.

Aortic and Coronary CTA

Conventional catheter-based diagnostic angiography examinations have been largely replaced by CTA acquired with high spatial and temporal resolution on MDCT. CTA has been used to depict not only large vessels such as the aorta but also small vessels such as the coronary, mesenteric, and peripheral run-off arteries. For thoracic CTA contrast enhancement, the aorta and coronary artery may be grouped and considered together because of their circulatory proximity.

Several recently published MDCT angiography studies have reported cardiac and coronary artery CTA imaging applications. Advances in MDCT and ECG-gating technology allow the acquisition of high-resolution, motion-free images of the heart and coronary arteries within a single short breath-hold.[98,99] A wide range of contrast administration and scan timing protocols were used for coronary CTA and cardiac imaging.[50–52,58,71,96,100–126] Contrast medium volumes ranging from 50 mL to 160 mL and injection rates ranging 3 to 5 mL/s have been used. This diversity in the protocols is partially a result of the rapid changes and evolution of cardiac and coronary CTA technology. As scan duration shortens from 30 to 40 seconds with 4-MDCT to 10 to 15 seconds with 64-MDCT, there is a trend of using less contrast medium for cardiac CTA, typically 75 to 100 mL with fast MDCT for an average-size adult.[110,112,114,115,119,121,122,124] Saline flush is invariably used. Recent technical development of wide-area detector CT (256- or 320-MDCT) with full cardiac coverage may allow for cardiac imaging in a single heart beat.[127–130] The ultrafast CT technology would further reduce the amount of contrast medium required for cardiac imaging at a "physiologic minimum" because the effect of scan duration is insignificant in the determination of iodine dose. However, with reduced amount of contrast medium, a precise determination of scan timing becomes more critical to achieve adequate contrast enhancement.

Contrast enhancement magnitude

The magnitude of CTA contrast enhancement depends on several patient-, contrast-, and scanner-related factors, including body weight, cardiac output, contrast medium volume, concentration, injection rate, type of contrast medium, saline flush, and scan speed. The magnitude of the CTA arterial enhancement increases directly proportional to the rate of iodine delivery (g I/s), which corresponds to the product of the contrast medium concentration (mg I/mL) and injection rate (mL/s) (see **Figs. 5–7**).

Attenuations of 250 to 300 HU (ie, net enhancement of 200–250 HU) for the aorta[21] and 300 to 350 HU for small arteries such as coronary arteries can be considered diagnostically adequate enhancement in CTA with fast MDCT.[58,71,117,131,132] To achieve these levels of contrast enhancement, the iodine dose (injection duration) should be adjusted for the patient's body size, iodine delivery rate, injection duration, and CT scan speed.

One scheme for determining injection duration for visceral parenchymal (eg, liver) or venous enhancement is to (1) estimate the total amount of iodine mass required to achieve a desired level of enhancement for the patient's body size (1 mg I/kg to generate 96 HU hepatic enhancement),[17] (2) choose a practical injection rate and contrast medium concentration, and (3) calculate the injection duration that corresponds to the iodine mass divided by the product of concentration and injection rate. This protocol results in a long injection duration for a large patient. Alternatively, when a fixed injection duration and concentration are used, a high injection rate should be used for a large patient to deliver a large amount of iodine. One advantage of using a fixed injection duration protocol rather than a fixed injection rate protocol is that scan timing can be more easily standardized.[133]

The calculation of optimal injection duration for arterial or CTA enhancement is more complicated than that for visceral parenchymal enhancement. This is because the degree of contrast enhancement is also heavily affected by the contrast medium delivery rate (see section on Injection rate). Based on a review of recently published studies on cardiac and coronary CTA enhancement,[12,50,58,71,125] it is possible to estimate the amount of contrast medium and injection rate to achieve a diagnostically adequate aortic (250–300 HU attenuation) and coronary artery enhancement (300–350 HU attenuation) for a 70-kg patient: (1) 45 g I injected at 1.2 g I/s (eg, 130 mL of 350 mg I/mL concentration at 3.5 mL/s) over 40 seconds for 4-row MDCT, (2) 35 g I injected at 1.4 g I/s (eg, 100 mL of 350 mg I/mL concentration at 4 mL/s) over 25 seconds for 16-row MDCT, and (3) 25 g I injected at 1.6 g I/s (eg, 75 mL of 350 mg I/mL concentration at 4.5–5.0 mL/s) over 15 seconds for 64-row MDCT, followed by a saline flush. Iodine doses larger than these estimated values are required for larger patients,[21,134,135] slower injection rates, and slower scan speed to maintain a consistent degree of contrast enhancement.

Our proposed scheme for formulating the injection duration for CTA applicable to different types

Table 1
Key contrast enhancement variables of 3 common thoracic CT protocols

	Typical Contrast Dose for 70-kg Patient (MDCT Type)	Typical Injection Rate for 70-kg Patient[a]	Injection Duration (ID)	Scan Duration (SD)	Fixed (Constant) Scan Delay	Variable Scan Delay[b]	Circulation-Adjusted Scan Delay[b]	Saline Flush
Thoracic aortic and coronary CTA	130 mL of 350 mg I/mL (4-MDCT) 100 mL (16-MDCT) 75 mL (64-MDCT)	3.5 mL/s (4-MDCT) 4 mL/s (16-MDCT) 4.5–5 mL/s (64-MDCT)	40 s (4-MDCT) 25 s (16-MDCT) 15 s (64-MDCT) or '15s + SD/2' or '10s + SD'	15–25 s (4-MDCT) 10–15s (16-MDCT) 5–10 s (64-MDCT) (longer for coronary)	20 s	ID+5-SD/2	ID+Tarr-7-SD/2 (Tarr at ascending aorta)	Essential
Pulmonary CTA	120 mL (for venogram or 4-MDCT) 100 mL of 350 mg I/mL (16-, 64-MDCT)	4–5 mL/s	25–30 s (4-MDCT) 20–25s (16-, 64-MDCT) or '15s + SD'	20–30 s (4-MDCT) 5–10 s (16-, 64-MDCT) 3–4 min (venogram)	15 s (4-, 16-MDCT) 20 s (64-MDCT)	ID+5-SD	ID+Tarr-5-SD (Tarr at main pulmonary artery)	Essential
Routine chest	70 mL of 300–350 mg I/mL	2–3 mL/s	30–40 s[c]	5–20 s	40–60 s[c]	ID+5-SD/2	ID+Tarr-7-SD/2 (Tarr at ascending aorta)	Not essential

Selection of the contrast concentration chosen arbitrarily. Different concentrations and volumes can be used to deliver the same amount of iodine.

[a] For a fixed injection duration protocol, the injection rate should be increased for a large patient to deliver a large amount of iodine or decreased for a small patient to deliver a small amount of iodine.

[b] For the background and rationale for the determination of scan delays, please refer to the corresponding clinical application section in the text.

[c] Given a wide range of fixed scan delays, the choice of scan delays depends on the diagnostic application: a shorter delay for arterial enhancement and a longer delay for soft-tissue and venous enhancement.

of MDCT scanners is to add a constant duration (ie, physiologic minimum injection duration to account for dispersive effects of the cardiopulmonary system on the contrast bolus) to half the scan duration. This empiric physiologic minimum duration will depend on the body size of the patient; it should be shorter in children than adults (we may use 5, 10, 15, or 20 seconds for different body sizes). For example, given a patient with body weight of 60 to 80 kg who receives contrast injected at 1.4 g I/s (4 mL/s of 350 mg I/s), the estimated injection duration is 15 seconds + 1/2 scan duration (ie, physiologic minimum duration = 15 seconds). When we use a fixed physiologic minimum duration for various body sizes to achieve a consistent degree of enhancement, the injection rate or the concentration of contrast medium should be adjusted proportional to the patient's body weight. Thus, a higher injection rate would be required for a large patient. With ultrafast CT scan and fast injections, the physiologic minimum duration may be pushed to 10 seconds for adults. For these cases, the authors propose an alternative approach of determining the injection duration to be 10 seconds + scan duration. However, special care must be taken to precisely determine scan timing to avoid aggressive reduction of contrast medium below a physiologic minimum to achieve adequate contrast enhancement.

Scan timing

A range of scanning delay values determined from the start of the injection, such as 15 to 30 seconds (choice primarily determined by scanner type and speed), have been used as fixed scan delays for aortic and coronary artery CTA. However, the precise determination of optimal scan delay is critical for fast MDCT and requires consideration of 3 key factors: (1) contrast medium injection duration, (2) contrast arrival time (T_{arr}), and (3) scan duration. For a prospective cardiac gating scan, the scan duration we defined corresponds to the time from the beginning to the end of the diagnostic scan (breath-hold duration), which is longer than each incremental duration when the x-ray tube is actually turned on for the CT data acquisition.

Our proposed scheme for computing scan delay (T_{DELAY}) has 2 steps: (1) determine the time to peak contrast enhancement (T_{PEAK}) in a target organ as a function of injection duration (T_{ID}) and contrast arrival time (T_{arr}); and (2) set the scan delay equal to the estimated peak enhancement time minus half the scan duration (T_{SD}) (see **Fig. 8**):

$$T_{DELAY} = T_{PEAK} - (1/2) \times T_{SD}$$

It is evident from this equation that for a given time to peak enhancement, scan delay should increase for shorter scan durations: that is, a longer delay with a faster scan (**Fig. 10**).

For a short injection of contrast medium (a test-bolus or injection duration <15 seconds), T_{PEAK} is dominated by T_{arr} with a fractional contribution of T_{ID}. This relationship may be expressed in a simple formula, $T_{PEAK} = T_{ID}/2 + T_{arr}$, which has been commonly used for the determination of the scan delay for magnetic resonance angiography.[3] For a typical injection of contrast medium for diagnostic CT applications (injection duration ≥ 15 seconds), T_{PEAK} is dominated by T_{ID} with a fractional contribution of T_{arr}: $T_{PEAK} = T_{ID} +$ fractional T_{arr}. As T_{ID} increases, the T_{arr} contribution reduces because a long injection perturbs the hemodynamics and accelerates the delivery of contrast medium delivery with shortened contrast arrival time, particularly in the upstream circulation before bolus dispersion is pronounced (ie, pulmonary artery and aorta). The normal range of the fractional T_{arr} is 0 to 5 seconds for pulmonary artery, 5 to 10 seconds for aorta, 20 to 30 seconds for portal vein, and 30 to 40 seconds for hepatic parenchyma.[3,24,50] T_{PEAK} for the pulmonary and aortic CTA is estimated by the sum of T_{ID} and T_{arr} (measured by the test-bolus or bolus-tracking methods) minus approximately 5 seconds (hemodynamic acceleration factor): $T_{ID} + T_{arr} - 5$.

In patients with normal circulation, peak arterial contrast enhancement is achieved shortly after the termination of a contrast medium injection.[3,30] In

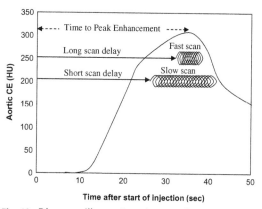

Fig. 10. Diagram illustrating the significance of scan duration in the determination of scan delay for maximal contrast enhancement. For a given duration of contrast enhancement or injection, the shorter the scan duration, the longer the additional delay needed to ensure that imaging takes place during the peak of aortic enhancement. Scan delay = peak enhancement time − (1/2) scan duration.

this case, the scan delay adjusted for the injection duration (variable delay) for the thoracic aortic and coronary CTA may be estimated as injection duration + 5 − (1/2) scan duration for an injection duration greater than 15 seconds or as 15 + (1/2) injection duration − (1/2) scan duration for an injection duration 15 seconds or less (for a short injection, the contrast transit time is governed more by intrinsic physiologic circulation time of contrast bolus than the injection duration).

When normal circulation cannot be assumed, scan delay should be individualized and can be formulated from the contrast arrival time (T_{arr}). After the T_{arr} is measured at the ascending aorta, the scan delay (circulation-adjusted delay) for the thoracic aorta and cardiac CTA can be determined with consideration of the injection duration and scan duration. When we use 12 seconds as the normal default value for T_{arr} at the aortic arch (a typical value in a patient with normal circulation), the time to peak aortic enhancement corresponds to injection duration + (T_{arr} − 12) + (5 seconds) or injection duration + T_{arr} − (7 seconds). Thus, the scan delay (circulation-adjusted delay) becomes injection duration + T_{arr} − 7 seconds − (1/2) scan duration. At T_{arr} = 12, the circulation-adjusted delay is equivalent to the variable delay, injection duration + 5 − (1/2) scan duration. T_{arr} would increase in patients with slow circulation. From the equation, scan delay can be computed: injection duration + T_{arr} − 7 − (1/2) scan duration. For example, for a 10-second scan with a 20-second injection, the scan delay would be 20 + T_{arr} − 7 − (10/2) or 'T_{arr} +8. Therefore, the scan delay is determined by adding 8 seconds to the T_{arr} measured from a test-bolus method. On the other hand, when a bolus-tracking method is used, T_{arr} is determined when the degree of contrast enhancement after the injection of a full bolus of contrast medium has exceeded a preset threshold. In our proposed scheme, the diagnostic scan will start at T_{arr} + 8, that is, 8 seconds of additional diagnostic delay after reaching the 50-HU enhancement threshold.[136]

CT Pulmonary Angiography

CT pulmonary angiography (CTPA) has become the first-line imaging study in the diagnosis of pulmonary embolism (PE),[137,138] and it has largely supplanted lung scintigraphy and conventional catheter-based pulmonary angiography for this purpose.[139] Following the evolution of CT techniques, a wide variation of CTPA protocols were reported in the literature.[94,140–147] Contrast medium volumes ranging from 80 to 150 mL and injection rates ranging from 2 to 5 mL/s were

used. However, with fast MDCT (scan duration <10 seconds), the contrast administration protocols have become unified with prevailing use of a fast injection of a small amount of contrast medium. Scanners slower than 16-MDCT are not recommended for CTPA because of the required prolonged injection and limited longitudinal resolution and image quality including respiratory motion artifacts.[94]

Contrast enhancement magnitude

Because the main clinical indication of CTPA is detection of pulmonary emboli, knowledge about the attenuation of pulmonary emboli is crucial for determining the level of appropriate CTPA enhancement. The mean attenuation for acute emboli was reported to be 33 HU (standard deviation 15 HU) and 87 HU (standard deviation 31 HU) for chronic emboli.[148] Similar ranges of attenuations for emboli including those in the peripheral extremity veins were published by other investigators.[149–151] Based on the mean and standard deviation values of emboli, the theoretic minimum attenuation of pulmonary artery required to detect acute and chronic emboli was computed as 211 HU.[94] However, CTPA attenuations higher than this minimum value are likely desirable for the detection of emboli in small distal pulmonary arteries subjected to increased partial volume averaging.[149]

Pulmonary artery attenuations of 300 to 350 HU (ie, 250–300 HU net contrast enhancement) may be considered as the preferred level of CTPA contrast enhancement. In recent CTPA contrast enhancement studies using 4-MDCT (20-second scan duration),[23,68] mean pulmonary vascular attenuations of 268 HU by 1.2 g I/s and 344 HU by 1.6 g I/s injections were obtained with a total of 36 g I (mean body weight of the patients, 72–75 kg). Saline flush was used for all patients. In a similar 4-MDCT study that used lower concentration contrast media,[152] however, a mean pulmonary attenuation of 255 HU was attained with a total of 24 g I injected at 3 mL/s (0.8 g I/s) over 30 seconds (no body weight information reported). In a recent study evaluating CTPA contrast enhancement with 16- and 64-MDCT,[153] mean pulmonary artery enhancement of 211 HU was achieved with 1.0 mL/kg of 350 mg I/mL (70 mL or 24.5 g I for a 70-kg patient) injected at 4 mL/s (1.4 g I/s) without saline flush. This study also showed that shorter scan duration of the 64-MDCT required less contrast medium than the 16-MDCT. From the review of these published studies, we estimate that, for a 70-kg patient, CTPA attenuation of 300 to 350 HU is likely achieved with 30 to 40 g I (smaller amount with faster scan) injected at 1.4 to 1.6 g I/s (100 mL of 350 mg I/mL injected at 4–5 mL/s at 16- and 64-MDCT).

To estimate the amount of contrast medium required for scans at different speeds, we may consider the injection duration to be 15 + scan duration with an injection rate of 4 to 5 mL/s for a 70-kg patient. For example, with a 5-second scan, the injection duration is 20 seconds. Given the practical limitations of injection at very high rates (>8–10 mL/s) including the exacerbated dissipation effect of fast injections, reflux into the inferior vena cava and challenge of precise scan timing, the injection duration should not be shorter than 15 seconds even with ultrafast MDCT. Larger patients will require larger amounts of contrast medium (by use of faster, longer, or higher concentration contrast medium injection) to obtain the desired degree of enhancement.

Several studies[151,154–157] demonstrated that the diagnosis of venous thromboembolism (VTE) increases in patients undergoing CTPA for PE with the addition of indirect CT venography of the pelvis and lower extremity. Adequate contrast enhancement for CT venography, however, may require an increased amount (by 20%–40%) of contrast medium, particularly when CTPA is performed with fast MDCT using a parsimonious amount of contrast medium. The amount of contrast medium required for contrast enhancement in CT venography is determined mainly by the patient's body weight (eg, 70-kg patient: 0.6 g I/kg; 120 mL of 350 mg I/mL) and is little affected by the injection rate. The benefit of a high injection rate, which helps improve pulmonary artery enhancement, is offset during the acquisition of CT venography because of the large pool of systemic venous blood diluting contrast medium and the long scan delay employed.[8,30]

Scan timing

The normal circulation transit time from the antecubital vein to the pulmonary artery is only 6 to 8 seconds.[158] Because of the proximity of the pulmonary circulation to the injection site, the temporal pattern of pulmonary artery contrast enhancement is closely associated with the injection duration and is more predictable than distal circulatory systems (aorta, peripheral run-off CTA). With a fast injection of contrast medium, the pulmonary arterial enhancement increases rapidly and quickly reaches near the plateau at 15 to 20 seconds. Hence, for most CTPA imaging studies, well-designed fixed scan delays (typically 15–20 seconds for 16- and 64-MDCT with a 20-second injection) are adequate. The enhancement at the peak may fluctuate during the cardiac cycle,

particularly as a result of in- and out-flow blood volume difference during systole.

An alternative to using a fixed scan delay is to use the completion of the injection as the reference for the scan delay. In this scheme (variable delay), regardless of the injection duration, the scan will be initiated as soon as completion of injection of contrast medium for a fast MDCT (scan duration of 5 seconds) scanner or 3 seconds before the completion of injection for a slower MDCT (scan duration <10 seconds). To make this "dump all and drive" approach practical, the injection duration should be a minimum of 15 seconds. A slower MDCT would require a longer injection, and the scan should start earlier (but no earlier than 15 seconds after the start of injection) before the completion of injection. When a long injection is used because of limited vascular access or a low injection rate, a long scan delay should be used.[94] In either case, the scan delay should be determined so that the CT scanning ends at 5 seconds (or 10 seconds using saline flush) after the completion of injection of contrast medium. This variable scan delay can be formulated as: injection duration + 5 − scan duration.

Although fixed scan delay approaches may work well in most CTPA studies, precise timing may be required when a tight contrast medium injection (duration <15 seconds) is used with fast MDCT or in patients with fast cardiac output, cardiac dysfunction, pulmonary artery hypertension, or compromised central or peripheral venous flow.[140,146] To individualize the scan delay, contrast arrival time (T_{arr}) is measured with a test-bolus[159] or a bolus-tracking technique[68,146,153,160] by placing an ROI over the main pulmonary artery or the right ventricle. The time delay for the diagnostic study is calculated by adding 4 to 6 seconds to the time to peak enhancement of the test-bolus (T_{arr}).[146,159] For the bolus-tracking method, the diagnostic CT scan is triggered when contrast enhancement over the ROI reaches the threshold of 100 HU. At the first monitoring scan obtained 10 seconds after the start of injection, this threshold would be exceeded in most patients unless a patient has a slow circulation or unless the injection is very slow for the patient's body size. The diagnostic scan starts after 5 to 10 additional seconds (longer for faster scan) required for the CT table to move, typically resulting in a scan delay of 15 to 20 seconds.[153]

Using the contrast arrival time (T_{arr}) measured earlier, the circulation-adjusted scan delay for CTPA may be determined as follows. Using 10 seconds as the normal default value for T_{arr}, the time to peak pulmonary enhancement corresponds to injection duration + (T_{arr} − 10). After the enhancement peak, the pulmonary enhancement declines rapidly as no additional contrast medium flows into the pulmonary artery.[50] Thus, it is desirable to complete the scan within 5 seconds after the peak. With this consideration, the scan delay can be computed as injection duration + (T_{arr} − 10) + 5 − scan duration. For example, a 5-second scan and a 20-second injection results in the scan delay, 20 + T_{arr} − 10 + 5 − 5 or T_{arr} +10. Therefore, the scan delay is determined by adding 10 seconds of diagnostic delay after the time of reaching the bolus-tracking threshold. In this example, at T_{arr} = 10, the scan delay is 20 seconds, which corresponds to the completion of the injection.

Precise timing for CT venography of the pelvis and lower extremities is not as critical as CTPA, but controversy remains.[146,161] Sufficiently high degrees of venous enhancement are observed for 2 to 4 minutes after the start of contrast medium administration.[162–165] Despite the maximal venous enhancement obtained at about 2 minutes after the start of injection, a scan delay of 3 to 4 minutes may be preferred to reduce mixing artifacts from unenhanced blood, particularly in patients with slow circulation.[163,165] Furthermore, a recent study suggested that, because CT venography of the pelvis during CTPA does not significantly improve the detection of VTE, CT venography may be limited to the lower extremities, thus reducing radiation dose.[157]

Routine Chest CT Imaging

Contrast enhancement is useful in routine chest CT for the characterization and differentiation of mass or lymphadenopathy from surrounding normal vascular, mediastinal, and hilar structures and the assessment of a wide range of vascular conditions such as aneurysm, dissection, bleeding, and malformation. Imaging of enhanced upper abdominal visceral organs is also an essential component for tumor staging. Thus, the objective of contrast enhancement in routine chest CT is to achieve a diagnostically adequate enhancement of the thoracic cardiovascular structures including the upper abdominal viscera. An additional desirable feature of contrast enhancement is minimizing artifacts caused by dense incoming or remaining contrast medium in the lumen of the thoracic veins.

During the past 3 decades of rapidly evolving CT technology, considerable variations in contrast administration protocols for routine chest CT scans have been reported. However, in the MDCT era, these protocols have become increasingly unified with reduced variability across different platforms. The scan delay for routine chest CT is determined by the clinical indications and the diagnostic target organs; typically, scanning early for the preferential enhancement of thoracic vessels versus scanning late for all-around enhancement of the soft-tissue and parenchyma structures of the thorax including the upper abdomen.

Contrast enhancement magnitude
Contrast enhancement of 150 to 200 HU in the thoracic vessels and cardiac chambers is considered diagnostically adequate for a routine chest CT.[166] For an average-sized adult, this magnitude of enhancement can be readily obtained with 60 to 90 mL of 350 to 370 mg I/mL contrast medium (a smaller volume may be used for faster scans and/or for smaller patients) injected at 2 to 3 mL/s in MDCT. The required amount of iodine dose adjusted for body weight would be 0.3 to 0.4 g I/kg (eg, 70 mL of 300–350 mg I/mL contrast medium for a 70-kg patient). When a combined chest and abdomen CT (chest scan followed by abdomen scan), a larger iodine dose (eg, 0.5 g I/kg) may be required for adequate enhancement of the abdominal visceral organs. The injection rate is determined based on an injection duration of 35 to 40 seconds for MDCT. Streak artifact from dense contrast medium is reduced using a saline flush and a long scan delay or using a low concentration contrast medium (eg, 150 mg I/mL).[79,166]

Scan timing
Given the clinical objective of achieving moderately high enhancement of the thoracic vessels and upper abdominal viscera, scan timing for routine chest CT may not have to be as precise as that for CTA (eg, pulmonary, aortic, and coronary CTA). Nevertheless, with MDCT, the scan timing for routine chest CT can be determined more precisely during a vascular (peak thoracic arterial enhancement and a narrow temporal window) or hepatic parenchymal (portal venous dominant enhancement and a broad temporal window) phase. CT scan can be acquired twice at 2 distinct phases (vascular and hepatic phases), but it may not be practical or clinically beneficial because of the resulting increased radiation. For given injection durations of 35 to 40 seconds, a range of fixed scan delays (40–60 seconds) is used for routine chest MDCT scan. The choice of scan delays depends on the diagnostic target organ: a shorter delay for thoracic vascular enhancement is typically used, whereas a longer delay is used for more hepatic and abdominal viscera.

Scan delays (variable scan delay) that allow variations in injection duration and scan duration in normal circulation may be formulated as injection duration + 5 − (1/2) scan duration for SDCT and MDCT. With a shorter injection duration (fast injection), the scan delay calculated from this formula will provide more arterial enhancement, whereas a longer injection results in a longer scan delay and less arterial enhancement.

For a circulation-adjusted scan delay with MDCT, the contrast arrival time (T_{arr}) is measured from an ROI placed over the thoracic aorta with 50-HU enhancement threshold. When we use 12 seconds as the normal default value for T_{arr} at the aortic arch (a typical value in a patient with normal circulation), the time to peak aortic enhancement corresponds to injection duration + (T_{arr} − 12) + (5 seconds) or injection duration + T_{arr} − (7 seconds). From the equation, the scan delay can be computed as injection duration + T_{arr} − (7 seconds) − (1/2) scan duration. For example, a 10-second scan with a 40-second injection results in a scan delay of 40 + T_{arr} − 7 − (10/2) or T_{arr} +28. Therefore, the scan delay is determined by adding 28 seconds of diagnostic delay after the time of reaching the bolus-tracking threshold. In this example, at T_{arr} = 12, the scan delay is 40 seconds, which corresponds to the completion of the injection. To improve the enhancement of the upper abdomen viscera, a 20-second additional delay may be included; injection duration + T_{arr} + 13 − (1/2) scan duration or T_{arr} + 48 in the earlier example.

SUMMARY AND FUTURE DIRECTIONS

MDCT, with its dramatically shorter image acquisition times, permits the acquisition of high spatial and temporal resolution images at multiple precisely defined phases of contrast enhancement. However, to fully realize the benefits of MDCT, protocols for contrast administration and scan timing must be modified by recognizing the specific objectives of each clinical imaging application and the characteristics of various MDCT scanners. Various patient-related and injection-related factors can affect the magnitude and timing of intravenous contrast medium enhancement. Although these factors are interrelated, some (body size, contrast volume, iodine concentration, saline flush) have more of an effect on enhancement magnitude, whereas others (cardiac output, contrast injection duration, contrast injection rate) have more of an effect on the temporal pattern of contrast enhancement. Injection duration should be considered for the determination of scan delay because it critically affects time to

peak enhancement. Individualized scan delay is more critical with MDCT than with SDCT. The contrast arrival time (T_{arr}) measured using test-bolus or bolus-tracking techniques can be integrated with the injection duration to predict peak enhancement time. Scan delay is then estimated such that the center of the scan is timed to the peak of contrast enhancement.

With MDCT, contrast administration and CT scan protocols have become more complex and challenging. In the future, the authors believe that these technical challenges will be overcome by means of computer modeling and intelligent software that facilitates communication between the injector and the scanner and that integrates the patient's demographic information from a clinical database, scan parameters, and injection parameters.

REFERENCES

1. Bae KT, Heiken JP, Brink JA. Aortic and hepatic contrast medium enhancement at CT. Part I. Prediction with a computer model. Radiology 1998;207:647–55.
2. Nakayama Y, Awai K, Funama Y, et al. Abdominal CT with low tube voltage: preliminary observations about radiation dose, contrast enhancement, image quality, and noise. Radiology 2005;237:945–51.
3. Bae KT. Peak contrast enhancement in CT and MR angiography: when does it occur and why? Pharmacokinetic study in a porcine model. Radiology 2003;227:809–16.
4. Kormano M, Partanen K, Soimakallio S, et al. Dynamic contrast enhancement of the upper abdomen: effect of contrast medium and body weight. Invest Radiol 1983;18:364–7.
5. Heiken JP, Brink JA, McClennan BL, et al. Dynamic incremental CT: effect of volume and concentration of contrast material and patient weight on hepatic enhancement. Radiology 1995;195:353–7.
6. Platt JF, Reige KA, Ellis JH. Aortic enhancement during abdominal CT angiography: correlation with test injections, flow rates, and patient demographics. AJR Am J Roentgenol 1999;172:53–6.
7. Han JK, Choi BI, Kim AY, et al. Contrast media in abdominal computed tomography: optimization of delivery methods. Korean J Radiol 2001;2:28–36.
8. Bae KT. Technical aspects of contrast delivery in advanced CT. Appl Radiol 2003;32(Suppl):12–9.
9. Ho LM, Nelson RC, Delong DM. Determining contrast medium dose and rate on basis of lean body weight: does this strategy improve patient-to-patient uniformity of hepatic enhancement during multi-detector row CT? Radiology 2007;243:431–7.

10. Kondo H, Kanematsu M, Goshima S, et al. Abdominal multidetector CT in patients with varying body fat percentages: estimation of optimal contrast material dose. Radiology 2008;249:872–7.

11. Yanaga Y, Awai K, Nakaura T, et al. Effect of contrast injection protocols with dose adjusted to the estimated lean patient body weight on aortic enhancement at CT angiography. AJR Am J Roentgenol 2009;192:1071–8.

12. Bae KT, Seeck BA, Hildebolt CF, et al. Contrast enhancement in cardiovascular MDCT: effect of body weight, height, body surface area, body mass index, and obesity. Am J Roentgenol 2008;190:777–84.

13. Livingston EH, Lee S. Body surface area prediction in normal-weight and obese patients. Am J Physiol Endocrinol Metab 2001;281:E586–91.

14. Bae KT, Heiken JP, Brink JA. Aortic and hepatic contrast medium enhancement at CT. Part II. Effect of reduced cardiac output in a porcine model. Radiology 1998;207:657–62.

15. Chu LL, Joe BN, Westphalen ACA, et al. Patient-specific time to peak abdominal organ enhancement varies with time to peak aortic enhancement at MR imaging. Radiology 2007;245:779–87.

16. Dean PB, Violante MR, Mahoney JA. Hepatic CT contrast enhancement: effect of dose, duration of infusion, and time elapsed following infusion. Invest Radiol 1980;15:158–61.

17. Heiken JP, Brink JA, McClennan BL, et al. Dynamic contrast-enhanced CT of the liver: comparison of contrast medium injection rates and uniphasic and biphasic injection protocols. Radiology 1993;187:327–31.

18. Chambers TP, Baron RL, Lush RM. Hepatic CT enhancement. Part I. Alterations in the volume of contrast material within the same patients. Radiology 1994;193:513–7.

19. Kopka L, Rodenwaldt J, Fischer U, et al. Dual-phase helical CT of the liver: effects of bolus tracking and different volumes of contrast material. Radiology 1996;201:321–6.

20. Han JK, Kim AY, Lee KY, et al. Factors influencing vascular and hepatic enhancement at CT: experimental study on injection protocol using a canine model. J Comput Assist Tomogr 2000;24:400–6.

21. Awai K, Hiraishi K, Hori S. Effect of contrast material injection duration and rate on aortic peak time and peak enhancement at dynamic CT involving injection protocol with dose tailored to patient weight. Radiology 2004;230:142–50.

22. Bae KT, Heiken JP. Scan and contrast administration principles for MDCT. Eur Radiol 2005;15(S5): E46–59.

23. Schoellnast H, Deutschmann HA, Berghold A, et al. MDCT angiography of the pulmonary arteries: influence of body weight, body mass index, and scan length on arterial enhancement at different iodine flow rates. AJR Am J Roentgenol 2006;187:1074–8.

24. Erturk SM, Ichikawa T, Sou H, et al. Effect of duration of contrast material injection on peak enhancement times and values of the aorta, main portal vein, and liver at dynamic MDCT with the dose of contrast medium tailored to patient weight. Clin Radiol 2008;63:263–71.

25. Berland LL, Lee JY. Comparison of contrast media injection rates and volumes for hepatic dynamic incremented computed tomography. Invest Radiol 1988;23:918–22.

26. Small WC, Nelson RC, Bernardino ME, et al. Contrast-enhanced spiral CT of the liver: effect of different amounts and injection rates of contrast material on early contrast enhancement. AJR Am J Roentgenol 1994;163:87–92.

27. Freeny PC, Gardner JC, vonIngersleben G, et al. Hepatic helical CT: effect of reduction of iodine dose of intravenous contrast material on hepatic contrast enhancement. Radiology 1995;197:89–93.

28. Megibow AJ, Jacob G, Heiken JP, et al. Quantitative and qualitative evaluation of volume of low osmolality contrast medium needed for routine helical abdominal CT. AJR Am J Roentgenol 2001;176:583–9.

29. Roos JE, Desbiolles LM, Weishaupt D, et al. Multidetector row CT: effect of iodine dose reduction on hepatic and vascular enhancement. Rofo 2004;176:556–63.

30. Bae KT, Heiken JP, Brink JA. Aortic and hepatic peak enhancement at CT: effect of contrast medium injection rate–pharmacokinetic analysis and experimental porcine model. Radiology 1998;206:455–64.

31. Tello R, Seltzer S. Effects of injection rates of contrast material on arterial phase hepatic CT. AJR Am J Roentgenol 1999;173:237–8.

32. Tublin ME, Tessler FN, Cheng SL, et al. Effect of injection rate of contrast medium on pancreatic and hepatic helical CT. Radiology 1999;210:97–101.

33. Garcia PA, Bonaldi VM, Bret PM, et al. Effect of rate of contrast medium injection on hepatic enhancement at CT. Radiology 1996;199:185–9.

34. Garcia P, Genin G, Bret PM, et al. Hepatic CT enhancement: effect of the rate and volume of contrast medium injection in an animal model. Abdom Imaging 1999;24:597–603.

35. Herts BR, O'Malley CM, Wirth SL, et al. Power injection of contrast media using central venous catheters: feasibility, safety, and efficacy. AJR Am J Roentgenol 2001;176:447–53.

36. Hittmair K, Fleischmann D. Accuracy of predicting and controlling time-dependent aortic

enhancement from a test bolus injection. J Comput Assist Tomogr 2001;25:287–94.

37. Sanelli PC, Deshmukh M, Ougorets I, et al. Safety and feasibility of using a central venous catheter for rapid contrast injection rates. AJR Am J Roentgenol 2004;183:1829–34.

38. Rivitz SM, Drucker EA. Power injection of peripherally inserted central catheters. J Vasc Interv Radiol 1997;8:857–63.

39. Behrendt FF, Bruners P, Keil S, et al. Impact of different vein catheter sizes for mechanical power injection in CT: in vitro evaluation with use of a circulation phantom. Cardiovasc Intervent Radiol 2009; 32:25–31.

40. Claussen CD, Banzer D, Pfretzschner C, et al. Bolus geometry and dynamics after intravenous contrast medium injection. Radiology 1984;153: 365–8.

41. Irie T, Suzuki S, Yamauchi T, et al. Prediction of the time to peak hepatic enhancement to optimize contrast-enhanced spiral CT. Acta Radiol 1995; 36:154–8.

42. Bader TR, Prokesch RW, Grabenwoger F. Timing of the hepatic arterial phase during contrast-enhanced computed tomography of the liver: assessment of normal values in 25 volunteers. Invest Radiol 2000;35:486–92.

43. Miles KA. Perfusion CT for the assessment of tumour vascularity: which protocol? Br J Radiol 2003;76 Spec No 1:S36–42.

44. Yeh BM, Kurzman P, Foster E, et al. Clinical relevance of retrograde inferior vena cava or hepatic vein opacification during contrast-enhanced CT. AJR Am J Roentgenol 2004;183:1227–32.

45. Foley WD, Hoffmann RG, Quiroz FA, et al. Hepatic helical CT: contrast material injection protocol. Radiology 1994;192:367–71.

46. Berland LL. Slip-ring and conventional dynamic hepatic CT: contrast material and timing considerations. Radiology 1995;195:1–8.

47. Hanninen EL, Vogl TJ, Felfe R, et al. Detection of focal liver lesions at biphasic spiral CT: randomized double-blind study of the effect of iodine concentration in contrast materials. Radiology 2000;216: 403–9.

48. Awai K, Imuta M, Utsunomiya D, et al. Contrast enhancement for whole-body screening using multidetector row helical CT: comparison between uniphasic and biphasic injection protocols. Radiat Med 2004;22:303–9.

49. Fleischmann D, Rubin GD. Quantification of intravenously administered contrast medium transit through the peripheral arteries: implications for CT angiography. Radiology 2005;236: 1076–82.

50. Utsunomiya D, Awai K, Sakamoto T, et al. Cardiac 16-MDCT for anatomic and functional analysis:

assessment of a biphasic contrast injection protocol. AJR Am J Roentgenol 2006;187:638–44.

51. Kerl JM, Ravenel JG, Nguyen SA, et al. Right heart: split-bolus injection of diluted contrast medium for visualization at coronary CT angiography. Radiology 2008;247:356–64.

52. Cao L, Du X, Li P, et al. Multiphase contrast-saline mixture injection with dual-flow in 64-row MDCT coronary CTA. Eur J Radiol 2009;69:496–9.

53. Fleischmann D, Rubin GD, Bankier AA, et al. Improved uniformity of aortic enhancement with customized contrast medium injection protocols at CT angiography. Radiology 2000;214:363–71.

54. Numburi UD, Chatzimavroudis GP, Stillman AE, et al. Patient-specific contrast injection protocols for cardiovascular multidetector row computed tomography. J Comput Assist Tomogr 2007;31: 281–9.

55. Bae KT, Tran HQ, Heiken JP. Multiphasic injection method for uniform prolonged vascular enhancement at CT angiography: pharmacokinetic analysis and experimental porcine model. Radiology 2000; 216:872–80.

56. Bae KT, Tran HQ, Heiken JP. Uniform vascular contrast enhancement and reduced contrast medium volume achieved by using exponentially decelerated contrast material injection method. Radiology 2004;231:732–6.

57. Awai K, Takada K, Onishi H, et al. Aortic and hepatic enhancement and tumor-to-liver contrast: analysis of the effect of different concentrations of contrast material at multi-detector row helical CT. Radiology 2002;224:757–63.

58. Becker CR, Hong C, Knez A, et al. Optimal contrast application for cardiac 4-detector-row computed tomography. Invest Radiol 2003;38:690–4.

59. Brink JA. Use of high concentration contrast media (HCCM): principles and rationale-body CT. Eur J Radiol 2003;45(Suppl 1):S53–8.

60. Fleischmann D. High-concentration contrast media in MDCT angiography: principles and rationale. Eur Radiol 2003;13(Suppl 3):N39–43.

61. Fleischmann D. Use of high-concentration contrast media in multiple-detector-row CT: principles and rationale. Eur Radiol 2003;13(Suppl 5):M14–20.

62. Fleischmann D. Use of high concentration contrast media: principles and rationale-vascular district. Eur J Radiol 2003;45(Suppl 1):S88–93.

63. Shinagawa M, Uchida M, Ishibashi M, et al. Assessment of pancreatic CT enhancement using a high concentration of contrast material. Radiat Med 2003;21:74–9.

64. Awai K, Inoue M, Yagyu Y, et al. Moderate versus high concentration of contrast material for aortic and hepatic enhancement and tumor-to-liver contrast at multi-detector row CT. Radiology 2004; 233:682–8.

65. Furuta A, Ito K, Fujita T, et al. Hepatic enhancement in multiphasic contrast-enhanced MDCT: comparison of high- and low-iodine-concentration contrast medium in same patients with chronic liver disease. AJR Am J Roentgenol 2004;183:157–62.

66. Suzuki H, Oshima H, Shiraki N, et al. Comparison of two contrast materials with different iodine concentrations in enhancing the density of the aorta, portal vein and liver at multi-detector row CT: a randomized study. Eur Radiol 2004;14:2099–104.

67. Yagyu Y, Awai K, Inoue M, et al. MDCT of hypervascular hepatocellular carcinomas: a prospective study using contrast materials with different iodine concentrations. AJR Am J Roentgenol 2005;184:1535–40.

68. Schoellnast H, Deutschmann HA, Fritz GA, et al. MDCT angiography of the pulmonary arteries: influence of iodine flow concentration on vessel attenuation and visualization. AJR Am J Roentgenol 2005;184:1935–9.

69. Marchiano A, Spreafico C, Lanocita R, et al. Does iodine concentration affect the diagnostic efficacy of biphasic spiral CT in patients with hepatocellular carcinoma? Abdom Imaging 2005;30:274–80.

70. Itoh S, Ikeda M, Achiwa M, et al. Multiphase contrast-enhanced CT of the liver with a multislice CT scanner: effects of iodine concentration and delivery rate. Radiat Med 2005;23:61–9.

71. Cademartiri F, Mollet NR, van der Lugt A, et al. Intravenous contrast material administration at helical 16-detector row CT coronary angiography: effect of iodine concentration on vascular attenuation. Radiology 2005;236:661–5.

72. Silvennoinen HM, Hamberg LM, Valanne L, et al. Increasing contrast agent concentration improves enhancement in first-pass CT perfusion. AJNR Am J Neuroradiol 2007;28:1299–303.

73. Konig M, Bultmann E, Bode-Schnurbus L, et al. Image quality in CT perfusion imaging of the brain. The role of iodine concentration. Eur Radiol 2007;17:39–47.

74. Behrendt FF, Mahnken AH, Stanzel S, et al. Intraindividual comparison of contrast media concentrations for combined abdominal and thoracic MDCT. AJR Am J Roentgenol 2008;191:145–50.

75. Keil S, Plumhans C, Behrendt FF, et al. MDCT angiography of the pulmonary arteries: intravascular contrast enhancement does not depend on iodine concentration when injecting equal amounts of iodine at standardized iodine delivery rates. Eur Radiol 2008;18:1690–5.

76. Muhlenbruch G, Behrendt FF, Eddahabi MA, et al. Which iodine concentration in chest CT? A prospective study in 300 patients. Eur Radiol 2008;18:2826–32.

77. Behrendt FF, Plumhans C, Keil S, et al. Contrast enhancement in chest multidetector computed tomography: intraindividual comparison of 300 mg/ml versus 400 mg/ml iodinated contrast medium. Acad Radiol 2009;16:144–9.

78. Rubin GD, Lane MJ, Bloch DA, et al. Optimization of thoracic spiral CT: effects of iodinated contrast medium concentration. Radiology 1996;201:785–91.

79. Kern MJ, Roth RA, Aguirre FV, et al. Effect of viscosity and iodine concentration of nonionic radiographic contrast media on coronary arteriography in patients. Am Heart J 1992;123:160–5.

80. Knollmann F, Schimpf K, Felix R. [Iodine delivery rate of different concentrations of iodine-containing contrast agents with rapid injection]. Rofo 2004;176:880–4 [in German].

81. Hopper KD, Mosher TJ, Kasales CJ, et al. Thoracic spiral CT: delivery of contrast material pushed with injectable saline solution in a power injector. Radiology 1997;205:269–71.

82. Dorio PJ, Lee FT Jr, Henseler KP, et al. Using a saline chaser to decrease contrast media in abdominal CT. AJR Am J Roentgenol 2003;180:929–34.

83. Haage P, Schmitz-Rode T, Hubner D, et al. Reduction of contrast material dose and artifacts by a saline flush using a double power injector in helical CT of the thorax. AJR Am J Roentgenol 2000;174:1049–53.

84. Irie T, Kajitani M, Yamaguchi M, et al. Contrast-enhanced CT with saline flush technique using two automated injectors: how much contrast medium does it save? J Comput Assist Tomogr 2002;26:287–91.

85. Schoellnast H, Tillich M, Deutschmann HA, et al. Abdominal multidetector row computed tomography: reduction of cost and contrast material dose using saline flush. J Comput Assist Tomogr 2003;27:847–53.

86. Cademartiri F, Mollet N, van der Lugt A, et al. Non-invasive 16-row multislice CT coronary angiography: usefulness of saline chaser. Eur Radiol 2004;14:178–83.

87. Schoellnast H, Tillich M, Deutschmann MJ, et al. Aortoiliac enhancement during computed tomography angiography with reduced contrast material dose and saline solution flush: influence on magnitude and uniformity of the contrast column. Invest Radiol 2004;39:20–6.

88. Schoellnast H, Tillich M, Deutschmann HA, et al. Improvement of parenchymal and vascular enhancement using saline flush and power injection for multiple-detector-row abdominal CT. Eur Radiol 2004;14:659–64.

89. Utsunomiya D, Awai K, Tamura Y, et al. 16-MDCT aortography with a low-dose contrast material protocol. AJR Am J Roentgenol 2006;186:374–8.

90. Lee CH, Goo JM, Bae KT, et al. CTA contrast enhancement of the aorta and pulmonary artery:

the effect of saline chase injected at two different rates in a canine experimental model. Invest Radiol 2007;42:486–90.

91. Behrendt FF, Bruners P, Keil S, et al. Effect of different saline chaser volumes and flow rates on intravascular contrast enhancement in CT using a circulation phantom. Eur J Radiol 2009, in press.

92. Kim DJ, Kim TH, Kim SJ, et al. Saline flush effect for enhancement of aorta and coronary arteries at multidetector CT coronary angiography. Radiology 2008;246:110–5.

93. Yamaguchi I, Kidoya E, Suzuki M, et al. Evaluation of required saline volume in dynamic contrast-enhanced computed tomography using saline flush technique. Comput Med Imaging Graph 2009;33:23–8.

94. Wittram C. How I do it: CT pulmonary angiography. Am J Roentgenol 2007;188:1255–61.

95. Bae KT. Test-bolus versus bolus-tracking techniques for CT angiographic timing. Radiology 2005;236:369–70; author reply 370.

96. Rist C, Nikolaou K, Kirchin MA, et al. Contrast bolus optimization for cardiac 16-slice computed tomography: comparison of contrast medium formulations containing 300 and 400 milligrams of iodine per milliliter. Invest Radiol 2006;41:460–7.

97. Mahnken AH, Rauscher A, Klotz E, et al. Quantitative prediction of contrast enhancement from test bolus data in cardiac MSCT. Eur Radiol 2007;17:1310–9.

98. Ohnesorge BM, Hofmann LK, Flohr TG, et al. CT for imaging coronary artery disease: defining the paradigm for its application. Int J Cardiovasc Imaging 2005;21:85–104.

99. Schoepf UJ, Becker CR, Ohnesorge BM, et al. CT of coronary artery disease. Radiology 2004;232:18–37.

100. Vogl TJ, Abolmaali ND, Diebold T, et al. Techniques for the detection of coronary atherosclerosis: multidetector row CT coronary angiography. Radiology 2002;223:212–20.

101. Nieman K, Cademartiri F, Lemos PA, et al. Reliable noninvasive coronary angiography with fast submillimeter multislice spiral computed tomography. Circulation 2002;106:2051–4.

102. Kopp AF, Schroeder S, Kuettner A, et al. Non-invasive coronary angiography with high resolution multidetector-row computed tomography. Results in 102 patients. Eur Heart J 2002;23:1714–25.

103. Pannu HK, Flohr TG, Corl FM, et al. Current concepts in multi-detector row CT evaluation of the coronary arteries: principles, techniques, and anatomy. Radiographics 2003;23(Spec No):S111–25.

104. Nikolaou K, Knez A, Sagmeister S, et al. Assessment of myocardial infarctions using multidetector-row computed tomography. J Comput Assist Tomogr 2004;28:286–92.

105. van Ooijen PM, Dorgelo J, Zijlstra F, et al. Detection, visualization and evaluation of anomalous coronary anatomy on 16-slice multidetector-row CT. Eur Radiol 2004;14:2163–71.

106. Kuettner A, Trabold T, Schroeder S, et al. Noninvasive detection of coronary lesions using 16-detector multislice spiral computed tomography technology: initial clinical results. J Am Coll Cardiol 2004;44:1230–7.

107. Kopp AF, Kuttner A, Trabold T, et al. Multislice CT in cardiac and coronary angiography. Br J Radiol 2004;77(Spec No 1):S87–97.

108. Hong C, Chrysant GS, Woodard PK, et al. Coronary artery stent patency assessed with in-stent contrast enhancement measured at multi-detector row CT angiography: initial experience. Radiology 2004;233:286–91.

109. Cademartiri F, Nieman K, van der Lugt A, et al. Intravenous contrast material administration at 16-detector row helical CT coronary angiography: test bolus versus bolus-tracking technique. Radiology 2004;233:817–23.

110. Hamoir XL, Flohr T, Hamoir V, et al. Coronary arteries: assessment of image quality and optimal reconstruction window in retrospective ECG-gated multislice CT at 375-ms gantry rotation time. Eur Radiol 2005;15:296–304.

111. Haberl R, Tittus J, Bohme E, et al. Multislice spiral computed tomographic angiography of coronary arteries in patients with suspected coronary artery disease: an effective filter before catheter angiography? Am Heart J 2005;149:1112–9.

112. Leber AW, Knez A, von Ziegler F, et al. Quantification of obstructive and nonobstructive coronary lesions by 64-slice computed tomography: a comparative study with quantitative coronary angiography and intravascular ultrasound. J Am Coll Cardiol 2005;46:147–54.

113. Datta J, White CS, Gilkeson RC, et al. Anomalous coronary arteries in adults: depiction at multidetector row CT angiography. Radiology 2005;235:812–8.

114. Achenbach S, Ropers D, Pohle FK, et al. Detection of coronary artery stenoses using multi-detector CT with 16 × 0.75 collimation and 375 ms rotation. Eur Heart J 2005;26:1978–86.

115. Nikolaou K, Knez A, Rist C, et al. Accuracy of 64-MDCT in the diagnosis of ischemic heart disease. AJR Am J Roentgenol 2006;187:111–7.

116. Husmann L, Alkadhi H, Boehm T, et al. Influence of cardiac hemodynamic parameters on coronary artery opacification with 64-slice computed tomography. Eur Radiol 2006;16:1111–6.

117. Cademartiri F, Mollet NR, Lemos PA, et al. Higher intracoronary attenuation improves diagnostic accuracy in MDCT coronary angiography. AJR Am J Roentgenol 2006;187:W430–3.

118. Cademartiri F, de Monye C, Pugliese F, et al. High iodine concentration contrast material for noninvasive multislice computed tomography coronary angiography: iopromide 370 versus iomeprol 400. Invest Radiol 2006;41:349–53.

119. Vrachliotis TG, Bis KG, Haidary A, et al. Atypical chest pain: coronary, aortic, and pulmonary vasculature enhancement at biphasic single-injection 64-section CT angiography. Radiology 2007;243: 368–76.

120. Yamamuro M, Tadamura E, Kanao S, et al. Coronary angiography by 64-detector row computed tomography using low dose of contrast material with saline chaser: influence of total injection volume on vessel attenuation. J Comput Assist Tomogr 2007;31:272–80.

121. Frydrychowicz A, Pache G, Saueressig U, et al. Comparison of reconstruction intervals in routine ECG-pulsed 64-row-MSCT coronary angiography in frequency controlled patients. Cardiovasc Intervent Radiol 2007;30:79–84.

122. Herzog C, Zwerner PL, Doll JR, et al. Significant coronary artery stenosis: comparison on per-patient and per-vessel or per-segment basis at 64-section CT angiography. Radiology 2007;244:112–20.

123. Tsai IC, Lee T, Tsai WL, et al. Contrast enhancement in cardiac MDCT: comparison of iodixanol 320 versus iohexol 350. AJR Am J Roentgenol 2008;190:W47–53.

124. Rist C, Becker CR, Kirchin MA, et al. Optimization of cardiac MSCT contrast injection protocols: dependency of the main bolus contrast density on test bolus parameters and patients' body weight. Acad Radiol 2008;15:49–57.

125. Nakaura T, Awai K, Yauaga Y, et al. Contrast injection protocols for coronary computed tomography angiography using a 64-detector scanner: comparison between patient weight-adjusted- and fixed iodine-dose protocols. Invest Radiol 2008;43: 512–9.

126. Johnson PT, Pannu HK, Fishman EK. IV contrast infusion for coronary artery CT angiography: literature review and results of a nationwide survey. AJR Am J Roentgenol 2009;192:W214–21.

127. Rybicki FJ, Otero HJ, Steigner ML, et al. Initial evaluation of coronary images from 320-detector row computed tomography. Int J Cardiovasc Imaging 2008;24:535–46.

128. Otero HJ, Steigner ML, Rybicki FJ. The "post-64" era of coronary CT angiography: understanding new technology from physical principles. Radiol Clin North Am 2009;47:79–90.

129. Kitagawa K, Lardo AC, Lima JA, et al. Prospective ECG-gated 320 row detector computed tomography: implications for CT angiography and perfusion imaging. Int J Cardiovasc Imaging 2009; 25(Suppl 2):P201–8.

130. Choi SI, George RT, Schuleri KH, et al. Recent developments in wide-detector cardiac computed tomography. Int J Cardiovasc Imaging 2009; 25(Suppl 1):23–9.

131. Cademartiri F, Maffei E, Palumbo AA, et al. Influence of intra-coronary enhancement on diagnostic accuracy with 64-slice CT coronary angiography. Eur Radiol 2008;18:576–83.

132. Fei X, Du X, Yang Q, et al. 64-MDCT coronary angiography: phantom study of effects of vascular attenuation on detection of coronary stenosis. AJR Am J Roentgenol 2008;191:43–9.

133. Awai K, Hori S. Effect of contrast injection protocol with dose tailored to patient weight and fixed injection duration on aortic and hepatic enhancement at multidetector-row helical CT. Eur Radiol 2003;13: 2155–60.

134. Macari M, Israel GM, Berman P, et al. Infrarenal abdominal aortic aneurysms at multi-detector row CT angiography: intravascular enhancement without a timing acquisition. Radiology 2001;220: 519–23.

135. Ho LM, Nelson RC, Thomas J, et al. Abdominal aortic aneurysms at multi-detector row helical CT: optimization with interactive determination of scanning delay and contrast medium dose. Radiology 2004;232:854–9.

136. Bae KT, Heiken JP. Computer modeling approach to contrast medium administration and scan timing for multislice CT. In: Marincek B, Ros PR, Reiser M, et al, editors. Multislice CT: a practical guide. Berlin (NY): Springer; 2000. p. 28–30.

137. Bhalla S, Lopez-Costa I. MDCT of acute thrombotic and nonthrombotic pulmonary emboli. Eur J Radiol 2007;64:54–64.

138. Remy-Jardin M, Pistolesi M, Goodman LR, et al. Management of suspected acute pulmonary embolism in the era of CT angiography: a statement from the Fleischner Society. Radiology 2007;245: 315–29.

139. Strashun AM. A reduced role of V/Q scintigraphy in the diagnosis of acute pulmonary embolism. J Nucl Med 2007;48:1405–7.

140. Yankelevitz DF, Shaham D, Shah A, et al. Optimization of contrast delivery for pulmonary CT angiography. Clin Imaging 1998;22:398–403.

141. Qanadli SD, Hajjam ME, Mesurolle B, et al. Pulmonary embolism detection: prospective evaluation of dual-section helical CT versus selective pulmonary arteriography in 157 patients. Radiology 2000;217: 447–55.

142. Ghaye B, Szapiro D, Mastora I, et al. Peripheral pulmonary arteries: how far in the lung does multi-detector row spiral CT allow analysis? Radiology 2001;219:629–36.

143. Raptopoulos V, Boiselle PM. Multi-detector row spiral CT pulmonary angiography: comparison

with single-detector row spiral CT. Radiology 2001; 221:606–13.

144. Remy-Jardin M, Tillie-Leblond I, Szapiro D, et al. CT angiography of pulmonary embolism in patients with underlying respiratory disease: impact of multislice CT on image quality and negative predictive value. Eur Radiol 2002;12:1971–8.

145. Tillie-Leblond I, Mastora I, Radenne F, et al. Risk of pulmonary embolism after a negative spiral CT angiogram in patients with pulmonary disease: 1-year clinical follow-up study. Radiology 2002;223:461–7.

146. Washington L, Gulsun M. CT for thromboembolic disease. Curr Probl Diagn Radiol 2003;32:105–26.

147. Schoepf UJ, Costello P. CT angiography for diagnosis of pulmonary embolism: state of the art. Radiology 2004;230:329–37.

148. Meaney TF, Raudkivi U, McIntyre WJ, et al. Detection of low-contrast lesions in computed body tomography: an experimental study of simulated lesions. Radiology 1980;134:149–54.

149. Brink JA, Woodard PK, Horesh L, et al. Depiction of pulmonary emboli with spiral CT: optimization of display window settings in a porcine model. Radiology 1997;204:703–8.

150. Cham MD, Yankelevitz DF, Shaham D, et al. Deep venous thrombosis: detection by using indirect CT venography. The pulmonary angiography-indirect CT Venography Cooperative Group. Radiology 2000;216:744–51.

151. Loud PA, Katz DS, Klippenstein DL, et al. Combined CT venography and pulmonary angiography in suspected thromboembolic disease: diagnostic accuracy for deep venous evaluation. AJR Am J Roentgenol 2000;174:61–5.

152. Bedard JP, Blais C, Patenaude YG, et al. Pulmonary embolism: prospective comparison of iso-osmolar and low-osmolarity nonionic contrast agents for contrast enhancement at CT angiography. Radiology 2005;234:929–33.

153. Bae KT, Tao C, Gurel S, et al. Effect of patient weight and scanning duration on contrast enhancement during pulmonary multidetector CT angiography. Radiology 2007;242:582–9.

154. Cham MD, Yankelevitz DF, Henschke CI. Thromboembolic disease detection at indirect CT venography versus CT pulmonary angiography. Radiology 2005; 234:591–4.

155. Stein PD, Fowler SE, Goodman LR, et al. Multidetector computed tomography for acute pulmonary embolism. N Engl J Med 2006;354: 2317–27.

156. Ghaye B, Nchimi A, Noukoua CT, et al. Does multidetector row ct pulmonary angiography reduce the incremental value of indirect CT venography compared with single-detector row CT pulmonary angiography? Radiology 2006;240:256–62.

157. Kalva SP, Jagannathan JP, Hahn PF, et al. Venous thromboembolism: indirect CT venography during CT pulmonary angiography–should the pelvis be imaged? Radiology 2008;246:605–11.

158. Leggett RW, Williams LR. A proposed blood circulation model for reference man. Health Phys 1995; 69:187–201.

159. Teigen CL, Maus TP, Sheedy PF 2nd, et al. Pulmonary embolism: diagnosis with contrast-enhanced electron-beam CT and comparison with pulmonary angiography. Radiology 1995;194:313–9.

160. Bae KT, Mody GN, Balfe DM, et al. CT depiction of pulmonary emboli: display window settings. Radiology 2005;236:677–84.

161. Katz DS, Loud PA, Bruce D, et al. Combined CT venography and pulmonary angiography: a comprehensive review. Radiographics 2002; 22(Spec No):S3–19 [discussion: S20–14].

162. Yankelevitz DF, Gamsu G, Shah A, et al. Optimization of combined CT pulmonary angiography with lower extremity CT venography. AJR Am J Roentgenol 2000;174:67–9.

163. Garg K, Kemp JL, Wojcik D, et al. Thromboembolic disease: comparison of combined CT pulmonary angiography and venography with bilateral leg sonography in 70 patients. AJR Am J Roentgenol 2000;175:997–1001.

164. Bruce D, Loud PA, Klippenstein DL, et al. Combined CT venography and pulmonary angiography: how much venous enhancement is routinely obtained? AJR Am J Roentgenol 2001; 176:1281–5.

165. Szapiro D, Ghaye B, Willems V, et al. Evaluation of CT time-density curves of lower-limb veins. Invest Radiol 2001;36:164–9.

166. Schnyder P, Meuli R, Wicky S. Injection technique. In: Remy-Jardin M, Remy J, editors. Spiral CT of the chest. Berlin: Springer; 1996. p. 57–100.

Acute Pulmonary Embolism

Jean Kuriakose, MBBS, MRCP, FRCR[a],
Smita Patel, MBBS, MRCP, FRCR[b],*

KEYWORDS

- CT pulmonary angiography • Pulmonary embolism
- CT venography • Radiation exposure

Imaging plays a crucial role in the diagnosis of pulmonary embolism (PE) and deep venous thrombosis (DVT), a spectrum of the same disease entity. PE is the third most common cause of cardiovascular death in the United States, following ischemic heart disease and stroke, with an annual incidence of 300,000 to 600,000 per year.[1,2] Despite the high prevalence, PE is difficult to diagnose, with only 43 to 53 patients per 100,000 being accurately diagnosed, and up to 70% of clinically unsuspected PE diagnosed at autopsy.[1,3] In the past few decades, the incidence of PE has decreased by 45%, whereas that of DVT is unchanged.[4,5] Death occurs in up to 90% of patients with unrecognized PE, whereas in treated patients PE accounts for less than 10% of deaths.[6,7]

Rapid and timely diagnosis of this life-threatening disease is important to improve patient outcome as the signs and symptoms as well as ancillary tests are nonspecific. The recent rapid growth in CT technology over the past decade has seen the emergence of CT pulmonary angiography (CTPA) as the single first line test in the diagnosis of PE because of its high diagnostic accuracy and ability to provide alternate diagnosis for diseases of the lung parenchyma, pleura, pericardium, aorta, heart, thoracic lymph nodes, and mediastinum.

The widespread availability and use of CTPA has made the diagnosis of PE easier in most cases, but has raised the need for optimal use of this technique in the appropriate patient population, in order to minimize unnecessary medical radiation exposure.

Pretest risk stratification using Wells criteria, clinical probability scores, assessing premorbid conditions, past history, and a thorough clinical examination should precede an appropriate, timely ,and accurate diagnostic test.[8,9] In some common scenarios like pregnancy and in critically ill patients, the diagnosis of PE still remains challenging.

DIAGNOSIS OF ACUTE PULMONARY EMBOLISM
Ventilation-Perfusion Scintigraphy

Combined ventilation and perfusion (V/Q) scintigraphy had been the imaging technique of choice for decades. A V/Q scan with normal findings essentially excludes pulmonary embolism with an NPV (Negative Predictive Value) close to 100%, thereby precluding the use of anticoagulation, whereas a high-probability scan is highly specific for the diagnosis of PE, allowing definitive treatment. In the original PIOPED (Prospective Investigation of Pulmonary Embolism Diagnosis) study only 14% of patients had a normal V/Q scan and 13% a high-probability V/Q scan, rendering a definitive diagnosis in only a small group of patients; most (73%) had an indeterminate (nondiagnostic) or low-probability test result.[10] This high degree of uncertainty makes initiation of definitive anticoagulant therapy difficult because

[a] Division of Cardiothoracic Radiology, Department of Radiology, University of Michigan Health System, 1500 East Medical Center Driver, Ann Arbor, MI, USA
[b] Department of Radiology, University of Michigan Health System, Cardiovascular Center - Room 5338, 1500 East Medical Center Drive, Ann Arbor, MI 48109-5868, USA
* Corresponding author.
E-mail address: smitap@med.umich.edu (S. Patel).

Radiol Clin N Am 48 (2010) 31–50
doi:10.1016/j.rcl.2009.10.002
0033-8389/09/$ – see front matter © 2010 Published by Elsevier Inc.

of risk of bleeding and necessitates additional tests to diagnose or exclude pulmonary embolism.

The criteria for reporting V/Q scans have improved significantly.[11] Recent use of V/Q scanning with SPECT allows 3-dimensional visualization of segments previously not identified on planar imaging, such as the medial basal segment of the right lower lobe. The lung segments are more clearly defined and can be viewed in any orthogonal plane, resulting in better detection and characterization of defects.[12] SPECT also improves image contrast, thus decreasing the rate of intermediate scan reports. Large-scale trials are needed to fully assess this modality and compare its performance with CTPA. Currently the definitive primary role of V/Q scanning is in patients where CTPA is contraindicated as in severe renal impairment or history of iodine or contrast allergy.

Catheter Pulmonary Angiography

Catheter pulmonary angiography has been considered as the reference test for the diagnosis of PE since the late 1960s. However, the invasive nature and expense of the study along with a small but definite risk in morbidity has contributed to its underutilization. Two studies, done 12 years apart in 1240 patients, showed that following an inconclusive V/Q scan result, catheter pulmonary angiography was performed in less than 15% of patients.[13,14] Many patients were treated with anticoagulants without a definitive result. Accurate diagnosis is important, as anticoagulants themselves account for significant morbidity (up to 6.5%), that increases with age and with comorbid conditions.[15,16]

With the newer generation of MDCT (multidetector CT) scanners, the role of catheter pulmonary angiography as the gold standard test has been questioned and is considered to be flawed, particularly at the subsegmental level.[17–19] The interobserver agreement at the subsegmental level on the original PIOPED study was reported to be only 66%.[10] In PIOPED II, in the 20 discordant cases, PE was missed at the lobar, segmental, and subsegmental levels in 13 patients; 8 of 13 were at the subsegmental level.[19] The current role of catheter pulmonary angiography is when CTPA is inconclusive, or when the clinical findings are discordant with CTPA results.

CT Pulmonary Angiography

Incidental detection of PE was first documented by Sinner in 1978.[20] The advent of single-detector helical CT in the early 1990s, made it possible to obtain volumetric datasets with good contrast in a single breath-hold, allowing diagnosis predominantly of central and segmental PE. With rapid evolvement of CT technology, the CT diagnosis of PE has been a subject of much research in the past couple of decades, and has resulted in CTPA becoming a first-line imaging test at many centers.[21] CTPA is a relatively safe, accurate, readily available and cost-effective noninvasive test that not only diagnoses PE, but also provides diagnosis of alternative pathologies in the thorax accounting for patient symptoms, particularly in the inpatient and emergency department settings.

Faster multidetector scanners have set the way for a potential new gold standard test. With newer 128 and higher slice scanners, the sensitivity and specificity is likely to increase albeit at a cost of increased radiation.

Advances in MDCT

MDCT has several advantages over SDCT (single detector CT) in the diagnosis of PE, which include improved z-axis resolution, shorter scan times, reduction in volume of contrast, and the ability to do a combined CTPA/CT venography (CTV) exam at the same setting with a single bolus of contrast.

Z-Axis Resolution

Advances in MDCT technology with improved gantry rotation speeds and increased detector width allow rapid acquisition of large volumetric datasets over a greater craniocaudal distance than with SDCT. While reduction in slice collimation with SDCT results in a longer breath hold and a likelihood of increased respiratory motion artifact, with MDCT reduction in slice thickness leads to better visualization of subsegmental pulmonary arteries, with 94% of fifth order and 74% of sixth order pulmonary arteries being visualized.[22–24] Reducing the reconstruction thickness decreases partial volume averaging and also results in better visualization of the obliquely oriented middle lobe and lingular arteries, in which an estimated 20% of emboli occur.[17] Reducing the slice thickness also improves the interobserver agreement for diagnosis of PE.[25]

Shorter Scan Acquisition Time

A shorter breath hold translates into decreased respiratory motion artifact which in turn results in less indeterminate studies and allows better visualization of the subsegmental pulmonary arteries. The scan range for SDCT typically ranges from 15 to 20 cm from the top of the aortic arch to the dome of the diaphragm, with a breath hold of 30 to 40 seconds or longer, whereas the entire chest can be scanned with 16-slice or higher generation

MDCT scanners at a shorter breath hold of 3 to 10 seconds.

Decrease in Contrast Volume

The shorter acquisition time enables a reduction in volume and tighter bolus of contrast for optimal opacification of the pulmonary arteries. With SDCT and early generation MDCT, contrast volumes of 120 mL or higher were commonly used, whereas on the current generation of MDCT scanners, studies can be performed with doses of 80 mL or less. A saline chase can also be used to further reduce the volume of contrast and to decrease beam hardening artifact from the SVC as is done for imaging of the coronary arteries.

CT Pulmonary Angiography Technique

With rapidly advancing MDCT technology, the techniques and protocols are continually evolving. Precise techniques vary between the different generation of scanners and between vendors. Table 1 suggests parameters for CTPA using different generations of MDCT scanners. The imaging acquisition on the current generation of scanners includes the entire lungs with resolution of 1.25 mm or less. The aim is to perform the study at thinnest slice collimation with a single short breath hold in full suspended respiration. With the 64-slice and higher generation scanners, it is possible to obtain the entire study with a breath hold of less than 5 seconds. In intubated patients, because of the short acquisition time, respiration can be suspended for the duration of the study. With such short breath holds, it does not matter whether the scan is acquired in a caudocranial or craniocaudal direction.

Power injectors are required for rapid contrast delivery to obtain adequate enhancement of the pulmonary arteries. An 18- to 20-gauge intravenous cannula is placed in the antecubital vein. The degree and quality of pulmonary arterial enhancement depends on the amount and concentration of contrast, injection rate, and the scan delay. On the 64-slice scanner we use 70 mL of contrast (Isovue 370, Bracco Diagnostics, New Jersey) for CTPA imaging of the chest alone, and for a combined CTPA/CTV study we use 120 mL of contrast (Isovue 370 Bracco Diagnostics) at 4 mL/s. A greater degree of arterial enhancement can be achieved by increasing the rate of contrast, independent of the concentration of iodine contrast medium.

Timing Bolus/Bolus Tracking

The timing of contrast bolus administration is critical to obtain optimal opacification of the pulmonary arteries. Incorrect timing is a common cause of suboptimal studies. A fixed scan delay of 20 to 25 seconds was used especially for SDCT and early generation of MDCT scanners, which leads to adequate opacification of the pulmonary arteries in at least 85% of patients with normal cardiac function. However, with the current generation of scanners, a timing bolus or bolus tracking method is more commonly used to optimize opacification of pulmonary arteries.

A timing bolus is usually performed by injecting 15 to 20 mL of intravenous contrast material and placing a region of interest in the pulmonary trunk to obtain a time-density curve from which the scan delay can be calculated. When comparing empirical delay with test bolus, Hartmann and colleagues reported that despite objective improvement in pulmonary artery enhancement, there was no significant difference in image quality.[26] Additionally, 16% of the studies had to be excluded because of uninterpretable time density curves.

Alternatively, bolus tracking method can be used with a cursor in the main pulmonary artery that triggers scanning at a preset threshold. For the 16-slice scanner, the scan is triggered when a threshold of 120 HU is reached and for the 64-slice scanner, at the first sight of contrast in the pulmonary artery. A timing or bolus tracking method should be used in patients with suspected or known cardiac dysfunction because the optimal scan delay time can be 40 seconds or more.

In larger patients, a larger volume of high-density contrast should be injected at a higher flow rate to improve the signal to noise, a higher kVP should be used, and images should be acquired at thicker collimation of 2.0 to 2.5 mm to decrease quantum mottle.

ECG Gating

The benefit of ECG gating in diagnostic PE evaluation is controversial.[27] Only 1% of subsegmental pulmonary arteries are inadequately visualized secondary to cardiac motion artifact using a 4-row scanner at 1-mm collimation.[22] The higher radiation dose secondary to ECG gating is therefore not justified. ECG gating in patients with high or irregular heart rates would lead to considerable artifacts. With MDCT scanners, 16-slice and higher, the addition of ECG gating to the CTPA study can be helpful when there is a need for a double/triple rule-out study to detect or exclude pathology within the pulmonary arteries, aorta, and/or the coronary arteries. Significant stenosis of coronary arteries or nonenhancement of the myocardium in patients with acute myocardial infarction may offer an alternative differential

Table 1
CT pulmonary angiography protocols with evolution of MDCT technology at our institution

Indication	Suspected Thromboembolic Disease			
Scan type	Lightspeed QXi 4-row	Lightspeed Ultra 8-row	Lightspeed 16 16-row thin/ultrathin collimation	VCT 64-row
Detector rows	4-row	8-row	16-row[a]	64-row[a]
Tube setting				
kVp	140	140	120	120
mA	380	380	400	500
Gantry speed (s):	0.8	0.7	0.7	0.6
Table speed (mm/rotation):	7.5	13.5	27.5[a]/13.75[a]	55
Pitch	1.5	1.35:1	1.375:1	1.375:1
Slice collimation (mm):	1.25	1.25	1.25[a]/0.625[a]	1.25/0.625
Breath-hold:	Suspended Respiration			
Anatomic coverage:	Mid diaphragm to lung apices (25 cm)			Entire lungs
Acquisition time (s):	27.6	13.8	7.0[a]/13.5[a]	3–5
Recon kernel:	Standard			
Reconstruction thickness (mm):	1.25	1.25	1.25/0.625	0.625
Effective slice thickness (mm):	2.5	1.6	1.6/0.8	
Reconstruction interval (mm):	0.625	0.625	0.625	0.625

Note that protocols vary depending on types of scanners and with different vendors.
[a] The 16-row and 64-row scanner allows for a choice of rapid acquisition using a 1.25-mm collimation, which is particularly useful in dyspneic patients, or thinner collimation for greater spatial resolution.

diagnosis on these studies. In patients with large central emboli or a large thrombus burden, right ventricular function can be assessed on ECG-gated studies, albeit at increased radiation exposure. Poor right ventricular function has prognostic implications in patients with significant pulmonary embolic disease.[28]

Image Interpretation

Given the large volume datasets and the increased number of images generated for these studies, CTPA is now routinely read off a dedicated work station or PACS system and not on hard copy images. The window level and width are adjusted on the fly while scrolling to optimally visualize the opacified pulmonary arterial lumen. At some institutions, coronal and sagittal reformats are routinely generated to aid fast review of the pulmonary arterial tree. In an interobserver study evaluating the utility of multiplanar reconstructions in CTPA, the authors report that generated sagittal and coronal reformats do not increase diagnostic accuracy, but do increase reader agreement and reader confidence, and may decrease interpretation time (Espinosa et al, presented at Society of Thoracic Radiology Annual Meeting, 2008).

The paddle wheel technique helps delineate the vessel and its branches in continuity as the artery radiates from the hilum, allowing visualization of the extent of thrombus burden on a single image (**Fig. 1**). There is no significant difference between the paddle wheel technique and axial images for detecting central PE.[29,30] However, for the diagnosis of peripheral pulmonary emboli, there is significantly lower sensitivity and specificity for the paddle wheel method alone without the concurrent use of axial images.[29]

CT FINDINGS OF PULMONARY EMBOLISM
Direct Findings

The diagnosis of PE is made on CT by direct visualization of a low attenuation filling defect that partially (**Fig. 2**) or completely occludes a contrast filled artery. A vessel "cut-off" sign is seen when the distal artery is not opacified owing to the presence of occlusive PE (**Fig. 3**). The involved artery could be significantly larger than the well-enhanced corresponding artery on the opposite side, particularly with occluded smaller-sized arteries (**Fig. 4**).[31] When PE partially occludes an artery, the "rim-sign" (**Fig. 2**A, C) is seen on short axis views of the vessel, when the low attenuation embolus is surrounded by a rim of high attenuation contrast, or the "railway-track"/"tram-track" sign, on the long axis view of the vessel (**Fig. 2**B).

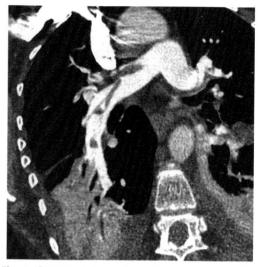

Fig. 1. Contrast-enhanced paddle wheel view depicts pulmonary emboli in the bilateral main pulmonary arteries, with embolus extending into the right lower lobe segmental and subsegmental arteries. Note that the vessels can be followed in a continuous manner from the hilum.

Indirect Findings

Pulmonary hemorrhage can occur as a result of PE and usually resolves within a week. Pulmonary infarction is seen more frequently in the lower lobes as wedge-shaped peripheral areas of consolidation with central low attenuation that do not enhance and represent uninfarcted secondary pulmonary lobules (see **Figs. 4** and **5**).[32] Air bronchograms are typically not seen in the areas of infarcted lung.[33,34] The vascular sign (**Fig. 4**A, B) increases the specificity for infarction and corresponds to acute embolus in a dilated vessel leading to the apex of the consolidation (see **Fig. 4**).[35,36] Other indirect signs of acute PE include areas of linear parenchymal bands, focal oligemia, atelectasis or small pleural effusions.[33] Although mosaic attenuation is more common with chronic PE, it can sometimes be seen with acute PE.

Acute large central pulmonary emboli can lead to right heart strain (**Fig. 6**). The effect of PE on the right heart can be assessed by dilatation of the right ventricle (RV) when the short axis diameter of the RV to left ventricle (LV) ratio is greater than one, straightening or deviation of the interventricular septum toward the LV and compression of the LV (**Fig. 6**) or acute enlargement of the central pulmonary arteries.[28,37,38] Signs of right heart strain need to be promptly communicated to the referring physician so that appropriate therapy can be implemented immediately to prevent circulatory collapse.

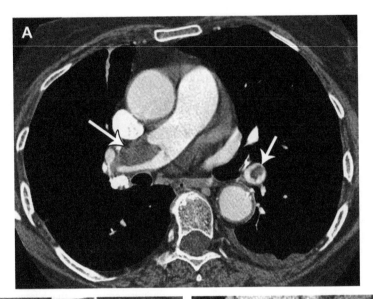

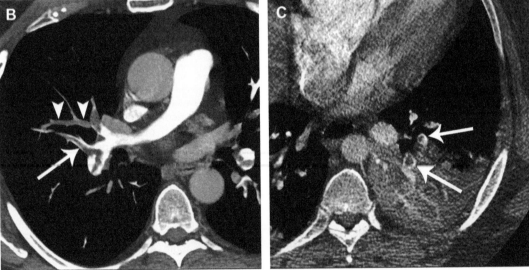

Fig. 2. "Rim-sign" and "railway-track" sign. (A) A low attenuation filling defect from nonocclusive embolus is completely surrounded by a rim of contrast on cross-sectional view of the left lower lobe pulmonary artery. Note large central PE in the right upper lobe artery. (B) On the long axis view of a segmental pulmonary artery, contrast is seen on either side of the nonocclusive embolus in the lateral segmental artery of the middle lobe. Occlusive thrombus is seen in the middle lobe medial segmental artery and its branches. (C) The "rim-sign" (arrows) can be identified even in the presence of consolidation in the right lower lobe.

ARTIFACTS
Technical

Respiratory motion artifact is a common cause for an indeterminate study. The use of 16-slice and higher generation scanners result in shorter breath holds. Routine use of oxygen via a nasal cannula and practicing breath holding with the patient before the acquisition can also help to reduce this artifact. Motion artifact can cause doubling of vessels creating a pseudo filling defect (Fig. 7).[39]

A common pitfall is poor contrast opacification of the pulmonary arteries. This may be because of poor cardiac function and can be overcome by delaying the trigger point by using bolus tracking or timing bolus. Improper coordination of the total contrast injection dose and injection flow rate may lead to a pseudo filling defect in the pulmonary artery that mimics pulmonary embolism (Fig. 8).

A soft tissue reconstruction algorithm should be used to avoid high attenuation around vessels that

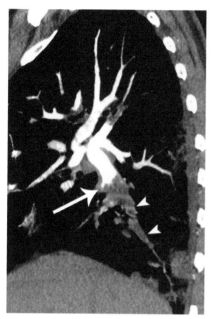

Fig. 3. Vessel cutoff sign of PE. Multiplanar sagittal oblique reformat of the lower lobe an abrupt cutoff (*long arrow*) of the contrast column from embolus that completely occludes the lobar artery in the artery and its distal branches (*short arrows*).

mimics PE. Image noise because of large body habitus increases the quantum mottle and makes it difficult to evaluate the subsegmental arteries. Increasing the collimation, volume, concentration, and rate of contrast helps to increase the signal-to-noise ratio.

Streak artifacts from beam hardening can occur from dense contrast material in the superior vena cava or of from a Swan Ganz balloon catheter in the pulmonary artery. This may obscure emboli or may mimic pulmonary embolism. Using a saline push immediately after the intravenous (IV) contrast injection and scanning in the caudal-to-cranial direction reduces the density of the contrast material in the SVC. A Swan-Ganz balloon catheter must ideally be pulled out of the pulmonary artery and placed in the heart or superior vena cava before CTPA acquisition in order to avoid this artifact.

A pulmonary arterial flow artifact called the stripe sign is caused by deep inspiration immediately before scanning that results in an inhomogeneous admixture of contrast material from the superior vena cava and unopacified blood from the inferior vena cava within the right atrium that leads to transient interruption of the contrast column in the pulmonary arteries.[40] This can be reduced by scanning in suspended inspiration.

Anatomical

Lymph nodes in the intersegmental region can be confused for emboli. This is less of a problem with thin collimation and active scrolling on the workstation. Low-density mucus-filled bronchi and pulmonary veins might also mimic filling defects. This can be differentiated from the corresponding artery by tracing the structure proximally to its origin.

Accuracy of CT Pulmonary Angiography

In the first prospective study by Remy-Jardin and colleagues[21] in 1992, single detector CTPA at 5-mm collimation was compared with catheter angiography, in an ideal group of patients with optimal contrast, with reported sensitivity of 100% and specificity of 96%, demonstrating promise for the use of this technique.[41] This study was followed by several studies that compared single-detector CTPA with catheter angiography as the reference test, with sensitivity ranging from 53% to 97% and specificity from 78% to 97%.[42] The wide variability in sensitivity and specificity partly reflects differences in technique and selection bias, as many of these studies were performed on selective patient groups rather than in consecutive patients with suspected PE. In a systematic literature review of accuracy for PE detection by Eng and coworkers, combined sensitivity for PE detection ranged from 66% to 93% and combined specificities from 89% to 97%.[43] Most of these studies were performed on SDCT. With continuously evolving technology, the true accuracy of the technique is difficult to know.

With the advent and evolution of MDCT techniques over the past decade, the higher spatial and temporal resolution of near isotropic data sets, with shorter breath holds at thinner collimation, has increased the sensitivity and specificity of MDCT for PE detection when compared with SDCT, with reported sensitivity ranging from 83% to 100%, and specificity from 89% to 97%.[18,23,44–46] The recently published PIOPED II study, which was mainly performed on four-slice MDCT scanners, that compared CT with a composite reference standard, a sensitivity of 83% and specificity of 96% was reported for CTPA.[18] When CTV was also performed, the sensitivity for the combined CTPA/CTV exam increased to 90%.[18]

Comparison of CT Pulmonary Angiography with Ventilation and Perfusion Scan

In a study of 179 patients by Blachere and colleagues a statistically significant greater accuracy for CTPA was reported (sensitivity, 94.1%;

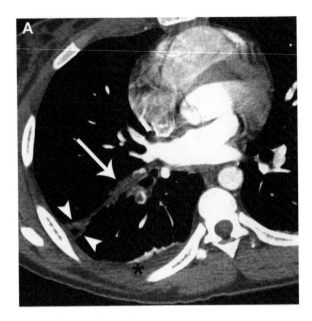

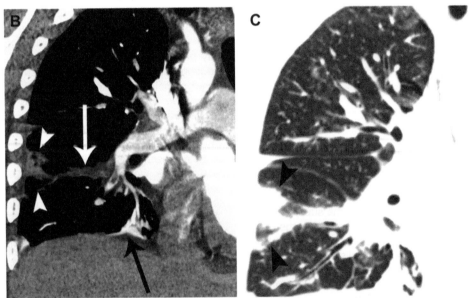

Fig. 4. Pulmonary infarct and the "vascular-sign". (*A*) Axial CT shows an occluded and dilated (*white arrow*) right lower lobe (RLL) pulmonary artery owing to the presence of PE. The vessel is enlarged (vascular sign) courses to the apex of a subpleural nonenhancing triangular opacity, which is an infarct (*arrowheads*). The asterisk indicates a small right pleural effusion. (*B*) Coronal reformatted image along the long axis of the vessel shows embolus (*white arrow*) occluding the RLL segmental pulmonary artery. Note the nonenhancing infarct along the lateral pleura (*arrowheads*), and enhancing atetectasis adjacent to the diaphragm (*black arrow*). (*C*) On lung window images the infarct is triangular in shape and has a broad base with the pleura (*arrowheads*).

specificity, 93.6%; positive predictive value [PPV], 95.5%; NPV, 96.2%) than for planar V/Q scans (sensitivity, 80.8%; specificity, 73.8%; PPV, 95.5%; NPV, 75.9%).[47] Similar results were reported by Grenier: sensitivities, specificities, and kappa values with helical CT and scintigraphy were 87%, 95%, and 0.85 and 65%, 94%, and 0.61, respectively.[48] Many believe these results are sufficient justification for CT pulmonary angiography to replace V/Q scintigraphy in the diagnostic algorithm for suspected acute pulmonary embolism. PIOPED II is the largest and most significant study that has assessed the use of MDCT in the diagnosis of PE in outpatients and inpatients, with reported sensitivity of 83% for CTPA, which is comparable to V/Q scanning.

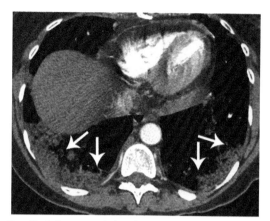

Fig. 5. Pulmonary infarction. Bilateral lower lobe infarction with wedge-shaped areas of peripheral consolidation (*arrows*) showing central lucencies, a reliable finding of infarction in the presence of PE. Air bronchograms are absent. The patient had extensive bilateral central and peripheral PE.

Comparison of CT Pulmonary Angiography and Catheter Angiography

Baile and coworkers[28] evaluated the accuracy of CTPA with catheter pulmonary angiography for the detection of subsegmental PE using post-mortem methacrylate casts of the pulmonary arteries in a porcine model. CT and pulmonary angiography were both performed. The sensitivity for 1-mm collimation helical CT of 87% (95% confidence interval [CI] 79%–93%) was the same as catheter angiography, 87% (95% CI 79%–93%) (P = .42).[49] Note that catheter angiography

did not show 100% sensitivity, but only 87%. In the PIOPED II study, in the 20 cases with discordant CTPA and catheter angiography results, an expert panel concluded that CTPA was accurate in 14 of 20 cases, with 13 cases false-negative and one false-positive on conventional catheter angiography and CT results were false-negative in 2/20 cases. In the remaining 4/20 cases, the panel thought that the CTPA was initially truly negative, however the subsequent pulmonary angiogram showed the presence of PE.[19] This resulted in the sensitivity for detection of PE of 87% with CT, and 32% with conventional angiography (P = 0.007). With better visualization of subsegmental pulmonary arteries on CT and greater interobserver agreement, investigators have questioned whether catheter pulmonary angiography should still be considered the gold standard test by which MDCT is judged.

Interobserver Agreement

For CTPA, interobserver agreement for the detection of acute PE is moderate to almost excellent, with kappa values ranging from 0.59 to 0.94.[39,45,50–54] Remy-Jardin and colleagues[41] report that using thinner collimation of 2 mm versus 3 mm, the kappa values improve, 0.98 versus 0.94 (P<.05).[53]

For subsegmental PE, interobserver agreement is significantly better with MDCT (k = 0.56–0.85) than with SDCT (k = 0.21–0.54), with worse agreement in the obliquely oriented arteries of the middle lobe and lingula.[55–57]

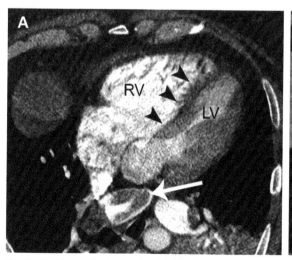
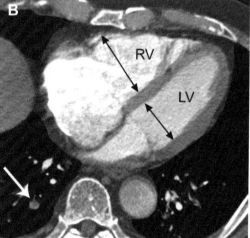

Fig. 6. Right ventricular strain. (*A*) The interventricular septum (*arrowheads*) is bowed toward the left ventricle (LV) and the LV is compressed. Note central PE in the RLL pulmonary artery (*arrow*). (*B*) In another patient with central and peripheral PE (*arrow*), the right atrium and right ventricle are dilated. The short axis diameter of the RV is greater than that of the LV.

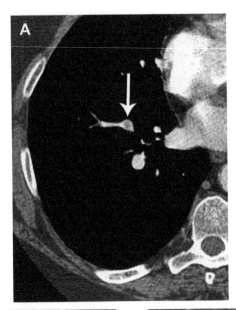

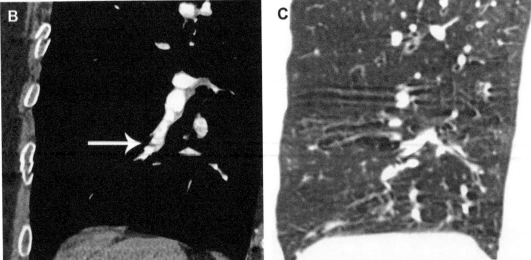

Fig. 7. Technical and interpretative pitfall. (A) Axial CT shows a filling defect (arrow) in a segmental RLL pulmonary artery suggestive of PE, discordant with clinical findings. (B) Coronal reformat at soft tissue window shows a horizontal linear filling defect (arrows) in the corresponding pulmonary artery, which was an artifact corresponding to the pseudofilling defect. Note step artifacts in the ribs from respiratory motion. (C) Lung window settings also show respiratory motion artifact.

For catheter angiography the interobserver agreement is moderate to poor at the subsegmental level. The interobserver agreement for central arteries is reported as 89%, whereas that for subsegmental pulmonary arteries is only 13% to 66%.[58–60]

Isolated Subsegmental Pulmonary Embolism

Ninety-four percent of segmental and 88% of subsegmental pulmonary arteries are well visualized using 16-MDCT (Patel and colleagues, 2003 Society for Computed Body Tomography and Magnetic Resonance annual meeting). There is not only improved visualization of the subsegmental pulmonary arteries using 1-mm collimation, but also improved interobserver agreement regarding the presence or absence of emboli.[25]

The prevalence of isolated subsegmental PE (ISSPE) varies from 3% to 36% at pulmonary angiography or CT (Fig. 9).[10,22,44,59,61,62] With better subsegmental artery visualization at MDCT, and the increased diagnosis of subsegmental PE, the question arises as to clinical significance of these

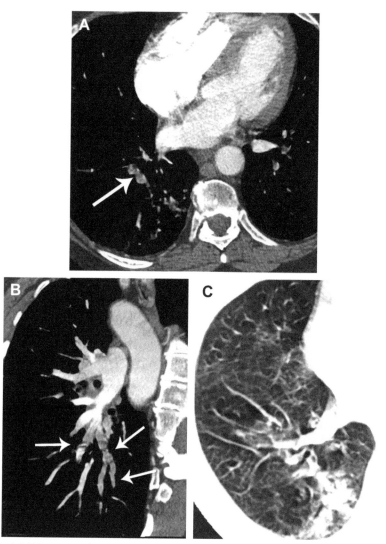

Fig. 8. Technical pitfall because of poor enhancement. (*A*) Axial CT shows low attenuation in the lower lobe pulmonary arteries mimicking PE. (*B*) Sagittal reformats show poor enhancement of the lower lobe pulmonary arteries because of poor bolus. This can be differentiated from vessel cut-off sign by the gradual and not abrupt margin of the contrast column. Respiratory motion artifact is also seen.

small emboli. Should we treat ISSPE? Subsegmental PE are common at autopsy, and when the pulmonary arteries are carefully examined, can be seen in 50% to 90% of patients, suggesting that these small emboli are usually asymptomatic and many resolve naturally.[1,63]

Currently there is no clear recommendation for treatment of ISSPE. Small PE can be clinically important and may benefit from anticoagulant therapy in patients with poor cardiopulmonary reserve, in those with coexistent DVT or a pro-thrombotic stage, in those with chronic pulmonary hypertension, and in cases of ISSPE with right ventricular dilatation, as the risk of death is increased in these patients.[21,38,64,65] When

treatment is withheld because of risks associated with anticoagulation, a lower extremity study is warranted to exclude a DVT.

EVIDENCE FOR MDCT IN THE DIAGNOSIS OF ACUTE PULMONARY EMBOLISM

A meta-analysis published in 2005 by Quiroz and colleagues found the overall negative likelihood ratio after a negative CTPA for PE was 0.07 (95% CI, 0.05–0.11); and the NPV was 99.1% (95% CI, 98.7%–99.5%).[66] The clinical validity of using a CT scan to rule out PE is similar to that reported for conventional pulmonary angiography, namely 1.0% to 2.8% for CT (including single-section,

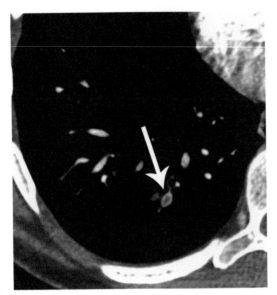

Fig. 9. Isolated subsegmental PE. An isolated nonocclusive filling defect is seen in a subsegmental branch of the right lower lobe posterior basal segmental artery compatible with PE.

multidetector, and electron-beam CT) versus 1.1% to 2.9% for conventional pulmonary angiography.[67,68] There have been a number of outcome studies following a negative CTPA with SDCT that report an average recurrence of VTE (venous thromboembolic disease) in 1.3% and that of fatal PE in 0.3%. Similar results are reported for outcome studies with MDCT. In the Christopher study, patients were classified as having a PE by using an algorithm of a dichotomized decision rule, D-dimer and CT (both SDCT and MDCT).[69] At 3-month follow-up in the 1505 untreated patients following a negative CTPA, a 1.1% risk of thromboembolic disease was reported. In a prospective management study in 756 ED (emergency department) patients with suspected PE, all patients with high clinical probability or non-high clinical probability and positive D-dimer, underwent both CTPA with MDCT and lower limb ultrasonography. Proximal DVT was found in only 3 of 318 patients (0.9%).[70] Righini and colleagues compared two diagnostic strategies that did or did not include lower extremity ultrasound along with D-dimer and MDCT. In the arm that did not use lower extremity ultrasound, the untreated patients with negative D-dimer and MDCT had a 3-month risk of VTE of only 0.3%.[71] These studies demonstrate that a negative MDCT in patients without a high clinical probability is adequate to exclude PE. Therefore, in most patients with suspected acute PE and no symptoms of DVT, especially in an outpatient setting, anticoagulation therapy can be safely withheld

after negative CTPA. The PIOPED II study suggests that in patients with high clinical probability and negative CTPA, further testing should be considered to exclude PE.[18]

Advantages

A significant advantage of CTPA is that it identifies additional findings like pneumothorax, pneumonia, lung cancer, pleural effusions, aortic dissection, pericardial effusion, mediastinitis, and so forth to account for patient symptoms. Alternative diagnosis rates can be seen in 25% to 67% of cases.[72,73] Of the negative CTPA studies in the emergency department, 7% had an alternative diagnosis that required specific and immediate action.[74] Aortic dissection and undiagnosed lung cancer were detected in about 7% of these cases. The incidental finding of clinically relevant disease is a powerful benefit of this modality.[75] There is improved visualization of the segmental and subsegmental pulmonary arteries using MDCT in patients with underlying pulmonary disease (**Fig. 2C**).[76] Cost analysis of different imaging algorithms show that per life saved, CT is the least expensive imaging modality.[77]

Disadvantages

CTPA is commonly used as a first-line imaging test for suspected acute PE. An increasing number of scans are performed especially in the ED setting, with a lower yield of positive PE test results. The high radiation dose is of concern particularly in the younger female patients, as it results in significant radiation dose to the female breast. The average whole-body doses for CTPA range from 2 to 10 mSv and that for V/Q, 0.6 to 1.5 mSv. CTPA causes significant breast radiation of at least 20 mGy (range 10 mGy–70 mGy).[78,79] This is equivalent to 10 to 25 two view mammograms or 100 to 400 chest radiographs. The Biological Effects of Ionizing Radiation, seventh report (BEIR VII) estimates that the lifetime attributable risk for breast cancer from a dose of 20 mGy is approximately 1 in 1200 for a woman aged 20, 1 in 2000 for a woman age 30, and 1 in 3500 for a woman age 40. That is, if a woman aged 30 has a CTPA with a breast dose of 20 mGy, there would be an additional 1/2000 chance of her developing breast cancer.[78] Studies using bismuth breast shields have shown radiation dose reductions of 34% to 57% to the breast, without significant decrease in image quality or diagnostic accuracy.[80]

Other dose-reduction strategies include increasing pitch, dose modulation of tube current, and lowering tube current–time product (milliampere–second) as well as using a lower kVP of 80 to 100 mSV.[81–83]

CT VENOGRAPHY

Most PE originate as thrombi in the lower extremity veins. These thrombi break off and propagate cranially to lodge in the pulmonary arteries. Sonography is the gold standard test for evaluating lower extremity DVT. Loud and colleagues first demonstrated the potential use for indirect CTV in combination with CTPA as a single exam.[84] Multiple studies followed that compared indirect CTV to sonography, with reported sensitivity and specificity greater than 95% in symptomatic patients. The development of indirect CTV has enabled a rapid and accurate combined evaluation for both DVT and PE with one exam.

A variety of techniques ranging from incremental to helical acquisition from the tibial plateaux to the iliac crests have been used, with similar accuracy results. Controversy remains between the use of helical versus incremental images with short skip intervals of 2 to 4 cm.[85] Helical scans minimize the likelihood of missing small DVT, but result in a higher radiation dose. Agreement with incremental discontinuous imaging is good but not perfect; however, the radiation dose is significantly reduced.

CT Venography Technique

CT venography is performed after a 2.5- to 4.0-minute delay following start of injection bolus for CTPA.[86] Eighty-five percent of patients are within 10% of their peak enhancement around this time, whereas in patients with peripheral vascular disease or poor cardiac output, the delays could vary from 145 to 210 seconds.[87,88] Scans are obtained from the tibial plateaus to the iliac crests at 5- to 10-mm collimation.

DVT is seen as a low attenuation filling defect partially or completely occluding the vein, with or without vessel dilatation. Additional findings include dense rim enhancement owing to contrast straining of the vasa vasorum (**Fig. 10**), perivenous soft tissue edema, and presence of collateral vessels.

Technical Pitfalls

Venous return depends on cardiac function, arterial inflow, and venous integrity. Flow artifacts owing to suboptimal contrast opacification and early scanning, can lead to streaming of contrast in the periphery of the vessel, mimicking DVT.[89] In patients with severe atherosclerotic disease, there are arterial inflow problems with delayed venous return, and poor opacification of veins. Streak artifacts from orthopedic hardware,

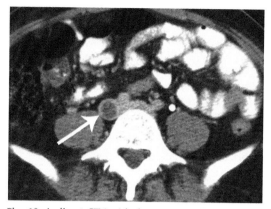

Fig. 10. Indirect CTV with deep venous thrombosis. A low-attenuation filling defect completely occludes the right common iliac vein (*arrow*).

vascular calcification, and contrast pooling in the urinary bladder can obscure portions of adjacent vein.[89]

Evidence for CT Venography

Multiple studies comparing indirect CTV to lower extremity ultrasound, the gold standard test, report sensitivities of 71% to 100%, specificity 97% to 100%, PPV 67% to 100%, and NPV 97% to 100%. In a large retrospective study by Loud and colleagues in 308 patients, the reported sensitivity was 97% and specificity 100%.[90] There were only two false negative and no false positive results. Among other prospective studies, the sensitivity ranges from 93% to 100% and specificity, 97% to 100%.[91–93] The interobserver agreement is also moderate to excellent kappa (0.59–0.88).[18,51,92]

The question arises whether the addition of CTV to the CTPA exam alters clinical management. In a study by Richman and colleagues in 800 ED patients, CTPA was positive in 5% of patients, combined CTPA/CTV in 4%, and CTV alone in 2%.[94] Several studies report an increased detection rate of 2% to 5% of VTE when CTV is added to the CTPA part of the exam. In PIOPED II, there was 95% concordance between ultrasound and CTV. Fourteen (8%) of 181 subjects had DVT alone and the addition of CTV to CTPA increased the overall sensitivity for VTE to 90% versus 83% for CTPA alone.[18] CT is better for diagnosing pelvic DVT and possibly nonobstructive DVT; however, patients with pelvic DVT often have a thrombus load in the leg veins.

Advantages

CTV can be combined with CTPA without requiring any additional intravenous contrast material and offers a one-stop comprehensive test in about 20 minutes. It is also superior for evaluating the inferior vena cava and iliac veins especially in obese patients and those with anomalous, duplicated, and complex venous anatomy.

Patients with recent surgery and with a cast in the lower extremity who are unable to undergo compression sonography can be assessed with CTV.

Disadvantages

The main disadvantage is the additional radiation incurred to the thighs and pelvis. Calculated radiation doses with helical CT range from 3.2 to 9.1 mSV, whereas with discontinuous axial images, radiation is reduced to 0.6 to 2.3 mSv.[85,95] Radiation dose can be minimized by the use of incremental sections, tube current modulation, and scanning only up to the acetabuli as incidence of DVT is low in the IVC (inferior vena cava) and pelvic veins, reported in only 3% in the PIOPED II study.[18] Given the high radiation doses, combined CTPA/indirect CTV should not be part of a routine test especially in the young female of childbearing years. The Fleischner Society Guidelines recommend the use of the combined test, when the emphasis is placed on a complete vascular exam.[79]

PULMONARY EMBOLISM IN PREGNANCY

Venous thromboembolic disease is challenging to diagnose, and is the second commonest cause of mortality in pregnancy following hemorrhage.[96] Even though the risk of radiation is high, the risk of fetal death is much greater if the mother has untreated PE.[97] The incidence of DVT is increasing and is significantly higher than in the nonpregnant female, whereas the incidence in PE between the two groups is not significantly different.[98] Controversy remains as to which is the best test to diagnose VTE in the pregnant female. Initial evaluation should begin with venous ultrasound of the lower extremities. If this is negative, then the question arises as to the preference for an imaging test that delivers the highest yield of a definitive test result, at the lowest radiation risk to the fetus. In the pregnant female, the likelihood of a normal V/Q is high (74%) and a high probability scan low (2%), with a significantly fewer number of patients (24%) having indeterminate scans compared with the general population with suspected VTE, probably because of young age and fewer comorbidities.[99]

The Fleischner society advocates CT as the first line imaging test in pregnancy following leg ultrasound. The fetal radiation exposure for CTPA varies from 3.3 mGy to 130.0 mGy; the dose increases at each trimester as the fetus enlarges and approaches the imaged area in the thorax.[100] The worst estimated absorbed dose for the fetus in the third trimester with CTPA is 130 mGy. The estimated fetal radiation dose for V/Q scanning is 100 to 370 mGy, ie, the dose may be more than three times greater than for CTPA. Based on the average background radiation to an adult, the equated dose to the fetus in utero for 9 months is about 1000 mGy.[101] So a third trimester CTPA delivers only about seven times less than the natural background radiation. All radiation to the fetus carries a potential risk. The absorbed dose to the fetus (0.2 to 0.3 mSv) is well below the level that would increase the risk of congenital abnormality.

Breast radiation dose from CTPA is an additional consideration. The female breast is extremely radiosensitive and a radiation dose of 100 cGy is associated with an increased risk of breast cancer of 40% in young Western women. Epidemiological studies have not detected a significantly increased risk of breast cancer below a dose of 20 cGy. Female breast radiation exposure during CTPA has been calculated at an effective minimum dose of 20 mGy (2 cGy)[64] and that for ventilation/perfusion scanning 0.28 mGy. These estimates are significantly below the level of 20 cGy, below which no effect on the breast can be demonstrated. This exposure should not be ignored and the use of breast shields may reduce this dose by up to 73%.[102]

Although CTPA is advocated as the initial imaging test after ultrasound of the legs, the quality of the scan may not be optimal in pregnant patients. Two recently published articles report a significantly lower enhancement of pulmonary arteries on CTPA in pregnant women with nondiagnostic rates of 7.5% or 27.5%.[103,104] This is thought to occur as a result of a combination of physiological factors: increased cardiac output, increased plasma volume, increased body weight, hyperdynamic circulation, and increased effects of a Valsalva maneuver. Contrast injection protocols need to be modified to address this problem. In pregnant women, the contrast material arrives early within the pulmonary arteries and the peak enhancement is lower. Therefore, the scan should be performed on the highest generation of scanners by using bolus tracking and increased concentration of the contrast material at higher rates of injection.[105] Scarsbrook and colleagues suggest radiation dose–reducing methods with CTPA such as reduced mAs, reduced kVp, increased pitch, increased detector and beam collimation, reducing z-axis range and field of view, and the use of abdominal shielding.[96]

Another consideration is the effect of contrast on a developing fetus, which has not been fully investigated. It is recommended that the infant has thyroid function testing within a week of birth because of the theoretical risk of contrast-induced hypothyroidism.[106]

Magnetic resonance angiography is another alternative to V/Q scanning and CTPA. MR is advantageous because the fetus is not exposed to ionizing radiation or to intravenous contrast material.

IMAGING ALGORITHM FOR DIAGNOSIS OF PE

Imaging algorithms vary, depending on the clinical probability (Fig. 11).

Low Pretest Probability

In the low and intermediate probability population, a cost-effective algorithm would be to perform a D-dimer. The value is in a negative test that effectively rules out significant VTE. If the test is positive, a diagnostic imaging study should be performed depending on local availability, easy access, cost, radiation, and clinician preference.

The chest x-ray (CXR) may be helpful to strategize management. If the CXR is abnormal, the patient should undergo CTPA. If the CXR is normal, either CTPA or V/Q scan can be done. The perfusion portion of the V/Q scan alone can be performed initially if there is radiation concern. The greatest drawback of the V/Q scan is the likelihood of intermediate probability scans which in a setting of a raised D-dimer necessitates another exam such as CTPA thereby increasing cost, radiation, and a delay in diagnosis.

High Pretest Probability

In high-risk cases and with strong pretest probability, D-dimer testing need not be performed because a negative D-dimer result in a patient with a high-probability clinical assessment may not exclude VTE. Depending on local preference, an early CTPA or V/Q scan can be performed if the CXR is normal. If the test is negative, the leg veins should be evaluated with compression sonography. If either CT angiography is positive or DVT is diagnosed, definitive treatment is recommended.

If the CTPA is nondiagnostic, the test can be repeated. If repeat examination is unlikely to alter image quality owing to known patient parameters (poor cardiac output, large patient habitus,

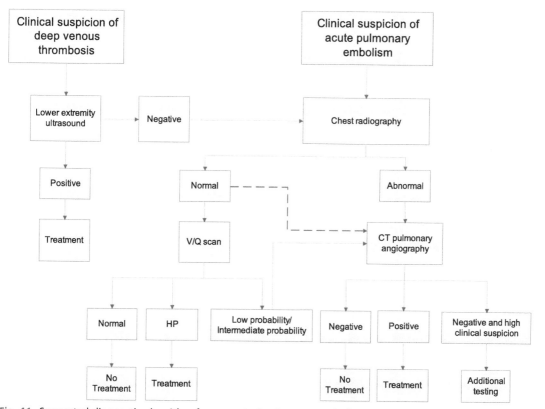

Fig. 11. Suggested diagnostic algorithm for suspected pulmonary embolism.

extensive respiratory motion), then pulmonary angiography can be performed. If both CT angiography and leg vein studies are negative or CTPA/CTV results are negative, options include serial venous ultrasound examinations, pulmonary digital subtraction angiography, and pulmonary scintigraphy.

In the critically ill patient, bedside echocardiogram to assess the right ventricle and for right heart strain and ultrasound examination of the legs can be performed until the patient is stabilized for further imaging tests. CTPA can be a challenging technique to perform in ICU patients because of respiratory motion, suboptimal bolus with poor cardiac reserve, and streak artifact from lines and tubes. However, in one series of 50 consecutive ICU patients with suspected pulmonary embolism, 76% of CT pulmonary angiography examinations were of diagnostic quality in this challenging group of patients.[107]

Future of Pulmonary Imaging

Research is now aimed at ways of radiation dose reduction of CT angiographic data and in computer-aided detection of luminal thrombus and perfusion defects. A large-scale study evaluating MR is under way (PIOPED III). With refinements in SPECT imaging, the role of SPECT V/Q scanning for PE diagnosis needs to be assessed.

Computer-aided detection (CAD) software is anticipated to become a promising supplement to the work and eyes of the radiologist in aiding detection of PE on CTPA. The high false-negative results demand technologic improvement to increase the sensitivity of the system.[108,109] The current role of CAD is that of a second reader particularly for inexperienced readers and for residents.

The Prospective Investigation of Pulmonary Embolism Diagnosis III (PIOPED III) that just completed enrollment will estimate the diagnostic accuracy of gadolinium-enhanced magnetic resonance angiography of the pulmonary arteries (Gd-MRA) and Gd-MRA combined with gadolinium-enhanced magnetic resonance venography (MRV) for the diagnosis of acute PE. If it proves to have high accuracy for diagnosis of PE, it would avoid radiation, which is a big problem with CT.

SUMMARY

CT pulmonary angiography has become a first-line imaging test for evaluation of PE because of its high accuracy, ease of use, and ready availability. PIOPED II supports the use of multidetector CT as a first-line test especially in outpatients. Technological advances continue to evolve, and with refinements in technology, we will continue to optimize imaging for PE detection. Ionizing radiation remains a concern particularly in the young and in pregnant patients, and methods to decrease these are being advocated. SPECT V/Q may play a bigger role in PE diagnosis in the future and the role of MR is yet to be determined in the PIOPED III study, with the potential of solving some of the issues regarding radiation in a select group of patients.

REFERENCES

1. Egermayer P. Follow-up for death or recurrence is not a reliable way of assessing the accuracy of diagnostic tests for thromboembolic disease. Chest 1997;111:1410–3.
2. Goldhaber SZ, Morpurgo M. Diagnosis, treatment, and prevention of pulmonary embolism. Report of the WHO/International Society and Federation of Cardiology Task Force. JAMA 1992;268:1727–33.
3. Stein PD, Beemath A, Olson RE. Trends in the incidence of pulmonary embolism and deep venous thrombosis in hospitalized patients. Am J Cardiol 2005;95:1525–6.
4. Patel S, Kazerooni EA. Helical CT for the evaluation of acute pulmonary embolism. AJR Am J Roentgenol 2005;185:135–49.
5. Silverstein MD, Heit JA, Mohr DN, et al. Trends in the incidence of deep vein thrombosis and pulmonary embolism: a 25-year population-based study. Arch Intern Med 1998;158:585–93.
6. Laporte S, Mismetti P, Decousus H, et al. Clinical predictors for fatal pulmonary embolism in 15,520 patients with venous thromboembolism: findings from the Registro Informatizado de la Enfermedad TromboEmbolica venosa (RIETE) Registry. Circulation 2008;117:1711–6.
7. Nijkeuter M, Hovens MM, Davidson BL, et al. Resolution of thromboemboli in patients with acute pulmonary embolism: a systematic review. Chest 2006;129:192–7.
8. Wells PS, Anderson DR, Rodger M, et al. Derivation of a simple clinical model to categorize patients' probability of pulmonary embolism: increasing the models utility with the SimpliRED D-dimer. Thromb Haemost 2000;83:416–20.
9. Wicki J, Perneger TV, Junod AF, et al. Assessing clinical probability of pulmonary embolism in the emergency ward: a simple score. Arch Intern Med 2001;161:92–7.
10. PIOPED Investigators The. Value of the ventilation/perfusion scan in acute pulmonary embolism. Results of the prospective investigation of pulmonary embolism diagnosis (PIOPED). JAMA 1990; 263:2753–9.

11. Freeman LM, Haramati LB. V/Q scintigraphy: alive, well and equal to the challenge of CT angiography. Eur J Nucl Med Mol Imaging 2009;36: 499–504.

12. Miles S, Rogers KM, Thomas P, et al. A Comparison of SPECT lung scintigraphy and CTPA for the diagnosis of pulmonary embolism. Chest 2009; published online before print June 12, 2009, doi: 10.1378/chest.09-0361.

13. Schluger N, Henschke C, King T, et al. Diagnosis of pulmonary embolism at a large teaching hospital. J Thorac Imaging 1994;9:180–4.

14. Sostman HD, Gottschalk A. The stripe sign: a new sign for diagnosis of nonembolic defects on pulmonary perfusion scintigraphy. Radiology 1982;142: 737–41.

15. Beyth RJ, Quinn LM, Landefeld CS. Prospective evaluation of an index for predicting the risk of major bleeding in outpatients treated with warfarin. Am J Med 1998;105:91–9.

16. Levine MN, Raskob G, Landefeld S, et al. Hemorrhagic complications of anticoagulant treatment. Chest 1998;114:511S–23S.

17. Ghaye B. Peripheral pulmonary embolism on multidetector CT pulmonary angiography. JBR-BTR 2007;90:100–8.

18. Stein PD, Fowler SE, Goodman LR, et al. Multidetector computed tomography for acute pulmonary embolism. N Engl J Med 2006;354:2317–27.

19. Wittram C, Waltman AC, Shepard JA, et al. Discordance between CT and angiography in the PIOPED II study. Radiology 2007;244:883–9.

20. Sinner WN. Computed tomographic patterns of pulmonary thromboembolism and infarction. J Comput Assist Tomogr 1978;2:395–9.

21. Torbicki A, Perrier A, Konstantinides S, et al. Guidelines on the diagnosis and management of acute pulmonary embolism: the Task Force for the Diagnosis and Management of Acute Pulmonary Embolism of the European Society of Cardiology (ESC). Eur Heart J 2008;29:2276–315.

22. Ghaye B, Szapiro D, Mastora I, et al. Peripheral pulmonary arteries: how far in the lung does multi-detector row spiral CT allow analysis? Radiology 2001;219:629–36.

23. Patel S, Kazerooni EA, Cascade PN. Pulmonary embolism: optimization of small pulmonary artery visualization at multi-detector row CT. Radiology 2003;227:455–60.

24. Remy-Jardin M, Remy J, Artaud D, et al. Peripheral pulmonary arteries: optimization of the spiral CT acquisition protocol [see comments]. Radiology 1997;204:157–63.

25. Schoepf UJ, Holzknecht N, Helmberger TK, et al. Subsegmental pulmonary emboli: improved detection with thin-collimation multi-detector row spiral CT. Radiology 2002;222:483–90.

26. Hartmann IJ, Lo RT, Bakker J, et al. Optimal scan delay in spiral CT for the diagnosis of acute pulmonary embolism. J Comput Assist Tomogr 2002;26:21–5.

27. Marten K, Engelke C, Funke M, et al. ECG-gated multislice spiral CT for diagnosis of acute pulmonary embolism. Clin Radiol 2003;58:862–8.

28. van der Meer RW, Pattynama PM, van Strijen MJ, et al. Right ventricular dysfunction and pulmonary obstruction index at helical CT: prediction of clinical outcome during 3-month follow-up in patients with acute pulmonary embolism. Radiology 2005;235: 798–803.

29. Brader P, Schoellnast H, Deutschmann HA, et al. Acute pulmonary embolism: comparison of standard axial MDCT with paddlewheel technique. Eur J Radiol 2008;66:31–6.

30. Chiang EE, Boiselle PM, Raptopoulos V, et al. Detection of pulmonary embolism: comparison of paddlewheel and coronal CT reformations—initial experience. Radiology 2003;228:577–82.

31. Remy J, Remy-Jardin M, Wattinne L, et al. Pulmonary arteriovenous malformations: evaluation with CT of the chest before and after treatment. Radiology 1992;182:809–16.

32. Revel MP, Triki R, Chatellier G, et al. Is it possible to recognize pulmonary infarction on multisection CT images? Radiology 2007;244:875–82.

33. Coche EE, Müller NL, Kim KI, et al. Acute pulmonary embolism: ancillary findings at spiral CT. Radiology 1998;207:753–8.

34. Shah AA, Davis SD, Gamsu G, et al. Parenchymal and pleural findings in patients with and patients without acute pulmonary embolism detected at spiral CT. Radiology 1999;211:147–53.

35. Balakrishnan J, Meziane MA, Siegelman SS, et al. Pulmonary Infarction: CT Appearance with Pathologic Correlation. J Comput Assist Tomogr 1989; 13:941–5.

36. Ren H, Kuhlman JE, Hruban RH, et al. CT of Inflation-fixed Lungs: Wedge-shaped Density and Vascular Sign in the Diagnosis of Infarction. J Comput Assist Tomogr 1990;14:82–6.

37. Findik S, Erkan L, Light RW, et al. Massive pulmonary emboli and CT pulmonary angiography. Respiration 2008;76:403–12.

38. Ghaye B, Ghuysen A, Willems V, et al. Severe pulmonary embolism:pulmonary artery clot load scores and cardiovascular parameters as predictors of mortality. Radiology 2006;239:884–91.

39. Perrier A, Howarth N, Didier D, et al. Performance of helical computed tomography in unselected outpatients with suspected pulmonary embolism. Ann Intern Med 2001;135:88–97.

40. Gosselin MV, Rassner UA, Thieszen SL, et al. Contrast dynamics during CT pulmonary angiogram: Analysis of an inspiration associated artifact. J Thorac Imaging 2004;19:1–7.

41. Remy-Jardin M, Remy J, Wattinne L, et al. Central pulmonary thromboembolism: diagnosis with spiral volumetric CT with the single-breath-hold technique—comparison with pulmonary angiography. Radiology 1992;185:381–7.

42. Safriel Y, Zinn H. CT pulmonary angiography in the detection of pulmonary emboli: a meta-analysis of sensitivities and specificities. Clin Imaging 2002; 26:101–5.

43. Eng J, Krishnan JA, Segal JB, et al. Accuracy of CT in the diagnosis of pulmonary embolism: a systematic literature review. Am J Roentgenol 2004;183. 1819–7.

44. Coche E, Verschuren F, Keyeux A, et al. Diagnosis of acute pulmonary embolism in outpatients: comparison of thin-collimation multi-detector row spiral CT and planar ventilation-perfusion scintigraphy. Radiology 2003;229:757–65.

45. Qanadli SD, Hajjam ME, Mesurolle B, et al. Pulmonary embolism detection: prospective evaluation of dual-section helical CT versus selective pulmonary arteriography in 157 patients. Radiology 2000;217: 447–55.

46. Winer-Muram HT, Rydberg J, Johnson MS, et al. Suspected acute pulmonary embolism: evaluation with multi-detector row CT versus digital subtraction pulmonary arteriography. Radiology 2004; 233:806–15.

47. Blachere H, Latrabe V, Montaudon M, et al. Pulmonary embolism revealed on helical CT angiography: comparison with ventilation-perfusion radionuclide lung scanning. Am J Roentgenol 2000;174:1041–7.

48. Grenier PA, Beigelman C. Spiral computed tomographic scanning and magnetic resonance angiography for the diagnosis of pulmonary embolism. Thorax 1998;53:S25–31.

49. Baile EM, King GG, Muller NL, et al. Spiral computed tomography is comparable to angiography for the diagnosis of pulmonary embolism. Am J Respir Crit Care Med 2000;161:1010–5.

50. Domingo ML, Marti-Bonmati L, Dosda R, et al. Interobserver agreement in the diagnosis of pulmonary embolism with helical CT. Eur J Radiol 2000;34: 136–40.

51. Garg K, Kemp JL, Russ PD, et al. Thromboembolic disease: variability of interobserver agreement in the interpretation of CT venography with CT pulmonary angiography. Am J Roentgenol 2001;176: 1043–7.

52. Mayo JR, Remy-Jardin M, Muller NL, et al. Pulmonary embolism: prospective comparison of spiral CT with ventilation-perfusion scintigraphy. Radiology 1997;205:447–52.

53. Remy-Jardin M, Remy J, Baghaie F, et al. Clinical value of thin collimation in the diagnostic workup of pulmonary embolism. Am J Roentgenol 2000; 175:407–11.

54. van Rossum AB, Treurniet FE, Kieft GJ, et al. Role of spiral volumetric computed tomographic scanning in the assessment of patients with clinical suspicion of pulmonary embolism and an abnormal ventilation/perfusion lung scan [comment]. Thorax 1996;51:23–8.

55. Brunot S, Corneloup O, Latrabe V, et al. Reproducibility of multi-detector spiral computed tomography in detection of sub-segmental acute pulmonary embolism. Eur Radiol 2005;15:2057–63.

56. Patel S, Kazerooni EA, Cascade PN. 16-slice MDCT optimization of small pulmonary artery visualization for pulmonary embolism detection vs 4-slice. Rancho Mirage, CA: MDCT. SCBT/MR Annual Meeting; March 2003.

57. Ruiz Y, Caballero P, Caniego JL, et al. Prospective comparison of helical CT with angiography in pulmonary embolism: global and selective vascular territory analysis. Interobserver agreement. Eur Radiol 2003;13:823–9.

58. Diffin DC, Leyendecker JR, Johnson SP, et al. Effect of anatomic distribution of pulmonary emboli on interobserver agreement in the interpretation of pulmonary angiography. Am J Roentgenol 1998; 171:1085–9.

59. Quinn MF, Lundell CJ, Klotz TA, et al. Reliability of selective pulmonary arteriography in the diagnosis of pulmonary embolism. Am J Roentgenol 1987; 149:469–71.

60. Stein PD, Henry JW, Gottschalk A. Reassessment of pulmonary angiography for the diagnosis of pulmonary embolism: relation of interpreter agreement to the order of the involved pulmonary arterial branch. Radiology 1999;210:689–91.

61. Eyer BA, Goodman LR, Washington L. Clinicians' response to radiologists' reports of isolated subsegmental pulmonary embolism or inconclusive interpretation of pulmonary embolism using MDCT. Am J Roentgenol 2005;184:623–8.

62. Stein PD, Henry JW. Prevalence of acute pulmonary embolism in central and subsegmental pulmonary arteries and relation to probability interpretation of ventilation/perfusion lung scans. Chest 1997;111:1246–8 [see comments].

63. Ryu JH, Olson EJ, Pellikka PA. Clinical recognition of pulmonary embolism: problem of unrecognized and asymptomatic cases. Mayo Clinic Proceedings 1998;73:873–9.

64. Perrier A, Bounameaux H. Accuracy or outcome in suspected pulmonary embolism. N Engl J Med 2006;354:2383–5.

65. Quiroz R, Kucher N, Schoepf UJ, et al. Right Ventricular Enlargement on Chest Computed Tomography. Prognostic Role in Acute Pulmonary Embolism. Circulation 2004:01.CIR.0000129302.0000190476.BC.

66. Quiroz R, Kucher N, Zou KH, et al. Clinical validity of a negative computed tomography scan in

patients with suspected pulmonary embolism: a systematic review. JAMA 2005;293:2012–7.

67. Henry JW, Relyea B, Stein PD. Continuing risk of thromboemboli among patients with normal pulmonary angiograms. Chest 1995;107:1375–8.

68. Novelline RA, Baltarowich OH, Athanasoulis CA, et al. The clinical course of patients with suspected pulmonary embolism and a negative pulmonary arteriogram. Radiology 1978;126:561–7.

69. van Belle A, Buller HR, Huisman MV, et al. Effectiveness of managing suspected pulmonary embolism using an algorithm combining clinical probability, D-dimer testing, and computed tomography. JAMA 2006;295:172–9.

70. Perrier A, Roy PM, Sanchez O, et al. Multidetector-row computed tomography in suspected pulmonary embolism. N Engl J Med 2005;352:1760–8.

71. Righini M, Le Gal G, Aujesky D, et al. Diagnosis of pulmonary embolism by multidetector CT alone or combined with venous ultrasonography of the leg: a randomised non-inferiority trial. Lancet 2008; 371:1343–52.

72. Cross JJ, Kemp PM, Walsh CG, et al. A randomized trial of spiral CT and ventilation perfusion scintigraphy for the diagnosis of pulmonary embolism [see comments]. Clin Radiol 1998;53:177–82.

73. Kim KI, Muller NL, Mayo JR. Clinically suspected pulmonary embolism: utility of spiral CT. Radiology 1999;210:693–7.

74. Richman PB, Courtney DM, Friese J, et al. Prevalence and significance of nonthromboembolic findings on chest computed tomography angiography performed to rule out pulmonary embolism: a multicenter study of 1,025 emergency department patients. Acad Emerg Med 2004;11:642–7.

75. Paul GK, Charles SW. Acute Pulmonary Embolism: Imaging in the Emergency Department. Radiol Clin North Am 2006;44:259–71.

76. Remy-Jardin M, Tillie-Leblond I, Szapiro D, et al. CT angiography of pulmonary embolism in patients with underlying respiratory disease: impact of multislice CT on image quality and negative predictive value. Eur Radiol 2002;12:1971–8.

77. Doyle NM, Ramirez MM, Mastrobattista JM, et al. Diagnosis of pulmonary embolism: a cost-effectiveness analysis. Am J Obstet Gynecol 2004;191: 1019–23.

78. Parker MS, Hui FK, Camacho MA, et al. Female breast radiation exposure during CT pulmonary angiography. Am J Roentgenol 2005;185:1228–33.

79. Remy-Jardin M, Pistolesi M, Goodman LR, et al. Management of suspected acute pulmonary embolism in the era of CT angiography: a statement from the Fleischner Society. Radiology 2007;245: 315–29.

80. Hurwitz LM, Yoshizumi TT, Goodman PC, et al. Radiation dose savings for adult pulmonary embolus 64-MDCT using bismuth breast shields, lower peak kilovoltage, and automatic tube current modulation. Am J Roentgenol 2009;192:244–53.

81. Coche E, Vynckier S, Octave-Prignot M. Pulmonary embolism: radiation dose with multi-detector row CT and digital angiography for diagnosis. Radiology 2006;240:690–7.

82. Heyer CM, Mohr PS, Lemburg SP, et al. Image quality and radiation exposure at pulmonary CT angiography with 100- or 120-kVp protocol: prospective randomized study. Radiology 2007; 245:577–83.

83. Schueller-Weidekamm C, Schaefer-Prokop CM, Weber M, et al. CT angiography of pulmonary arteries to detect pulmonary embolism: improvement of vascular enhancement with low kilovoltage settings. Radiology 2006;241:899–907.

84. Loud PA, Grossman ZD, Klippenstein DL, et al. Combined CT venography and pulmonary angiography: a new diagnostic technique for suspected thromboembolic disease. Am J Roentgenol 1998; 170:951–4.

85. Goodman LR, Stein PD, Beemath A, et al. CT venography for deep venous thrombosis: continuous images versus reformatted discontinuous images using PIOPED II data. Am J Roentgenol 2007;189:409–12.

86. Bruce D, Loud PA, Klippenstein DL, et al. Combined CT Venography and Pulmonary Angiography: How Much Venous Enhancement Is Routinely Obtained? Am. J. Roentgenol 2001;176: 1281–5.

87. Szapiro D, Ghaye B, Willems V, et al. Evaluation of CT time-density curves of lower-limb veins. Invest Radiol 2001;36:164–9.

88. Yankelevitz DF, Gamsu G, Shah A, et al. Optimization of combined CT pulmonary angiography with lower extremity CT venography. Am J Roentgenol 2000;174:67–9.

89. Ghaye B, Szapiro D, Willems V, et al. Pitfalls in CT venography of lower limbs and abdominal veins. Am J Roentgenol 2002;178:1465–71.

90. Loud PA, Katz DS, Bruce DA, et al. Deep venous thrombosis with suspected pulmonary embolism: detection with combined CT venography and pulmonary angiography. Radiology 2001;219:498–502.

91. Begemann PG, Bonacker M, Kemper J, et al. Evaluation of the deep venous system in patients with suspected pulmonary embolism with multi-detector CT: a prospective study in comparison to Doppler sonography. J Comput Assist Tomogr 2003;27: 399–409.

92. Coche EE, Hamoir XL, Hammer FD, et al. Using dual-detector helical CT angiography to detect deep venous thrombosis in patients with suspicion of pulmonary embolism: diagnostic value and additional findings. Am J Roentgenol 2001;176:1035–9.

93. Loud PA, Katz DS, Klippenstein DL, et al. Combined CT venography and pulmonary angiography in suspected thromboembolic disease: diagnostic accuracy for deep venous evaluation. Am J Roentgenol 2000;174:61–5.

94. Richman PB, Wood J, Kasper DM, et al. Contribution of indirect computed tomography venography to computed tomography angiography of the chest for the diagnosis of thromboembolic disease in two United States emergency departments. J Thromb Haemost 2003;1:652–7.

95. Goodman LR, Sostman HD, Stein PD, et al. CT venography: a necessary adjunct to CT pulmonary angiography or a waste of time, money, and radiation? Radiology 2009;250:327–30.

96. Scarsbrook AF, Evans AL, Owen AR, et al. Diagnosis of suspected venous thromboembolic disease in pregnancy. Clin Radiol 2006;61:1–12.

97. Matthews S. Short communication: imaging pulmonary embolism in pregnancy: what is the most appropriate imaging protocol? Br J Radiol 2006;79:441–4.

98. Stein PD, Hull RD, Kayali F, et al. Venous thromboembolism in pregnancy: 21-year trends. Am J Med 2004;117:121–5.

99. Chan WS, Ray JG, Murray S, et al. Suspected pulmonary embolism in pregnancy: clinical presentation, results of lung scanning, and subsequent maternal and pediatric outcomes. Arch Intern Med 2002;162:1170–5.

100. Winer-Muram HT, Boone JM, Brown HL, et al. Pulmonary embolism in pregnant patients: fetal radiation dose with helical CT. Radiology 2002; 224:487–92.

101. Committee to Assess Health Risks from Exposure to Low Levels of Ionizing Radiation, National Research Council. Health risks from exposure to low levels of ionizing radiation: BEIR VII Phase 2, 2006. Available at: http://wwwlnapledu./books/030909156X/html. Accessed October 10, 2009.

102. Hurwitz LM, Yoshizumi TT, Goodman PC, et al. Radiation Dose Savings for Adult Pulmonary Embolus 64-MDCT Using Bismuth Breast Shields, Lower Peak Kilovoltage, and Automatic Tube Current Modulation. Am. J. Roentgenol 2009;192: 244–53.

103. Andreou AK, Curtin JJ, Wilde S, et al. Does pregnancy affect vascular enhancement in patients undergoing CT pulmonary angiography? Eur Radiol 2008;18:2716–22.

104. Jm UK-I, Freeman SJ, Boylan T, et al. Quality of CT pulmonary angiography for suspected pulmonary embolus in pregnancy. Eur Radiol 2008;18: 2709–15.

105. Schaefer-Prokop C, Prokop M. CTPA for the diagnosis of acute pulmonary embolism during pregnancy. Eur Radiol 2008;18:2705–8.

106. Webb JA, Thomsen HS, Morcos SK. The use of iodinated and gadolinium contrast media during pregnancy and lactation. Eur Radiol 2005;15:1234–40.

107. Kelly AM, Patel S, Kazerooni EA. CT pulmonary angiography for acute pulmonary embolism in ICU patients: Clinical Experience. 2002 [abstract] Radiology 2002:225(P):385.

108. Maizlin ZV, Vos PM, Godoy MB, et al. Computer-aided Detection of Pulmonary Embolism on CT Angiography: Initial Experience. J Thorac Imaging 2007;22: 324–9. 310.1097/RTI.1090b1013e31815b31889ca.

109. Walsham AC, Roberts HC, Kashani HM, et al. The use of computer-aided detection for the assessment of pulmonary arterial filling defects at computed tomographic angiography. J Comput Assist Tomogr 2008;32:913–8.

Multidetector Computed Tomographic Pulmonary Angiography: Beyond Acute Pulmonary Embolism

Kristopher W. Cummings, MD*, Sanjeev Bhalla, MD

KEYWORDS

- MDCT • Pulmonary embolism • CTEPH
- Pulmonary angiography

Although multidetector computed tomographic (MDCT) pulmonary angiography (CTPA) has found widespread use in the evaluation for acute pulmonary embolism, advances in technology have allowed for its application in realms that were previously exclusive to conventional pulmonary angiography. Evaluation of chronic thromboembolic pulmonary hypertension (CTEPH) and pulmonary arteriovenous malformations (PAVMs) are 2 specific diagnostic applications that are addressed in this article. Understanding how CTPA can be used in both conditions enables the reader to realize the power of this technique for evaluation of the pulmonary arteries and their relationship with other vessels. With its multiplanar capabilities, MDCTPA can be used for a comprehensive pulmonary artery evaluation, decreasing the need for conventional angiography.

CHRONIC THROMBOEMBOLIC PULMONARY HYPERTENSION

Each year, approximately 600,000 cases of acute pulmonary embolism are diagnosed in the United States.[1] Although most cases demonstrate resolution with anticoagulation therapy, autopsy studies and prospective studies have indicated a 3% to 4% incidence of symptomatic CTEPH after an acute pulmonary embolism.[1–4] The diagnosis requires a high degree of clinical suspicion and is often delayed because of the nonspecific presenting complaints, including decreased exercise tolerance and progressive dyspnea. Large perfusion defects on ventilation-perfusion scintigraphy, extensive clot burden, elevated pulmonary artery pressures on echocardiography at the time of acute presentation, idiopathic pulmonary embolism, and splenectomy have all been cited as risk factors for subsequent development of CTEPH.[3,5]

The pathogenesis and underlying mechanisms of CTEPH are incompletely understood. Most theories favor an inciting embolic event leading to incomplete resorption, endothelialization, and scar formation. However, nearly 50% of patients with diagnosed CTEPH have no prior documented history of venous thromboembolism, presumably because of previously asymptomatic episodes of pulmonary embolism.[6,7] Although physical obstruction of central pulmonary vessels is likely to play a role in the pathogenic process, it is known

Funding/Grant support: none.
Cardiothoracic Imaging, Mallinckrodt Institute of Radiology, Barnes-Jewish Hospital, 510 South Kingshighway Boulevard, Campus Box 8131, St Louis, MO 63110, USA
* Corresponding author.
E-mail address: cummingsk@mir.wustl.edu (K.W. Cummings).

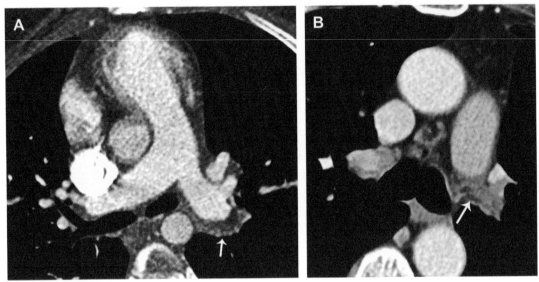

Fig. 1. (*A, B*) Left main pulmonary artery occlusions due to chronic organizing thrombus in 2 different patients. Low attenuation thrombus (*arrows*) results in rapid tapering and occlusion of the left main pulmonary arteries of 2 different patients with prior pulmonary embolus. The convex leading margin of the contrast column results in a pouch deformity.

that patients with CTEPH also develop a peripheral small vessel arteriopathy that is histologically identical to that seen in idiopathic pulmonary hypertension affecting both regions of the lung with and without evidence of prior thromboemboli.[6,8] This peripheral vasculopathy is believed to be a major reason for persistently elevated pulmonary vascular resistance in 10% to 15% of patients who have undergone pulmonary endarterectomy.[6]

MDCT has emerged as an important tool in the diagnosis and preoperative assessment of CTEPH. Although conventional angiography has traditionally been the study of choice, newer studies have established the equivalence or even superiority of MDCT with pulmonary angiography for the diagnosis of central clot burden and the equivalence for segmental and subsegmental vessel occlusion.[9–11] These studies suggest

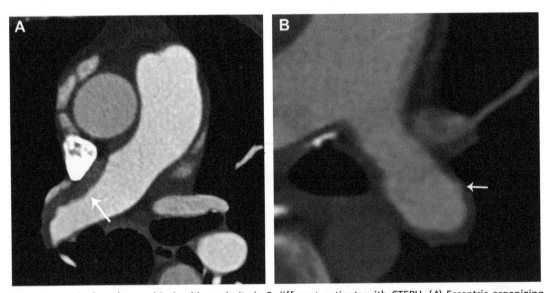

Fig. 2. Eccentric thrombus and intimal irregularity in 2 different patients with CTEPH. (*A*) Eccentric organizing thrombus (*arrow*) is seen extending from the right main pulmonary artery into lobar branches causing luminal narrowing in a patient with chronic pulmonary emboli. (*B*) Subtle intimal irregularity (*arrow*) in the left main pulmonary artery in a different patient with CTEPH.

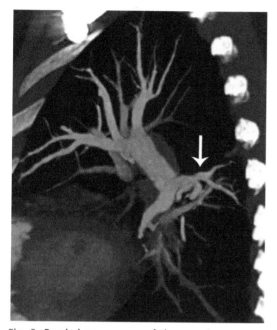

Fig. 3. Beaded appearance of the superior segment left lower lobe pulmonary artery in a patient with CTEPH. Thin MIP image in oblique sagittal plane demonstrates a beaded appearance (*arrow*) at the pulmonary arterial branch indicating prior thromboembolic injury.

superiority of angiography for nonocclusive segmental and subsegmental thrombus, although the use of thin maximum intensity projection (MIP) images and multiplanar viewing are likely to improve the accuracy of CTPA with higher detector row scanners. Data from comparison of computed tomography (CT) and pulmonary angiography for acute pulmonary embolism, limited comparative evidence of CT and angiography for chronic pulmonary embolism, and the avoidance of complications associated with an invasive procedure combine to make CTPA a first-line diagnostic consideration for suspected chronic thromboembolic disease. At the authors' institution, contrast-enhanced CT imaging is performed with approximately 100 mL of 350 mg/mL nonionic intravenous contrast (Optiray 350, Covidien, Mansfield, MA) injected at a rate of 4 mL/s using a collimation of 0.6 mm, slice thickness of 1 mm, and pitch of 1 (SOMATOM Sensation 64, Siemens Healthcare, Erlangen, Germany). Bolus tracking software is used with the region of interest placed at the main pulmonary artery, and data is acquired in a caudal to cranial direction to limit respiratory motion artifact at the lung bases where embolic events are more common. This protocol is identical to that used for acute pulmonary embolism at the authors' institution. In most

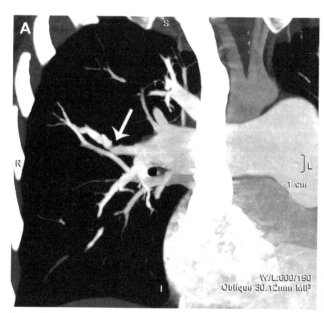
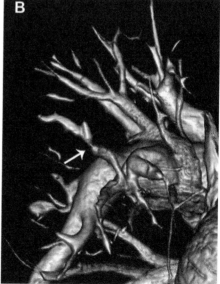

Fig. 4. Focal stenosis in a pulmonary arterial branch in a patient with CTEPH. Coronal thin MIP (*A*) and 3-dimensional volume-rendered (*B*) images demonstrate focal pulmonary arterial branch narrowing (*arrows*) with mild peripheral vessel dilatation.

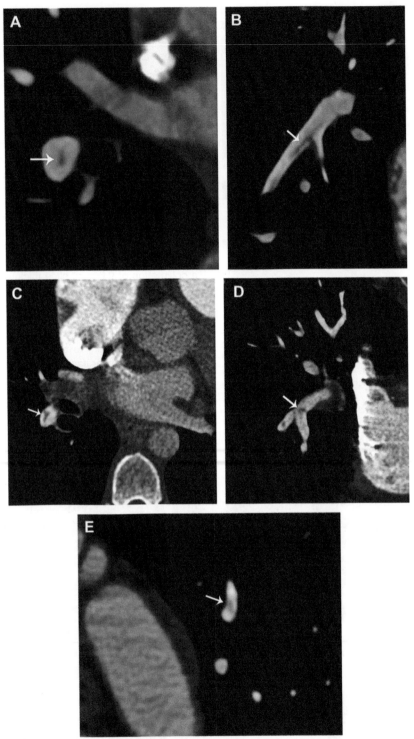

Fig. 5. Intravascular pulmonary arterial webs in 3 different patients with CTEPH. Contrast-enhanced axial (*A*) and oblique multiplanar reconstruction (*B*) images demonstrate a thin web-like filling defect (*arrows*) in the right lower lobe pulmonary artery. In a different patient (*C, D*) a similar defect (*arrows*) is seen. A third patient (*E*) has a short band (*arrow*) in a left upper lobe pulmonary arterial branch.

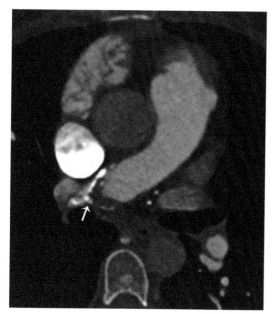

Fig. 6. Calcification of organizing thrombus in a patient with CTEPH. Contrast-enhanced CT image demonstrates chronic occlusion of the right main pulmonary artery with partially calcified thrombus (*arrow*).

examinations, the authors observed adequate opacification of the thoracic aorta for evaluation of systemic collaterals, although some institutions make specific contrast volume or timing adjustments to ensure systemic arterial enhancement. One-millimeter soft tissue reconstructions are performed, and the data is interpreted on a 3-dimensional workstation where the study is viewed in axial, sagittal, and coronal planes, including the use of multiplanar thin (4–7 mm) MIP images.

MDCT pulmonary angiographic findings can be divided into vascular, nonvascular, and cardiac categories. Pulmonary artery occlusion, eccentric narrowing or mural thrombus, intravascular webs, and beaded or tortuous vessels are all findings similar to those seen at conventional angiography. Although abrupt occlusion of a pulmonary artery by acute embolus results in a concave contrast margin, the margin of the contrast column in a chronically occluded vessel is convex, resulting in a "pouch" deformity (**Fig. 1**).[12] The peripheral pulmonary artery in this region is often attenuated and smaller than the adjacent bronchus, which is a finding that is best appreciated on lung window settings. As organization and endothelialization of thrombus occurs, the lumen may be eccentrically narrowed or may demonstrate luminal irregularity (**Fig. 2**). This can result in beaded or rapidly tapering pulmonary vessels (**Fig. 3**). Central recanalization in an occlusive thrombus can result in the appearance of a focal stenosis (**Fig. 4**).[13] Webs or bands, thin linear filling defects within the contrast stream over a short segment, are attached to the vessel wall at 1 or 2 points and are indicators of chronic embolic disease (**Fig. 5**).[14] Use of a wide window setting is needed to avoid obscuration of these defects by a dense contrast column. Rarely, calcification can be seen in chronic, organizing thrombus

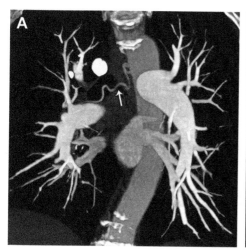
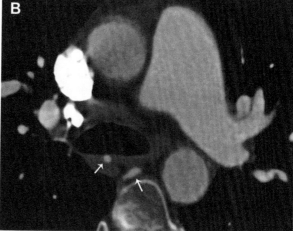

Fig. 7. Bronchial artery enlargement in 2 different patients with CTEPH. Oblique coronal MIP (*A*) and axial (*B*) CT images demonstrate enlarged bronchial arteries (*arrows*) arising from the descending thoracic aorta in the region of the carinal bifurcation.

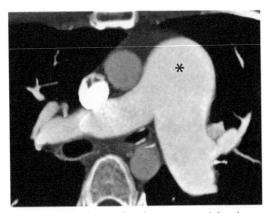

Fig. 8. Main and central pulmonary arterial enlargement in a patient with CTEPH. The main pulmonary artery (*asterisk*) is more than twice the size of the ascending aorta in this patient with marked pulmonary arterial hypertension.

(Fig. 6). Extensive calcification should prompt consideration of other entities, such as Eisenmenger syndrome or mitral disease.

As in certain chronic inflammatory conditions or disease that limits pulmonary arterial flow, systemic collateral blood flow to the lung via enlarged bronchial, transpleural (intercostal), internal mammary, or phrenic arteries develops in chronic thromboembolic disease.[15,16] In one study, up to 47% of patients with CTEPH had dilated bronchial arteries (Fig. 7). Enlarged bronchial arteries are rarely seen in cases of acute pulmonary embolism or primary pulmonary hypertension.[16–19] Bronchial enlargement has been positively correlated with more central thromboembolic disease burden.[20] This is likely the explanation for the finding of lower postoperative mortality in patients with dilated bronchial arteries who undergo pulmonary thromboendarterectomy (PTE).[21] Similar to other conditions with elevated pulmonary arterial pressures, dilatation of the main and central pulmonary arteries can also be seen in CTEPH (Fig. 8). When the main pulmonary artery measures 30 mm or more, orthogonal to its long axis, or when the ratio of the main pulmonary artery diameter to the ascending aortic diameter is greater than 1 mm, then there is a strong correlation with elevated pulmonary artery pressures.[22,23]

Mosaic lung attenuation, areas of sharply demarcated lower and higher differential attenuation at lung window settings on MDCT, has been reported in more than 70% of cases of CTEPH.[17,24,25] The darker areas, a result of the vascular obstruction related to thromboemboli or a distal arteriopathy, correspond to areas of relatively decreased perfusion and often demonstrate attenuated pulmonary vessels in comparison with the adjacent bronchi (Fig. 9). The areas of higher attenuation have normal or increased perfusion and may have arterial enlargement. Mosaicism is much more commonly seen in CTEPH than in primary pulmonary hypertension, and it has been found to be a predictor of persistently elevated pulmonary vascular resistance after PTE, making it a possible marker for distal arteriopathy if found in the setting of little central disease.[17,24] One must use caution in attributing mosaic attenuation to small vessel disease and CTEPH in the absence

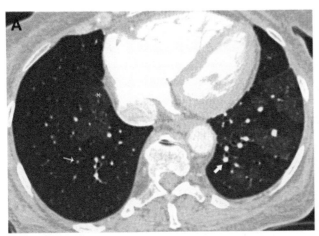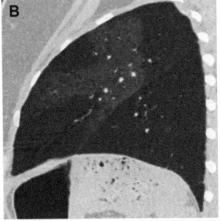

Fig. 9. Mosaic lung attenuation in patients with CTEPH. Axial CT image on lung window settings (*A*) demonstrates areas of differential attenuation, with the lighter areas (*asterisk*) representing regions of preserved pulmonary arterial perfusion. The pulmonary arterial branch size was also decreased (*thin arrow*) in certain of areas of "darker" or underperfused lung where the normal pulmonary arterial to bronchial diameter ratio is maintained in other regions (*thick arrow*). A minimum intensity projection sagittal image (*B*) in a patient with mosaic lung attenuation also demonstrates a paucity of pulmonary vasculature in the left lower lobe.

of additional evidence of chronic pulmonary emboli, as small airways disease is common and gives a similar appearance. An exhalation sequence, which demonstrates accentuation of the darker regions of air trapping in small airways disease, can help to differentiate the 2 entities if there is uncertainty.

Nonvascular findings at MDCT of CTEPH include parenchymal opacities and bronchiectasis. Peripheral parenchymal opacities are frequently seen in cases of CTEPH (Fig. 10).[17] These areas are believed to represent the sequela of prior parenchymal infarctions, although the typical wedge-shaped pleural-based appearance may evolve over time and become irregular as scar formation occurs. Cylindrical bronchiectasis at the segmental and subsegmental levels can be seen in CTEPH.[26] This is accentuated by the

adjacent pulmonary arterial vessels, which are frequently diminutive or absent because of occlusion and scarring.

Rapid acquisition thin collimation MDCT also demonstrates secondary morphologic and/or physiologic cardiac changes in CTEPH. Chronically elevated pulmonary arterial pressures result in right ventricular enlargement and muscular hypertrophy (Fig. 11). A right to left ventricular maximal diameter ratio of greater than 1 and the presence of interventricular septal flattening or bowing leftward are signs of enlargement and elevated pulmonary arterial pressures.[27] Disease progression and further elevation in pressures result in right atrial dilatation, and tricuspid regurgitation, as evidenced by reflux of contrast into a dilated inferior vena cava and hepatic veins (Fig. 12). Patency of the foramen ovale may also

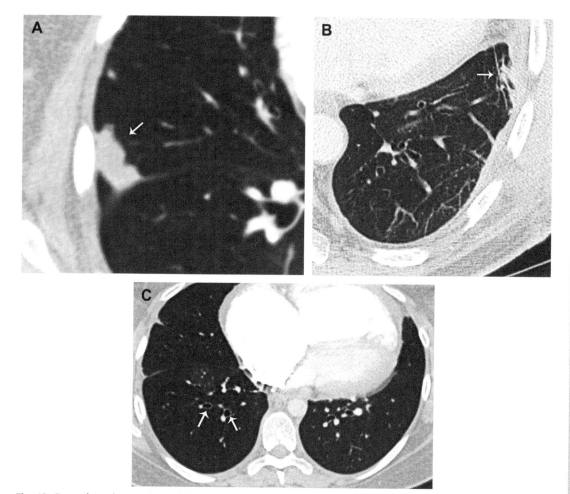

Fig. 10. Parenchymal opacities and bronchiectasis in 2 different patients with CTEPH. (A) Peripheral parenchymal opacity (arrow) representing scarring from prior infarction and (C) cylindrical bronchiectasis (arrows) are seen in a patient with CTEPH. A different patient (B) also has evidence of pleural thickening and peripheral parenchymal scarring (arrow) from prior infarction.

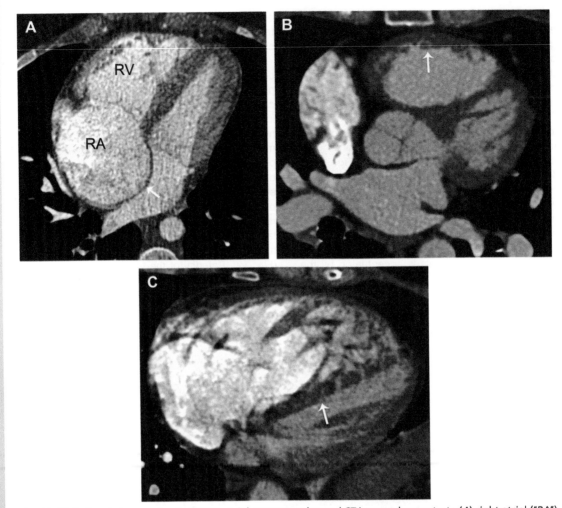

Fig. 11. Right heart changes due to CTEPH. Axial contrast-enhanced CT images demonstrate (*A*) right atrial ("RA") and right ventricular ("RV") enlargement and leftward bowing of the interatrial septum due to elevated right artrial pressures (*arrow*). (*B*) right ventricular hypertrophy (*arrow*). In a different patient (*C*), there is flattening of the interventricular septum (*arrow*) in addition to right heart chamber enlargement.

be observed on nongated MDCT in patients with CTEPH and elevated right heart pressures, as evidence by differential contrast extending from the right atrium toward the left atrium at the fossa ovalis.

Another benefit of MDCT over conventional pulmonary angiography is the ability of MDCT to demonstrate alternative explanations for pulmonary arterial hypertension in those patients not found to have evidence of chronic thromboembolic disease. As thin collimation and reconstruction intervals are used to evaluate the pulmonary vasculature, the pulmonary parenchyma is also evaluated in a fashion analogous to high-resolution CT protocols, allowing for detection of interstitial lung disease or emphysema. Intracardiac shunts, such as atrial and ventricular septal defects, can be detected. Occasionally,

congenital abnormalities, such as partial anomalous pulmonary venous return, have been discovered during MDCT evaluation to exclude CTEPH.

MDCT also plays a crucial role in the selection of patients for PTE, which is the only curative treatment for chronic thromboembolic pulmonary hypertension. At experienced centers where mortality rates range from 4% to 10%, selected patients undergo surgical removal of organized thrombus and the inner portion of the arterial wall in the main, lobar, segmental, and even subsegmental pulmonary vessels.[28] During the interpretation of MDCT cases of CTEPH, it is important for the radiologist to convey the degree of central (main, lobar, or proximal segmental) disease versus distal (peripheral segmental and subsegmental) disease, because central disease is more easily accessible surgically and demonstrates the best

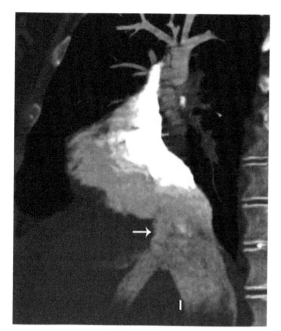

Fig. 12. Tricuspid regurgitation with inferior vena cava and hepatic vein enlargement. Oblique sagittal MIP CT image demonstrates marked enlargement of the inferior vena cava (*arrow*) and engorged hepatic veins in this patient with CTEPH and tricuspid regurgitation.

response to PTE. Those patients with little apparent central disease and significantly elevated pulmonary vascular resistance measurements are at higher risk for poor surgical outcome.[28]

PAVMS

Just as MDCT for chronic pulmonary embolism illustrates the ability of CTPA to image the intrinsic properties of the pulmonary arteries, CTPA for PAVMs is a good example of how this technique can demonstrate the intricate relationships of the pulmonary arteries with other vascular structures. PAVMs are rare direct vascular communications that occur between pulmonary arterial and venous channels. Any discussion on PAVMs must include the disorder known as hereditary hemorrhagic telangiectasia (HHT) or the Osler-Weber-Rendu syndrome, an autosomal dominant condition with variable penetrance resulting in the formation of numerous visceral AVMs, mucocutaneous telangiectasia, and frequently recurrent episodes of epistaxis, as approximately 80% of patients with a PAVM have HHT.[29] Although HHT is a relatively rare disorder with prevalence estimates of 1/5000 to 1/10,000, 15% to 45% of patients have PAVMs.[29,30] Many of the clinical complications of this disorder are related to the presence of PAVMs. Due to the underlying right-to-left shunting, hypoxia and dyspnea on exertion are common presenting complaints. Stroke, transient ischemic attack, and brain abscesses are well-known complications that are also believed to be

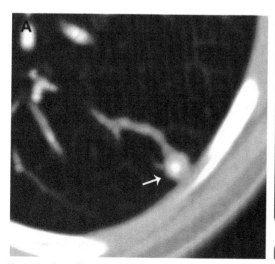
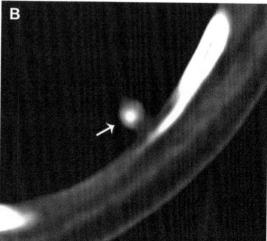

Fig. 13. Granuloma mimicking a PAVM. Thin MIP lung window setting image (*A*) demonstrates a peripheral nodule (*arrow*) with a feeding arterial vessel. Noncontrast axial CT image (*B*) demonstrates central calcification (*arrow*) typical of healed granulomatous infection. No draining vein was present.

a direct result of shunting. Rarer complications such as pulmonary hemorrhage, hemothorax, and migraine headaches have also been encountered. Presumably related to increased cardiac output and decreased vascular wall stability associated with hormonal changes, the risk of life-threatening hemorrhagic complications is increased during pregnancy.[30,31]

PAVMs may also be encountered in patients with prior chest trauma or surgery, infections such as schistosomiasis, and surgically created cavopulmonary shunts (Glenn shunt), but some patients may not have a known cause. As the authors' institution has a large patient population with congenital heart disease, PAVMs are frequently encountered in patients who have undergone cavopulmonary shunts to direct systemic venous blood from the upper body to the pulmonary arterial circulation, most commonly in patients with single ventricle anatomy. Up to 25% of patients have been reported to develop PAVMs after cavopulmonary anastomosis.[32] Exclusion of admixture with hepatic venous blood is believed to play a key role in the development of

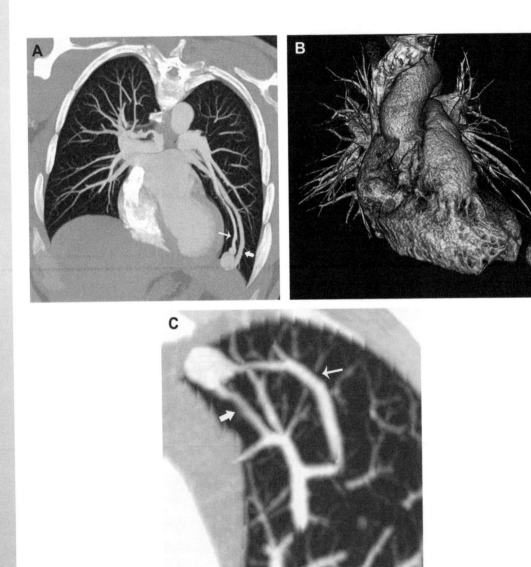

Fig. 14. Simple PAVMs in 2 patients with HHT. Oblique coronal thin MIP lung window setting (A) and 3-dimensional volume rendered (B) CT images demonstrate a simple lingular PAVM with single feeding artery (*thin arrow, A*) and single draining vein (*thick arrow, A*) filling a large vascular nidus (*arrow, B*). Axial thin MIP image (C) in a different patient demonstrates a simple PAVM with feeding artery (*small arrow*) and draining vein (*thick arrow*).

PAVMs, as surgical restoration of hepatic blood flow to the pulmonary arterial circulation can cause regression of PAVMs.[33]

Contrast transthoracic echocardiography (with agitated saline) is the test of choice for initial screening of patients with HHT, because it has a reported sensitivity of more than 90% for detection of intrapulmonary shunting related to PAVMs.[34] Injection of agitated saline solution demonstrates the presence of contrast, which should normally be filtered by the lung, in the left heart within 3 to 4 heartbeats. Although conventional pulmonary angiography was once considered the gold standard for evaluation of PAVMs, it has been supplanted by MDCT for screening. In initial studies, the sensitivity of MDCT was greater than that of pulmonary angiography, approaching 98%.[35] This higher sensitivity has also been shown in newer studies involving digital subtraction pulmonary angiography (DSPA); MDCT had a mean whole-lung sensitivity of up to 83% compared with 70% for DSPA.[36] The ability to avoid an invasive procedure has important implications for patients with HHT and their family members who will need screening and follow-up examinations.

At the authors' institution, all evaluations for PAVMs begin with MDCT. Initially, a low-dose precontrast examination (120 kV, 30 mA) of the chest is performed to delineate any calcified granulomas that might subsequently be confused for AVMs on contrast-enhanced and MIP images because of the frequent presence of a feeding artery (Fig. 13). Contrast-enhanced CT imaging is then performed with approximately 100 mL of Optiray 350, a nonionic intravenous contrast injected at a rate of 4 mL/s using a collimation of 0.6 mm, slice thickness of 1 mm, and pitch of 1 (Siemens 64 detector row scanner). Bolus tracking software is used with the region of interest placed at the main pulmonary artery, and data is acquired in a cranial to caudal direction. Data is transferred to a 3-dimensional workstation where interpretation occurs using soft tissue and lung window settings in multiple planes and thin (3–4 mm) multiplanar and oblique MIP lung window images to best display and characterize any feeding artery and draining vein.

By definition, a feeding pulmonary artery and a draining pulmonary vein must be present to classify a lesion as a PAVM on MDCT (Fig. 14). Lesions frequently have an enhancing nodular focus or nidus intervening between the feeding and draining vessels, although sometimes this focus is only a ground glass opacity likely representing a microscopic telangiectasia (Fig. 15). Simple PAVMs are fed by a single pulmonary artery and drained by a single pulmonary vein. Complex PAVMs have more than 1 feeding artery and 1 or more draining veins, and they have been estimated to represent 20% of lesions.[37] Lesions are more frequently seen in the lower lobes and have a predilection for the outer, subpleural lung parenchyma.[38,39] Multiple or diffuse PAVMs are more commonly seen in HHT and in patients with cavopulmonary shunts (Fig. 16). Measurement of the diameter of the feeding arterial branch is more important than the actual size of the nidus, because lesions with feeding arteries of 3 mm or greater in size are treated with embolotherapy.[40] The decision about where along the feeding pulmonary artery this diameter should be

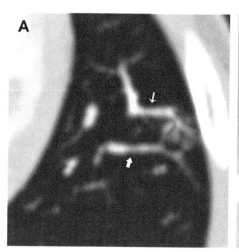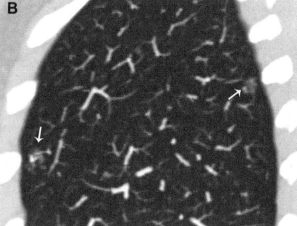

Fig. 15. Telangiectatic PAVMs. Thin axial MIP image (A) demonstrates a single feeding artery (thin arrow) and a single draining vein (thick arrow) to a ground glass nidus. Sagittal thin MIP image (B) demonstrates additional foci of ground glass (arrows) indicating telangiectatic PAVMs.

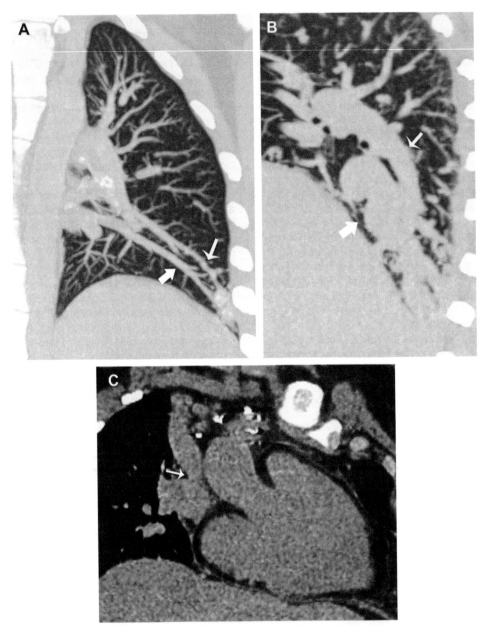

Fig. 16. PAVMs in a patient with double outlet right ventricle and Glenn shunt. Oblique coronal (*A*) and sagittal (*B*) thin MIP images demonstrate PAVMs with enlarged feeding arteries (*thin arrows, A* and *B*) and draining veins (*thick arrows, A* and *B*). (*C*) Glenn shunt (*arrow*) directs systemic venous return from the superior vena cava to the right pulmonary artery. Note is made that intravenous contrast is not required for PAVM assessment.

measured is somewhat arbitrary, but the measurement should occur as close to the nidus as possible beyond any parenchymal branches. Although intravenous contrast material is routinely used in the authors' protocol to allow confirmation of enhancement of the nidus and to allow 3-dimensional mapping of the feeding and draining vessels, with advanced MDCT and thin collimation, intravenous contrast is not required for detection of PAVMs given the inherent contrast between dense pulmonary vessels and less-dense lung parenchyma.

Embolotherapy has replaced surgical resection as the standard treatment of patients with PAVMs having feeding arteries of size 3 mm or more, given that 50% of patients have a stroke, brain abscess, or other complications without intervention.[41] MDCT plays an important role in follow-up

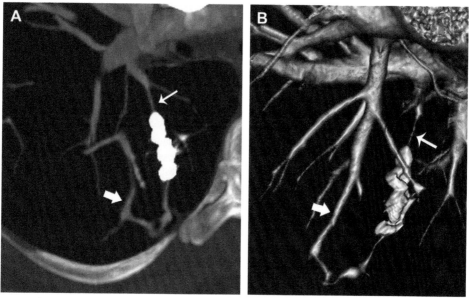

Fig. 17. Recanalized PAVM in the right lower lobe. Thin MIP soft tissue window (*A*) and 3-dimensional volume-rendered (*B*) images demonstrate persistent enhancement of the feeding pulmonary artery (*thin arrows*) and draining pulmonary vein (*thick arrows*) in a PAVM, which has previously undergone coil embolization.

evaluation of these patients, as recanalization or re-perfusion of PAVMs after embolotherapy has been reported in up to 20% of cases (**Fig. 17**).[42] On follow-up examinations after treatment, the nidus should decrease in size and the embolized feeding artery should fail to demonstrate enhancement. The draining vein may continue to show enhancement on postcontrast studies, a finding that, by it-self, does not indicate treatment failure as it can also be seen with retrograde filling of the vein. Treated lesions may develop reperfusion due to the enlargement of previously unseen feeding pulmonary arteries or the development of systemic perfusion (**Fig. 18**).[42] Follow-up examinations are needed as growth of nonoccluded PAVMs may occur and reach size thresholds for treatment.[43]

The authors routinely image the abdomen in the arterial phase for assessment of hepatic

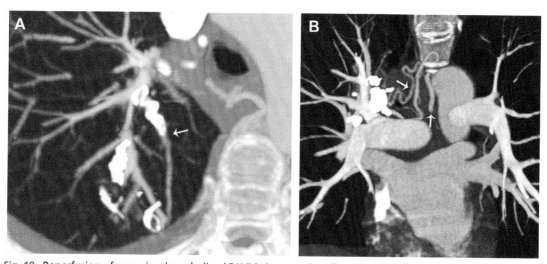

Fig. 18. Reperfusion of a previously embolized PAVM via systemic collaterals. Thin MIP axial CT image (*A*) demonstrates persistent enhancement of a feeding pulmonary artery distal to an embolization coil (*arrow*). On a coronal thin MIP image (*B*) the arterial supply to reperfuse this PAVM is seen to arise from systemic bronchial artery enlargement (*arrows*).

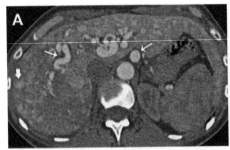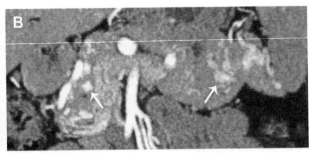

Fig. 19. Abdominal AVMs in 2 patients with HHT. Axial thin MIP CT image (*A*) demonstrates enlarged, tortuous hepatic arteries and celiac axis (*thin arrows*) and parenchymal contrast blushes (*thick arrow*) indicating diffuse hepatic AVMs. Coronal thin MIP CT image (*B*) in a different patient reveals diffuse pancreatic parenchymal replacement by AVMs seen as focal areas of arterial contrast blushing (*arrows*).

arteriovenous malformations (AVMs) (**Fig. 19**). These can be seen as areas of arterial contrast blushing, early enhancement of hepatic or portal veins, and transient hepatic attenuation difference. Enlargement and tortuosity of the celiac and hepatic arteries are also strongly suggestive of hepatic AVMs. In addition, pancreatic and gastrointestinal lesions may be detected.

SUMMARY

Technologic advancements that allow for rapid acquisition and very thin collimation reconstruction of images on MDCT have provided opportunities for the expansion of noninvasive diagnostic imaging of the pulmonary arteries beyond evaluation for acute pulmonary embolus. MDCT now plays a crucial role in the diagnosis and treatment planning for CTEPH and PAVMs. Both indications demonstrate the power of this technique to image the pulmonary arteries themselves and their relationship with other vascular structures. The additional use of multiplanar and 3-dimensional techniques has allowed CTPA to continue expanding its use, reserving conventional angiography for problem solving and embolotherapy.

REFERENCES

1. Tapson VF, Humbert M. Incidence and prevalence of chronic thromboembolic pulmonary hypertension: from acute to chronic pulmonary embolism. Proc Am Thorac Soc 2006;3(7):564–7.
2. Fedullo PF, Auger WR, Kerr KM, et al. Chronic thromboembolic pulmonary hypertension. Semin Respir Crit Care Med 2003;24:273–86.
3. Pengo V, Lensing AW, Prins MH, et al. Incidence of chronic thromboembolic pulmonary hypertension after pulmonary embolism. N Engl J Med 2004; 350(22):2257–64.
4. Dalen JE, Albert JS. Natural history of pulmonary embolism. Prog Cardiovasc Dis 1975;17:259–70.
5. Jais X, Ioos V, Jardim C, et al. Splenectomy and chronic thromboembolic pulmonary hypertension. Thorax 2005;60(12):1031–4.
6. Auger WR, Kim NH, Kerr KM, et al. Chronic thromboembolic pulmonary hypertension. Clin Chest Med 2007;28(1):255–69.
7. Fedullo PF, Auger WR, Kerr KM, et al. Chronic thromboembolic pulmonary hypertension. N Engl J Med 2001;345(20):1465–72.
8. Moser KM, Bloor CM. Pulmonary vascular lesions occurring in patients with chronic major vessel thromboembolic pulmonary hypertension. Chest 1994;105(5):1619–20.
9. Tardivon AA, Musset D, Maitre S, et al. Role of CT in chronic pulmonary embolism: comparison with pulmonary angiography. J Comput Assist Tomogr 1993;17(3):345–51.
10. Pitton MB, Kemmerich G, Herber S, et al. [Chronic thromboembolic pulmonary hypertension: diagnostic impact of multislice-CT and selective pulmonary DSA]. Rofo 2002;174(4):474–9 [in German].
11. Bergin CJ, Sirlin CB, Hauschildt JP, et al. Chronic thromboembolism: diagnosis with helical CT and MR imaging with angiographic and surgical correlation. Radiology 1997;204:695–702.
12. Wittram C, Kalra MK, Maher MM, et al. Acute and chronic pulmonary emboli: angiography-CT correlation. Am J Roentgenol 2006;186(6 Suppl 2):S421–9.
13. Auger WR, Fedullo PF, Moser KM, et al. Chronic major-vessel thromboembolic pulmonary artery obstruction: appearance at angiography. Radiology 1992;182:393–8.
14. Korn D, Gore I, Blenke A, et al. Pulmonary arterial bands and webs: unrecognized manifestation of organized pulmonary emboli. Am J Pathol 1962;40: 129–51.
15. Ley S, Kreitner KF, Morgenstern I, et al. Bronchopulmonary shunts in patients with chronic

thromboembolic pulmonary hypertension: evaluation with helical CT and MR imaging. Am J Roentgenol 2002;179:1209–15.

16. Remy-Jardin M, Duhamel A, Deken V, et al. Systemic collateral supply in patients with chronic thromboembolic and primary pulmonary hypertension: assessment with multi-detector row helical CT angiography. Radiology 2005;235(1):274–81.

17. Heinrich M, Uder M, Tscholl D, et al. CT findings in chronic thromboembolic pulmonary hypertension. Chest 2005;127:1606–13.

18. Hasegawa I, Boiselle PM, Hatabu H. Bronchial arterial dilatation on MDCT scans of patients with acute pulmonary embolism: comparison with chronic or recurrent pulmonary embolism. AJR Am J Roentgenol 2004;182:67–72.

19. Endrys J, Hayat N, Cherian G. Comparison of bronchopulmonary collaterals and collateral blood flow in patients with chronic thromboembolic and primary pulmonary hypertension. Heart 1997;78:171–6.

20. Shimizu H, Tanabe N, Terada J, et al. Dilatation of bronchial arteries correlates with extent of central disease in patients with chronic thromboembolic pulmonary hypertension. Circ J 2008;72(7): 1136–41.

21. Kauczor HU, Schwickert HC, Mayer E, et al. Spiral CT of bronchial arteries in chronic thromboembolism. J Comput Assist Tomogr 1994;18:855–61.

22. Frazier AA, Galvin JR, Franks TJ, et al. From the archives of AFIP: pulmonary vasculature: hypertension and infarction. Radiographics 2000;20(2): 491–524.

23. Ng CS, Wells AU, Padley SPG. A CT sign of chronic pulmonary arterial hypertension: the ratio of main pulmonary artery to aortic diameter. J Thorac Imaging 1999;14:270–8.

24. Sherrick AD, Swensen SJ, Hartman TE. Mosaic pattern of lung attenuation on CT scans: frequency among patients with pulmonary artery hypertension of different causes. AJR Am J Roentgenol 1997; 169:79–82.

25. King MA, Bergin CJ, Yeung DW, et al. Chronic pulmonary thromboembolism: detection of regional hypoperfusion with CT. Radiology 1994;191:359–63.

26. Remy-Jardin M, Remy J, Louvegny S, et al. Airway changes in chronic pulmonary embolism: CT findings in 33 patients. Radiology 1997;203(2):355–60.

27. Castaner E, Gallardo X, Ballesteros E, et al. CT diagnosis of chronic pulmonary thromboembolism. Radiographics 2009;29:31–53.

28. Thistlethwaite PA, Kaneko K, Madani MM, et al. Technique and outcomes of pulmonary endarterectomy surgery. Ann Thorac Cardiovasc Surg 2008; 14(5):274–82.

29. Cottin V, Dupuis-Girod S, Lesca G, et al. Pulmonary vascular manifestations of hereditary hemorrhagic telangiectasia (Rendu-Osler Disease). Respiration 2007;74(4):361–78.

30. Faughnan ME, Granton JT, Young LH. The pulmonary vascular complications of hereditary haemorrhagic telangiectasia. Eur Respir J 2009;33: 1186–94.

31. Ference BA, Shannon TM, White RI, et al. Life-threatening pulmonary hemorrhage with pulmonary arteriovenous malformations and hereditary hemorrhagic telangiectasia. Chest 1994;106: 1387–90.

32. Mathur M, Glenn WW. Long-term evaluation of cava-pulmonary artery anastomosis. Surgery 1973;74: 899–916.

33. Duncan BW, Desai S. Pulmonary arteriovenous malformations after cavopulmonary anastomosis. Ann Thorac Surg 2003;76:1759–66.

34. Nanthakumar K, Graham AT, Robinson TI, et al. Contrast echocardiography for detection of pulmonary arteriovenous malformations. Am Heart J 2001;141:243–6.

35. Remy J, Remy-Jardin M, Wattinne L, et al. Pulmonary arteriovenous malformations: evaluation with CT of the chest before and after treatment. Radiology 1992;182:809–16.

36. Nawaz A, Litt HI, Stavropoulos W, et al. Digital subtraction pulmonary arteriography versus multidetector CT in the detection of pulmonary arteriovenous malformations. J Vasc Interv Radiol 2008;19: 1582–8.

37. White RI, Mitchell SE, Barth KH, et al. Angioarchitecture of pulmonary arteriovenous malformations: an important consideration before embolotherapy. AJR Am J Roentgenol 1983;140(4):681–6.

38. Khurshid I, Downie GH. Pulmonary arteriovenous malformation. Postgrad Med J 2002;78:191–7.

39. Cottin V, Chinet T, Lavole A, et al. Pulmonary arteriovenous malformations in hereditary hemorrhagic telangiectasia: a series of 126 patients. Medicine 2007;86(1):1–17.

40. White RI. Pulmonary arteriovenous malformations: how do I embolize? Tech Vasc Interv Radiol 2007; 10(4):283–90.

41. White RI, Pollak JS, Wirth JA. Pulmonary arteriovenous malformations: diagnosis and transcatheter embolotherapy. J Vasc Interv Radiol 1996;7: 787–804.

42. Remy-Jardin M, Dumont P, Brillet PY, et al. Pulmonary arteriovenous malformations treated with embolotherapy: helical CT evaluation of long-term effectiveness after 2–21 year follow-up. Radiology 2006;239(2):576–85.

43. Pollack JS, Saluja S, Thabet A, et al. Clinical and anatomic outcomes after embolotherapy of pulmonary arteriovenous malformations. J Vasc Interv Radiol 2006;17:35–44.

MDCT Evaluation of Acute Aortic Syndrome

Seung Min Yoo, MD, PhD[a], Hwa Yeon Lee, MD, PhD[b], Charles S. White, MD[c],*

KEYWORDS

- Acute aortic syndrome • Aortic dissection
- Intramural hematoma • Penetrating atherosclerotic ulcer
- Multidetector CT (MDCT)

Acute aortic syndrome (AAS) comprises aortic dissection (AD), intramural hematoma (IMH), penetrating atherosclerotic ulcer (PAU), and unstable aortic aneurysm. Because the highest mortality of AAS, particularly AD, occurs during the first 48 hours after onset of symptoms, prompt diagnosis and immediate initiation of appropriate therapy is essential for a favorable outcome.[1] Unfortunately, several studies have reported that a delay in diagnosis of more than 24 hours after admission occurs in up to 39% of patients with AD.[2,3] This is mainly because of a significant overlap of clinical symptoms between AAS and acute coronary syndrome (ACS) or pulmonary embolism (PE). In addition, the annual incidence of AAS, ACS, and PE has been estimated at 0.5 to 3.0, 440.0, and 69.0 per 100,000 in the United States, respectively.[4,5] This relatively rare occurrence of AAS compared with ACS and PE increases the likelihood of delayed diagnosis or misdiagnosis of AAS as ACS or PE. Although radiologists are not directly involved with history taking or physical examination of patients with suspicious AAS, a precise understanding of both the pretest probability and typical clinical symptoms and signs of AAS is valuable for radiologists to get the broadest perspective of AAS.

Current multidetector CT (MDCT) equipped with state-of-the art tube and detector technology, and optimal temporal and spatial resolution has become widely available globally. With appropriately obtained MDCT data in patients who have findings suspicious for AAS, the diagnostic accuracy of MDCT is nearly 100%.

This article provides a summary of AAS, focusing especially on MDCT technique and findings of AAS, as well as recent concepts regarding the subtypes of AAS, consisting of AD, IMH, PAU, and unstable aortic aneurysm.

AORTIC DISSECTION
Pathogenesis of Aortic Dissection

The exact mechanism of AD still remains unclear.[6] AD is characterized by intimal rupture and subsequent formation of a false lumen parallel to the original aortic lumen. An entry tear is likely to be a primary event for development of most AD. In some cases, intramural hemorrhage in the media followed by intimal rupture may also be an initiating event. Most patients with AD have hypertension. The most common sites of entry tear are the right lateral wall of the ascending aorta and the descending aorta just distal to the left subclavian artery, where the shearing stress against the aortic wall generated by hypertensive blood flow is maximal. Once an entry tear is made, propagation of AD ensues along the aortic lumen, either in an

[a] Department of Diagnostic Radiology, 351 Yatop-dong Bundang-gu, CHA Medical University Hospital, Bundang 463-712, Korea
[b] Department of Diagnostic Radiology, 65-207 Hangang-ro 3 ga Youngsan-gu, Chung-Ang University College of Medicine, Seoul 140-757, Korea
[c] Department of Diagnostic Radiology, 22 S. Greene St, University of Maryland, Baltimore, MD 21201, USA
* Corresponding author.
E-mail address: cwhite@umm.edu (C.S. White).

Radiol Clin N Am 48 (2010) 67–83
doi:10.1016/j.rcl.2009.09.006

antegrade or retrograde fashion. When an ascending aortic dissection propagates into the aortic arch and descending aorta, the dissection often extends along the greater curvature of the aortic arch, resulting in frequent involvement of aortic arch branches (**Fig. 1**).[7] The term intimal flap is a misnomer. As the dissection flap is composed of intima and the inner two-thirds of media, intimomedial flap is a more appropriate terminology. The thickness of the outer wall of false lumen is only one-third of the intimomedial flap and one-quarter of the original aortic wall. The outer wall of the false lumen is thus vulnerable to aortic rupture.[7,8] Surgeons operating on AD often describe this structure as paper-thin. Most aortic ruptures occur in the vicinity of the entry tear. The presence and location of the high-density hematoma on pre–contrast-enhanced CT suggests the site of aortic rupture. Hemopericardium or right hemothorax indicates rupture of the ascending aorta, whereas hemomediastinum and left hemothorax suggest rupture of the aortic arch and descending aorta, respectively (**Fig. 2**).[7]

Predisposing Factors

Predisposing factors related to AD are hypertension, aortic disease (eg, bicuspid aortic valve, aortic coarctation, and aortic aneurysm),[9] connective tissue diseases of the aorta (eg, Marfan's syndrome and Ehler-Danlos syndrome),[10,11] direct trauma to the aortic wall,[12] cocaine abuse,[13] and pregnancy.[14]

Most AD occurring in young patients is related to Marfan's syndrome.[9] Cocaine use may result in rapid increase of blood pressure, making cocaine users vulnerable to intimal tear. AD occurring in young women is often associated with pregnancy-induced hypertension during the third trimester or labor.[15]

CLINICAL FINDINGS OF AORTIC DISSECTION AND CHOICE OF IMAGING MODALITIES

Typical AD has been associated with severe chest or back pain of sudden onset with a tearing or ripping quality in an older patient (ie, sixth or seventh decade) who has hypertension.[3] However, ripping or tearing chest pain may not be a typical descriptor in patients with AD. According to a study performed by the International Registry of Acute Aortic Dissection (IRAD), the incidence of tearing or ripping pain (51%) was less frequent than that of sharp pain (64%) in patients with AD.[4] The location of pain is related to the site of AD: patients with ascending AD are more likely to have anterior chest pain, whereas those with descending aortic dissection more often complain of posterior chest, back, or abdominal pain. A migratory nature of the pain (16.6%) and radiation of pain (28.3%) to the interscapular region, back, or abdomen are fairly typical of AD.[4]

Focal neurologic signs or symptoms, and a pulse deficit or pressure difference between the two extremities are also characteristic of AD. For example, in a patient with severe chest pain of sudden onset, a nonpalpable unilateral extremity pulse is highly suggestive of AD, regardless of the nature of the pain (**Fig. 3**).

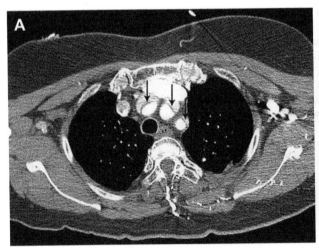
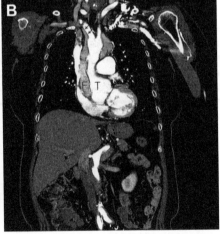

Fig. 1. Extension of intimomedial flap into all of three aortic arch branches in 67-year-old woman with Stanford type A aortic dissection. (*A*) Intimomedial flap (*arrows*) is noted in brachiocephalic, left common carotid, and left subclavian artery on contrast-enhanced axial CT image at the level of left brachiocephalic vein. (*B*) Intimomedial flap (*arrows*) extending into brachiocephalic artery is clearly noted on coronal MPR image. The contrast enhancement of true lumen (T) is higher than that of false lumen (F) owing to slow flow of the false lumen.

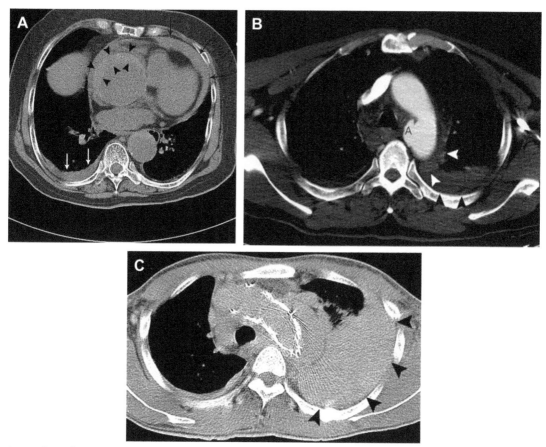

Fig. 2. The different locations of intrathoracic hematoma may suggest the site of aortic rupture. (*A*) Right hemo-thorax (*white arrows*) and hemopericardium (*black arrows*) of high attenuation are seen in a patient with ruptured Stanford type A dissection on pre–contrast-enhanced axial CT image at the level of left atrium. Note the high attenuation of ascending aortic wall (*black arrowheads*) owing to partial thrombosis of false lumen. (*B*) Mediastinal hemorrhage (*white arrowheads*) is demonstrated on contrast-enhanced axial CT image at the level of aortic arch in a patient with traumatic aortic pseudoaneurysm (*A*) at the aortic isthmus. Left pleural effu-sion (*black arrowheads*) is also noted. (*C*) Left hemothorax (*arrowheads*) of high attenuation is noted on pre–contrast-enhanced axial CT image at the level of aortic arch in a patient in whom aortic stent-graft was inserted owing to ruptured Stanford type B dissection.

Acute aortic regurgitation is one of the most deleterious consequences of AD. A new diastolic murmur at the apex may therefore suggest AD.

With respect to imaging, mediastinal widening or displacement of aortic intimal calcifications away from the outer aortic wall on chest radiog-raphy can be an important clue of AD, although these signs are not specific.[4,16]

Von Kodolitsch and colleagues[16] reported a clin-ical prediction model of AD. In their study, there were three independent predictors of AD: chest pain of abrupt onset with a tearing or ripping nature, or both, a pulse or blood pressure differen-tial, and substantial mediastinal widening on chest radiograph. The presence of one of these variables was detected in 96% of patients with AD. The pretest probability of AD was low (7%) in the absence of three variables, intermediate with one of characteristic chest pain or mediastinal widening (31%), and high (>83%) in patients with either pulse or blood pressure differential, or any combination of three variables. Therefore, these variables can provide an important guide for further imaging evaluation.

MDCT has both advantages and disadvantages with respect to other imaging techniques such as ultrasound and MRI for the evaluation of AD. Because of the inability of transthoracic echocar-diography (TTE) to visualize the aorta beyond the root, transesophageal echocardiography (TEE) is mainly used for assessment of AD. A major advan-tage of TEE is its portability, which is useful in unstable patients. The disadvantages of TEE are operator dependency, limited acoustic window,

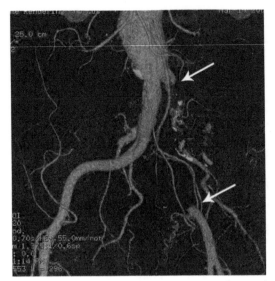

Fig. 3. Total occlusion of left common iliac and external iliac artery owing to false lumen thrombosis in a patient with Stanford type B dissection. Volume rendering (VR) image intuitively shows total occlusion (*arrows*) of left common iliac and external iliac artery. Left common femoral artery is opacified by collateral circulation. This patient had a sudden onset of sharp chest pain and a loss of left femoral pulse.

innate blind spot (ie, the distal ascending aorta and proximal aortic arch due to the air in the trachea), and inability to visualize the entire aorta. By contrast, a major strength of MDCT is the ability to image aortic branch vessels as well as the entire

aorta without any limitations encountered on TEE. Another advantage of MDCT over TEE is the ability to make alternative extracardiac diagnoses such as PE. Because of a relatively long examination time and difficulty in monitoring the unstable patients in the magnetic field, the role of MRI in the evaluation of acute AD is limited.[7] MRI is mainly used for follow-up of chronic AD rather than MDCT to avoid radiation exposure and the use of contrast material. Therefore, the choice of imaging modality for evaluating AD should be individualized according to the specific clinical situations.

MULTIDETECTOR CT TECHNIQUE IN THE ASSESSMENT OF AORTIC DISSECTION

The 64-slice MDCT has become widely used and can provide iso-volumetric, 3-dimensional information without loss of spatial resolution during a single breath-hold. Because of a diagnostic accuracy approaching 100%, MDCT has become the first-line imaging study for evaluating patients with suspicious AD.[7]

Various postprocessing techniques such as multiplanar reformation (MPR), maximum intensity projection (MIP), and volume rendering (VR) help to facilitate understanding of complex aortic pathology and to expedite communication with surgeons and attending physicians.[17]

The standard protocol for evaluating AAS should include a pre–contrast-enhanced CT to recognize the presence of IMH and high-density blood in the

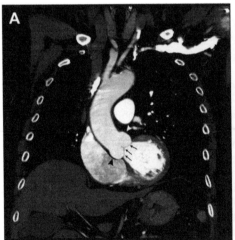
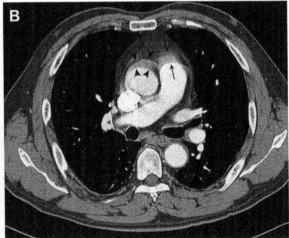

Fig. 4. The advantages of ECG-gated aortic CT and differential point between intimomedial flap and aortic pulsation artifact. (*A*) Artifact-free ascending aortic root (*arrowheads*) and normal coaptation of aortic valves (*arrows*) are noted on coronal MPR image of mid-diastolic phase. (*B*) Aortic (*arrowheads*) and pulmonary arterial motion artifact (*arrows*) are noted on non-ECG gated axial CT image at the level of right main pulmonary artery. Simultaneous visualization of crescent-shaped low attenuation in both ascending aorta and pulmonary artery suggests motion artifact rather than aortic dissection.

pericardium, pleural space, or mediastinum, indicating aortic rupture. Pre–contrast-enhanced CT with low-dose technique accompanied by thick collimation (collimation, 1.5 mm; slice thickness, 5 mm; reconstruction interval, 5 mm) may be used to reduce total radiation dose.[18,19] In addition, the scan range of pre–contrast-enhanced CT can be restricted from the lung apex to upper abdomen, instead of a full-scan range from the thoracic inlet to femoral head.[20]

The scan range of contrast-enhanced CT is from the thoracic inlet to femoral head in our institution to exclude involvement of major aortic arch branches and both iliac arteries.[21] However, if there is no evidence of AD during scanning of the thorax and upper abdomen (ie, at least at the level of celiac axis), further scanning should be stopped to avoid unnecessary radiation exposure.

There is no standard iodine concentration for a dedicated MDCT protocol of AD. In general, a body weight–adapted iodine concentration accounting for flow rate of 1.0 to 1.6 g per second is sufficient to opacify the entire aorta in most patients.[17,22] For example, in a nonobese patient, an iodine concentration of 3 to 4 mL of 300 mg I/mL per second (ie, 0.9–1.2 g per second) may be adequate, whereas in a patient with higher body mass index, 5 mL of 300 mg I/mL per second (ie, 1.5 g per second) may be necessary to obtain satisfactory opacification of the aorta.

The starting time point for a contrast-enhanced scan can be best achieved using a bolus tracking method.[19] When the CT attenuation value in the ascending aorta reaches 100 Hounsfield Units, scanning starts with a scan delay time of 5 to 7 seconds. A saline chaser technique with a dual-head injector is used to reduce the amount of

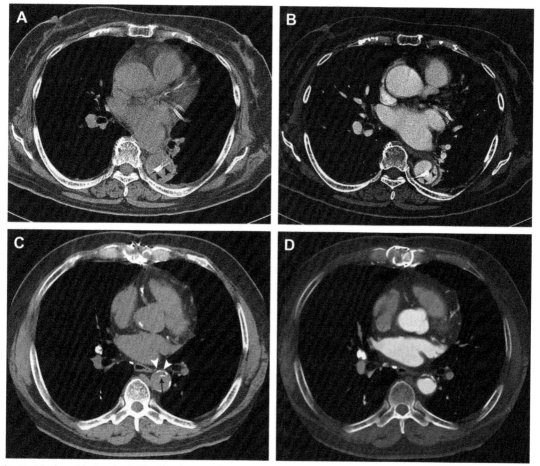

Fig. 5. Displaced intimal calcification in a patient with Stanford type B dissection and calcification at the top of mural thrombus in an asymptomatic patient. Displaced intimal calcification (*arrowheads*) is noted on pre-enhanced (*A*) and contrast-enhanced (*B*) axial CT image at the level of left atrium. Calcifications lying on intima (*arrowheads*) and top of mural thrombus (*arrow*) are noted on preenhanced (*C*) and contrast-enhanced (*D*) axial CT image at the level of left atrium.

contrast material while maintaining the flow rate of contrast material. It is feasible to obtain adequate opacification of the entire aorta if contrast material is administered at least as long as scan time plus the scan delay time. For example, if scan time and scan delay time are 15 and 5 seconds, respectively, a 20-second injection of contrast material followed by a 50-mL saline chase is sufficient. With 64-slice MDCT, it is possible to scan the entire aorta with submillimeter collimation (collimation, 0.625 mm; slice thickness, 0.625 mm; reconstruction interval, 0.3 mm) within a single breath-hold, thus making high-resolution 3-dimensional reconstruction and other postprocessing displays possible.

ECG-GATED MULTIDETECTOR CT FOR AORTIC DISSECTION

Artifacts caused by the pendular or circular motion of aortic root may simulate an intimomedial flap of AD, particularly in the ascending aorta. With an ECG-gated acquisition, the aortic motion artifact can be completely eliminated (**Fig. 4A**), thus increasing diagnostic confidence.[17,23] Other advantages of retrospectively ECG-gated aortic CT include precise evaluation of involvement of coronary arteries by intimomedial flap extension, detection of myocardial perfusion defect as evidence of ischemia, indirect assessment of aortic regurgitation based on lack of coaptation of the aortic valve leaflets, calculation of left ventricular ejection fraction, and evaluation of ventricular wall motion.[17,24] As the entry tear is often perpendicular to the long axis of the aorta, it can be better visualized on an ECG-gated multiplanar reformatted image.[17] These advantages may help in deciding therapeutic strategy and presurgical prognosis.

However, in most cases, aortic motion artifact is not a major diagnostic problem because it can be differentiated from intimomedial flap.[25] Motion artifact is often limited to one or two slices and is accompanied by pulmonary artery motion

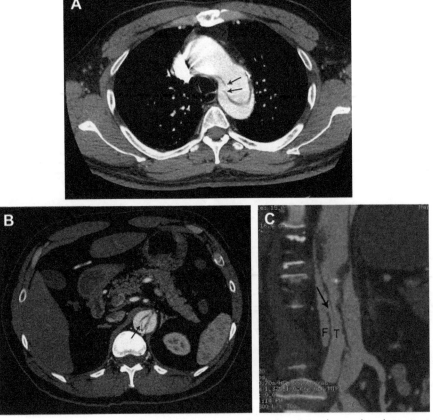

Fig. 6. Entry and reentry tear in a patient with Stanford type B dissection. Entry (*arrows*) and reentry tear (*arrow*) are noted on contrast-enhanced axial CT image at the level of aortic arch (*A*) and upper pole of left kidney (*B*), respectively. (*C*) Curved multiplanar reformatted image (MPR) shows reentry tear (*arrow*) to connect true lumen (T) with false lumen (F) in distal abdominal aorta more intuitively.

(Fig. 4B). A study with four-slice MDCT in a tertiary referral hospital indicated no false positive case caused by aortic motion artifact among 373 cases of AD.[26] Therefore, the use of ECG-gated MDCT is controversial. In particular, a major disadvantage of retrospective ECG-gated acquisition is increased radiation exposure. Therefore, it may be advisable to limit use of ECG-gated acquisition to cases in which a non–ECG-gated scan mandates further investigation (eg, equivocal involvement of coronary artery by the intimomedial flap or aortic regurgitation).

MULTIDETECTOR CT FINDINGS OF AORTIC DISSECTION

The following information should be provided when interpreting MDCT in patients with AD: extent of AD (ie, Stanford classification); site of entry tear; side branch involvement such as coronary, carotid, subclavian, celiac, superior mesenteric, inferior mesenteric, renal, and iliac artery; the presence of aortic rupture; differentiation between the true and false lumen; the size of false lumen diameter as a predictor for aortic rupture.

Inwardly displaced intimal calcification can be a sign of AD on precontrast MDCT (Fig. 5A, B). However, this finding may be confused with calcified mural thrombus in patients without AD (Fig. 5C, D).[21]

An intimomedial flap is the major finding demonstrated on contrast-enhanced MDCT. Identification of the precise location of the entry tear is important because current endovascular stent-graft therapy targets the exclusion of the entry tear. The entry tear is often at the most proximal location of the intimomedial flap and can be identified on contrast-enhanced MDCT in most cases. Conversely, a reentry tear is usually in the descending thoracic or abdominal aorta, or iliac arteries (Fig. 6),[17] and is not frequently identified because it typically consists of a minute defect or defects. The Stanford classification is based on the extent of intimomedial flap. By definition, a Stanford type A dissection involves the ascending aorta regardless of involvement of descending aorta, whereas a type B dissection affects only the descending aorta. A Stanford Type B dissection is more frequent in radiological and surgical series of AD, whereas Type A dissection is more prevalent in autopsy series.[8] This discrepancy is because substantial numbers of patients with type A dissection die before reaching the hospital. As a Stanford type A dissection is frequently associated with deadly complications such as pericardial tamponade, acute aortic regurgitation, or the involvement of aortic arch branch,

aortic replacement is the mainstay of therapy. The worst outcome is expected in patients with Stanford type A dissection treated conservatively because of old age or severe comorbidity. Conversely, Stanford type B dissection is usually managed conservatively because emergent operation is associated with a mortality rate of up to 40%. However, operative or interventional treatment is mandatory for the following situations: uncontrollable hypertension and the presence of symptoms or signs such as intractable pain or shock suggesting impending rupture.

Endovascular stent-graft repair is an emerging therapeutic option in patients with complicated Stanford type B dissection. This procedure is aimed at the complete exclusion of the false lumen by sealing up the entry tear site with a stent-graft. Candidates for aortic stent-graft placement include those with a sufficient landing zone without excessive aortic tortuosity (ie, proximal neck of more than 5 mm distal to left subclavian artery) and adequate vascular access (ie, iliac arterial diameter larger than 9 mm). However, in the absence of long-term follow-up data and complications such as retrograde extension of the dissection flap into the ascending aorta or endoleak occurring after insertion of aortic stent-graft (Fig. 7), the exact role of aortic stent-graft in patients with acute type B dissection remains to be elucidated.[27–29]

The differentiation between the true and false lumen is extremely important because major side branches originating from the false lumen may be

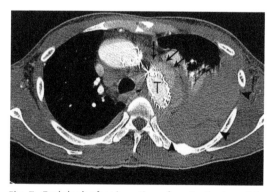

Fig. 7. Endoleak after insertion of aortic stent-graft in a patient with ruptured Stanford type B dissection. Aortic stent-graft was emergently inserted in 40-year-old man because of symptoms and signs of rupture. The presence of contrast material (*arrows*) within false lumen is noted on axial CT image at the level of tracheal carina obtained after interventional procedure, consistent with endoleak. Left hemothorax (*arrowheads*) is also noted. The patient died 2 days after CT as a result of shock. Note aortic stent-graft in true (T) lumen.

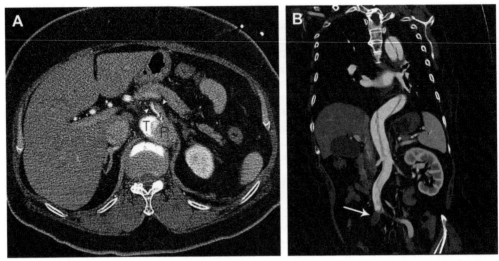

Fig. 8. Static obstruction in patients with Stanford type B dissection. (*A*) The proximal portion of celiac trunk (*arrowheads*) originating from true lumen (T) is severely narrowed by thrombosis of false lumen (F) on contrast-enhanced axial CT at the level of upper pole of left kidney in a patient with Stanford type B dissection. (*B*) Static obstruction of right common iliac artery (*arrow*) caused by thrombosis of false lumen is noted on coronal curved MPR image in a patient with Stanford type B dissection. Note the intimomedial flap in aorta.

occluded after stent-graft insertion, especially in cases without a reentry tear.[7]

There are two kinds of side branch involvement: static versus dynamic obstruction. Static obstruction can occur if the intimomedial flap directly extends into the affected side branch (**Fig. 8**). A possible solution for this complication is to insert a stent into the true lumen of the involved side branch. Conversely, dynamic obstruction indicates that the ostium of the affected side branch or aortic lumen before the side branch is occluded by an overlaying flap on the lumen (**Fig. 9**). This type of side branch involvement is caused by marked increase of false lumen pressure compared with that of the true lumen.[30] Stent-graft insertion into the severely compressed true lumen with or without fenestration of the intimomedial flap is the only good therapeutic option for dynamic obstruction of the branch vessel.

A simple way to discriminate true lumen from the false lumen is to demonstrate its communication with the uninvolved aortic segment. The larger

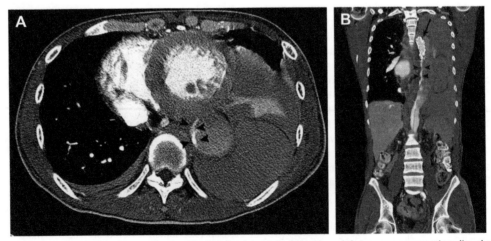

Fig. 9. Dynamic obstruction in a patient with Stanford type B dissection. (*A*) Severe compression (ie, dynamic obstruction) of true lumen (*arrowheads*) owing to high pressure of false lumen (F) is noted on contrast-enhanced axial CT image at the level of left ventricle in a patient with Stanford type B dissection. Note large amount of left hemothorax. (*B*) Dynamic obstruction (*arrowheads*) is also demonstrated on coronal MPR image. Note aortic stent-graft (*arrow*) inserted proximal to the site of dynamic obstruction.

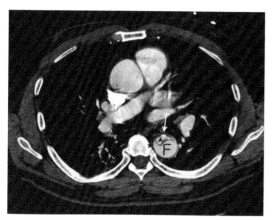

Fig. 10. Differentiation between true and false lumen in a patient with Stanford type B dissection. Beak sign (*arrowheads*) and larger lumen sign are noted in false lumen (F) on contrast-enhanced axial CT image at the level of mid-descending aorta. Intimal calcification (*arrow*) on the wall of true lumen is noted.

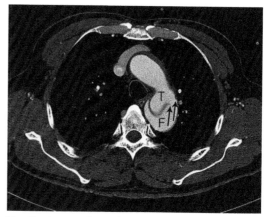

Fig. 12. A case of Stanford type B dissection showing intimomedial rupture sign. Both free ends (*arrows*) of intimomedial flap direct toward the false lumen (F) from true lumen (T) on contrast-enhanced axial CT image at the level of aortic arch.

lumen (**Fig. 10**) is typically the false lumen because the pressure in the false lumen is higher than that of true lumen.[7,18,21] In some cases, the velocity of blood flowing through the small true lumen is higher than that of large false lumen, resulting in lesser opacification of the false lumen (see **Fig. 1**).[7,18] The false lumen may show a beak sign manifested as an acute angle between the intimomedial flap and outer false lumen on axial CT images.[7,18,21] Intraluminal thrombus is more frequently encountered in the false lumen (46%) rather than true lumen (6%) owing to slow flow in the acute setting.[31] Although it has a low

sensitivity, the cobweb sign (**Fig. 11**) is typical of the false lumen, and corresponds to strands from incompletely torn connective tissue of the aortic media.[32] The intimomedial rupture sign (**Fig. 12**) is also helpful to distinguish the true lumen from false lumen. This sign refers to the discontinued ends of intimomedial flap at the site of entry tear

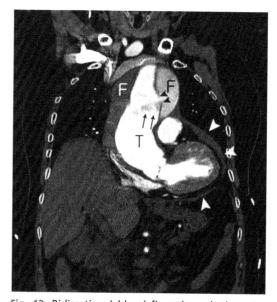

Fig. 13. Bidirectional blood flow through the entry tear in a patient with Stanford type A dissection. The presence of contrast material noted in false lumen (F) indicates flow direction from true lumen to false lumen through the entry tear (*black arrowheads*) on coronal MPR image. Conversely, low attenuation (*arrows*) noted in true lumen (T) suggests flow direction from false lumen to true lumen. Note hemopericardium (*white arrowheads*).

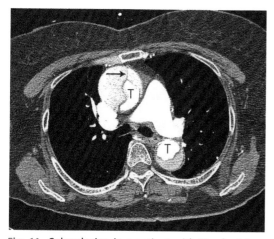

Fig. 11. Cobweb sign in a patient with Stanford type A dissection. Cobweb (*arrow*) is noted in false lumen of ascending aorta on contrast enhanced axial CT image at the level of main pulmonary artery. Attenuation of true lumen (T) is denser than that of false lumen due to slow flow of false lumen.

that point toward false lumen.[33] It is indicative of the direction of blood flow through entry tear from true to false lumen. However, the direction of blood flow through the entry tear can be bidirectional or reversed depending on the cardiac phase (Fig. 13).[15] Intimal calcification occurs along the wall of the true lumen or true lumen side of intimomedial flap (see Fig. 10).

Consistent with Laplace's law, a large false lumen is more likely to be associated with aortic rupture than a small false lumen.

INTRAMURAL HEMATOMA

Similar to classic AD, the pathogenesis of IMH is not fully understood. Hypertension is a major predisposing factor of IMH as it is for classic AD. Although IMH can be caused by blunt trauma of the aortic wall or penetrating atherosclerotic ulcer (PAU),[6] two major pathophysiological mechanisms of IMH are bleeding of the vasa vasorum and intimal tear with complete thrombosis of false lumen. Spontaneous rupture of the vasa vasorum that supplies the aortic media is a primary event of first theory. Cases of IMH observed without an intimal tear at autopsy or during surgery support this theory. According to the second theory, IMH results from complete thrombosis of false lumen in an otherwise classic AD with an entry tear. Several recent reports suggest that most IMH results from an entry tear similar to classic AD[34–37] rather than bleeding of the vasa vasorum. Park

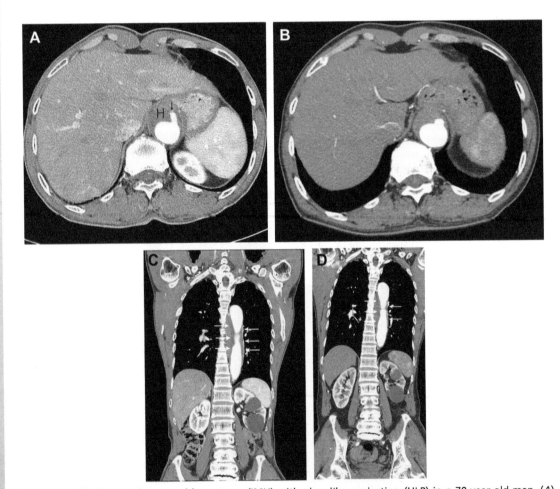

Fig. 14. Stanford type B intramural hematoma (IMH) with ulcer-like projection (ULP) in a 70-year-old man. (A) IMH (H; maximal thickness, 18 mm) with ULP (arrow; depth, 16 mm; width, 7 mm) is noted in descending thoracic aorta on contrast-enhanced axial CT image at the level of upper pole of left kidney. The lack of atherosclerotic change in the aortic lumen may suggest the diagnosis of IMH with intimal tear rather than IMH with PAU. However, definite differentiation between the two entities is difficult. (B) On follow-up CT performed on 15 months later, ULP (depth, 6.5 mm; width, 8 mm) is slightly decreased compared with A. (C) Coronal MPR image performed on same day with A shows extent of intramural hematoma (arrows) more intuitively. (D) On coronal MPR image performed on same day as B, thickness of IMH (arrows) is also decreased compared with C.

and colleagues[34] reported that intimal defects were identified during surgery in 27 patients (73.0%) among 37 patients with type A IMH, whereas preoperative CT detected intimal defects in only 13 patients (35.1%). Therefore, small intimal defects were identified in only 14 cases during surgery. As a result, they proposed that most IMH develops from intimal tear, not from bleeding of the vasa vasorum. They also suggested that it is unlikely that intimal defect is a secondary event followed by vasa vasorum bleeding. If intimal defect were a secondary event, the incidence of detection of intimal defects during surgery should have increased as the time interval between initial CT and surgery increases. However, no such increase was observed. They

postulated that a small entry tear without a reentry tear is likely to form IMH,[38] whereas a large entry tear with reentry tear would predispose to the formation of classic AD.

Several reports indicate that IMH associated with an ulcerlike projection (ULP) has less favorable outcome (ie, complications such as overt AD or rupture) compared with IMH without ULP, regardless of when the ULP is visualized.[39,40] ULP seems to be a more reasonable terminology to describe this entity than PAU or intimal tear, as it is often not confirmed pathologically. Because of the prognostic implications, radiologists should give special attention to detecting ULP when evaluating patients with IMH. ULP has been considered to represent the site of the entry

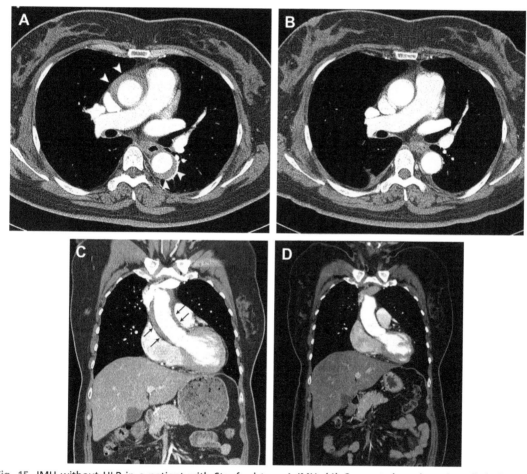

Fig. 15. IMH without ULP in a patient with Stanford type A IMH. (*A*) Crescent shaped aortic wall thickening (*arrowheads*) (diameter, 8 mm) is noted in ascending and descending aorta without the evidence of ULP or aortic rupture on contrast-enhanced axial CT image at level of right main pulmonary artery. Maximal aortic diameter including false lumen is within normal range (37 mm). The combination of these findings may suggest benign prognosis of this IMH. (*B*) IMH involving ascending and descending aorta is nearly disappeared on follow-up axial CT image performed 10 months later. (*C*) Coronal MPR image performed on same day as *A* shows intramural hematoma (*arrows*) involving ascending aorta. (*D*) Marked improvement of IMH is noted on coronal MPR image performed on same day with *B*.

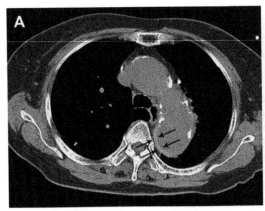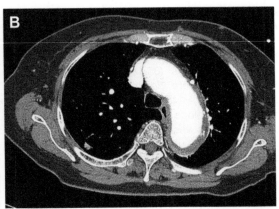

Fig. 16. Typical high attenuation of IMH on pre–contrast-enhanced CT in a patient with Stanford type B intramural hematoma. (A) High-density thickening of aortic wall (arrows) is noted on pre–contrast-enhanced axial CT image at the level of aortic arch. (B) After administration of contrast materials, IMH does not show contrast enhancement.

tear or a PAU.[41–44] IMH can be preoperatively divided into IMH with ULP (Fig. 14) and IMH without ULP (Fig. 15) based on CT findings, although this may be changed at surgery. IMH with ULP can be further subdivided into IMH with intimal tear and IMH with PAU pathologically.

The treatment for IMH is essentially the same as classic AD. However, there is debate about the optimal treatment of type A IMH. Some studies reported that the prognosis of type A IMH is more favorable than that of Stanford type A dissection[45,46]; however, most of the studies that recommended conservative treatment of type A IMH did not disclose the size of the aorta or thickness of the IMH. In one study that recommended a conservative approach,[45] the mean diameter of the aorta and thickness of the IMH were unusually small (35 mm and 5.5 mm, respectively), making such a conclusion difficult to generalize.[34] Park and colleagues[34] suggested that type A IMH be treated by surgery unless all of the following criteria are satisfied: no aortic aneurysm (ie, aortic diameter less than 5 cm); small thickness of IMH (ie, less than 10 mm); no evidence of aortic rupture such as pericardial, mediastinal, or pleural hemorrhage; and no intimal defect in the proximal aorta on CT (see Fig. 15).

The major CT finding on pre–contrast-enhanced CT is crescentic or ring-shaped high attenuation of the aortic wall (Fig. 16).[6,7,18,21] Aortic wall thickening demonstrated on contrast-enhanced CT may be missed without special attention or alternatively may be confused with atheromatous mural thrombus.[6,7] Although wall thickening of a long segment in a nondilated aorta and a smooth internal border favor IMH rather than mural thrombus,[18,21] a pre–contrast-enhanced CT is highly recommended for definitive diagnosis of IMH.

Several CT findings are associated with an adverse outcome of IMH. Sueyoshi and colleagues[39] suggested that new ULP occurring on follow-up CT is predictive of an adverse outcome. Thickness of IMH greater than 11 mm was associated with progression of IMH to frank aortic dissection.[46] Normal aortic diameter more likely led to a good prognosis for IMH.[47] However, the natural history of IMH varies from complete resolution to formation of aortic aneurysm or pseudoaneurysm, overt dissection, or aortic rupture.[48] Therefore, patients in whom IMH is not operated on should be followed closely to detect complications.

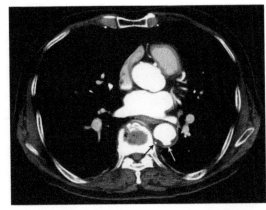

Fig. 17. Intimal calcification in an asymptomatic patient with atheromatous ulcer. Although atheromatous ulcer (white arrow) has a similar appearance with PAU, atheromatous ulcer does not extend over intimal calcification (black arrow) and expected aortic margin on contrast-enhanced axial CT image at the level of left atrium. This is an important differential point to distinguish atheromatous ulcer from PAU.

PENETRATING ATHEROSCLEROTIC ULCER

Clinical manifestations of PAU are quite similar to classic AD although the former tends to occur in elderly patients with severe atherosclerosis and hypertension. By definition, PAU forms when ulcerated atherosclerotic plaque breaks down the internal elastic lamina and propagates into the media, often resulting in IMH. The most common site of PAU is the middle or lower thoracic descending aorta. Therefore, the typical CT finding of PAU is ULP in the middle or lower descending thoracic aorta often accompanied by IMH and severe atherosclerotic change of aortic wall.[49]

PAU should be differentiated from atheromatous ulcer in which ulceration is confined within intima. The location of intimal calcification can be helpful in this situation.[6] Atheromatous ulcer (Fig. 17) often overlies the expected aortic contour and calcified intima, whereas PAU extends outwardly beyond the expected aortic margin and calcified intima.[6,7,18] However, if there is a calcified mural thrombus, differentiation between two entities can be challenging.

Park and colleagues[34] suggested that CT findings of IMH with an entry tear cannot be reliably differentiated from IMH with PAU. In most studies of the natural history of PAU, the diagnosis of PAU was not confirmed pathologically,[50–53] thus making inclusion of some cases of IMH with intimal tear highly probable.

In addition, a precise understanding of the natural history of PAU is further complicated because a variable proportion of asymptomatic cases of PAU were included in most previous studies. As a result, the natural history of PAU is reported to range from fairly benign[50,51] to extremely malignant.[52,54] Therefore, a well-designed prospective study in which PAU is confirmed

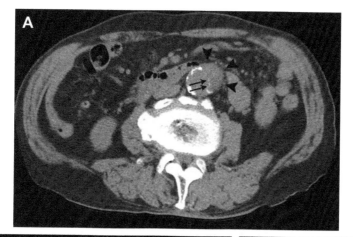

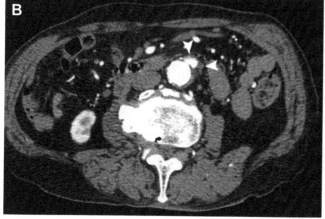
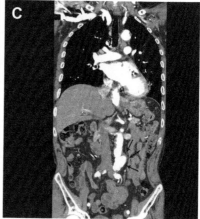

Fig. 18. Abdominal saccular pseudoaneurysm in an asymptomatic patient. Abdominal saccular pseudoaneurysm (*arrowheads*) is noted on pre–contrast (*A*) and contrast-enhanced (*B*) axial CT image at the level of distal abdominal aorta. Note the low attenuation of aortic wall thickening or mural thrombus (T) and intimal calcification (*arrows*) overlying saccular pseudoaneurysm. (*C*) Coronal MPR image also shows distal abdominal saccular pseudoaneurysm (*arrows*).

pathologically is needed to elucidate its natural history and prognosis as well as CT features that distinguish IMH with PAU from IMH with intimal tear.

CT features of asymptomatic PAU can be similar or identical to that of saccular pseudoaneurysm. It is often accompanied by aortic wall thickening of low attenuation on pre–contrast-enhanced CT (**Fig. 18**), which corresponds to chronic IMH or mural thrombus, whereas IMH of high attenuation on pre–contrast-enhanced CT is often demonstrated in PAU cases presented with AAS. Therefore, it is rational to classify asymptomatic PAU separately from PAU with acute IMH which is a subtype of AAS.

There is also debate about the relationship between the size of PAU and natural history.[55] One study suggested that a depth (>10 mm) and diameter of ulcer (>20 mm) are independent predictors of lesion progression such as further thickening of IMH, progression into overt AD, or aortic rupture on follow-up CT.[52] In contrast, Cho and colleagues[53] suggested that there are no predictors of adverse outcomes except for aortic rupture at presentation. Therefore, interval change on follow-up CT rather than size of the PAU on initial CT is likely to be more reliable in determining treatment options or prognosis.[49]

As IMH with PAU tends to occur in elderly patients with comorbidities, it is usually treated conservatively unless accompanied by impending or frank rupture. With recent advances in interventional technique, stent-graft insertion may be the best option in such patients.

THE ROLE OF TRIPLE RULE-OUT PROTOCOL IN PATIENTS WITH UNSPECIFIED ACUTE CHEST PAIN

Rapid and accurate diagnosis of AAS can be life saving, as the highest mortality occurs in the initial 48 hours. Unfortunately, studies reported that a delayed diagnosis of more than 24 hours after admission occurs in up to 39% of AD.[2,3] This is mainly caused by a significant overlap of clinical symptoms among AAS and ACS or PE, and relatively infrequent occurrence of AAS.[4,5] Accordingly, emergency department (ED) physicians and cardiologists risk misdiagnosing AAS as ACS or PE (**Fig. 19**). As the treatment of AAS is quite different from ACS or PE, catastrophic results may occur if patients with AAS mistakenly receive anticoagulant therapy such as heparin or a thrombolytic agent.

As AAS cannot always be reliably differentiated from ACS and PE on clinical grounds, an accurate, noninvasive imaging modality is desirable to make this distinction.[56,57] A triple rule-out protocol, essentially an ECG-gated study of the entire thorax aimed at these three diagnoses can be valuable. However, because of the fairly high radiation dose, the triple rule-out protocol should be performed only in patients with unspecified acute chest pain in whom the potential benefit justifies the radiation dose.[57,58]

UNSTABLE AORTIC ANEURYSM

Thoracic aortic aneurysm is diagnosed when the diameter of the aorta exceeds 5 cm.[18] The size

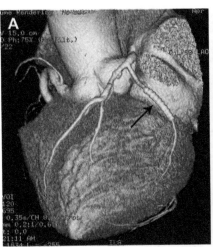
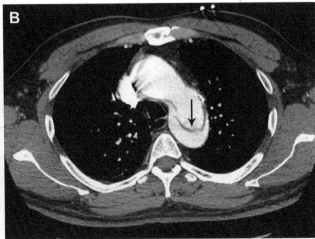

Fig. 19. A case of delayed diagnosis of AD as ACS. Volume rendering (VR) image (*A*) shows a coronary stent (*arrow*) inserted in proximal left circumflex artery on coronary CT angiography performed on 10 months before the onset of symptoms. Because of the history of coronary heart disease and nonspecific nature of chest pain in this patient, the ED physician considered non-ST elevated myocardial infarction (NSTEMI) or unstable angina (UA) as a first diagnostic concern. However, contrast-enhanced axial CT image (*B*) performed 48 hours after the onset of symptoms at the level of aortic arch demonstrates Stanford type B dissection (*arrow*).

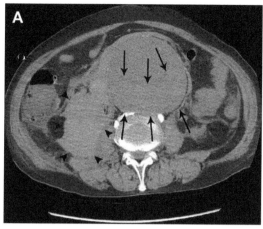 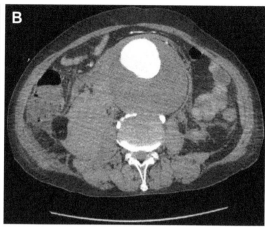

Fig. 20. Ruptured abdominal aortic aneurysm in a 69-year-old man. Abdominal aortic aneurysm about 10 cm in diameter is noted on pre–contrast (A) and post–contrast (B) enhanced axial CT image at the level of distal abdominal aorta. Faint high attenuation of aneurysmal wall (arrows) is consistent with crescent sign. Note hematoma (arrowheads) of high attenuation around right psoas muscle which indicates rupture of aortic aneurysm.

threshold for surgical repair of a thoracic aortic aneurysm in the ascending and descending aorta is 5.5 cm and 6.5 cm, respectively.[59] As the diameter of thoracic aortic aneurysm increases, the risk of aortic rupture increases according to Laplace's law. Rapid increase in the size of the thoracic aortic aneurysm (ie, aortic diameter increase more than 1 cm per year) also strongly correlates with aortic rupture.[60] Endovascular stent-graft repair is an alternative therapeutic option in patients with a large aortic aneurysm accompanied by multiple comorbidities. Thoracic aortic aneurysm often does not produce symptoms by itself, but may be associated with vague chest pain resulting from compression of adjacent structures.

In contrast, unstable aortic aneurysm is characterized by severe chest pain. High attenuation of the aneurysmal aortic wall on pre–contrast-enhanced CT (ie, crescent sign) indicates hemorrhage or hematoma into aortic wall (ie, impending aortic rupture) (Fig. 20).[61] Three-dimensional post-processing techniques help to measure accurately the size of aortic aneurysm and to discriminate which aneurysms have suitable anatomy for aortic stent-graft insertion.[27,62]

SUMMARY

MDCT plays an important role in the rapid and accurate diagnosis of AAS. Precise understanding of the current concepts and various CT features of subtypes of AAS is helpful in diagnosing AAS and improving patient outcome.

REFERENCES

1. Hirst AE Jr, Johns VJ Jr, Kime SW Jr. Dissecting aneurysms of the aorta: a review of 505 cases. Medicine 1958;37:217–79.
2. Viljanen T. Diagnostic difficulties in aortic dissection. Retrospective study of 89 surgically treated patients. Ann Chir Gynaecol 1986;75:328–32.
3. Klompas M. Does this patient have an acute thoracic aortic dissection? JAMA 2002;287:2262–72.
4. Hagan PG, Nienaber CA, Isselbacher EM, et al. The international registry of acute aortic dissection (IRAD): new insights into an old disease. JAMA 2000;283:897–903.
5. Abcarian PW, Sweet JD, Watabe JT, et al. Role of a quantitative D-dimer assay in determining the need for CT angiography of acute pulmonary embolism. AJR Am J Roentgenol 2004;182: 1377–81.
6. Macura KJ, Corl FM, Fishman EK, et al. Pathogenesis in acute aortic syndromes: aortic dissection, intramural hematoma, and penetrating atherosclerotic aortic ulcer. AJR Am J Roentgenol 2003; 181:309–16.
7. Chiles C, Carr JJ. Vascular diseases of the thorax: evaluation with multidetector CT. Radiol Clin North Am 2005;43:543–69.
8. Roberts WC. Aortic dissection: anatomy, consequences, and causes. Am Heart J 1981;101: 195–214.
9. Larson EW, Edwards WD. Risk factors for aortic dissection: a necropsy study of 161 cases. Am J Cardiol 1984;53:849–55.
10. Murdoch JL, Walker BA, Halpern BL, et al. Life expectancy and causes of death in the Marfan syndrome. N Engl J Med 1972;286:804–8.

11. Matter SG, Kumar AG, Lumsden AB. Vascular complications in Ehlers-Danlos syndrome. Am Surg 1994;60:827–31.

12. Rogers FB, Osler TM, Shackford SR. Aortic dissection after trauma: case report and review of the literature. J Trauma 1996;41:906–8.

13. Rashid J, Eisenberg MJ, Topol EJ. Cocaine-induced aortic dissection. Am heart J 1996;132:1301–4.

14. Pumphrey CW, Fay T, Weir I. Aortic dissection during pregnancy. Br Heart J 1986;55:106–8.

15. Khan IA, Nair CK. Clinical, diagnostic, and management perspectives of aortic dissection. Chest 2002; 122:311–28.

16. von Kodolitsch Y, Schwartz AG, Nienaber CA. Clinical prediction of acute aortic dissection. Arch Intern Med 2000;160:2977–82.

17. Manghat NE, Morgan-Hughes GJ, Roobottom CA. Multi-detector row computed tomography: imaging in acute aortic syndrome. Clin Radiol 2005;60(12): 1256–67.

18. Bhalla S, West OC. CT of nontraumatic thoracic aortic emergencies. Semin Ultrasound CT MR 2005;26:281–304.

19. Salvolini L, Renda P, Fiore D, et al. Acute aortic syndromes: role of multi-detector row CT. Eur J Radiol 2008;65:350–8.

20. Batra P, Bigoni B, Manning J, et al. Pitfalls in the diagnosis of thoracic aortic dissection at CT angiography. Radiographics 2000;20:309–20.

21. Castaner E, Andreu M, Gallardo X, et al. CT in nontraumatic acute thoracic aortic disease: typical and atypical features and complications. Radiographics 2003;23:S93–110.

22. Johnson TR, Nikolaou K, Wintersperger BJ, et al. Optimization of contrast material administration for electrocardiogram-gated computed tomographic angiography of the chest. J Comput Assist Tomogr 2007;31:265–71.

23. Roos JE, Willmann JK, Weishaupt D, et al. Thoracic aorta: motion artifact reduction with retrospective and prospective electrocardiography-assisted multi-detector row CT. Radiology 2002;222: 271–7.

24. Morgan-Hughes GJ, Marshall AJ, Roobottom CA. Refined computed tomography of the thoracic aorta: the impact of electrocardiographic assistance. Clin Radiol 2003;58:581–8.

25. Yoshida S, Akiba H, Tamakawa M, et al. Thoracic involvement of type A aortic dissection and intramural hematoma: diagnostic accuracy-comparison of emergency helical CT and surgical findings. Radiology 2003;228:430–5.

26. Hayter RG, Rhea JT, Small A, et al. Suspected aortic dissection and other aortic disorders: multi-detector row CT in 373 cases in the emergency setting. Radiology 2006;238:841–52.

27. Fattori R, Napoli G, Lovato L, et al. Descending thoracic aortic diseases: stent-graft repair. Radiology 2003;229:176–83.

28. Therasse E, Soulez G, Giroux MF, et al. Stent-graft placement for the treatment of thoracic aortic diseases. Radiographics 2005;25:157–73.

29. Iezzi R, Cotroneo AR, Marano R, et al. Endovascular treatment of thoracic aortic diseases: Follow-up and complications with multi-detector computed tomography angiography. Eur J Radiol 2008;65:365–76.

30. Williams DM, Lee DY, Hamilton BH, et al. The dissected aorta: part III. Anatomy and radiologic diagnosis of branch-vessel compromise. Radiology 1997;203:37–44.

31. Lepage MA, Quint LE, Sonnad SS, et al. Aortic dissection: CT features that distinguish true lumen from false lumen. AJR Am J Roentgenol 2001;177: 207–11.

32. Williams DM, Joshi A, Dake MD, et al. Aortic cobwebs: an anatomic marker identifying the false lumen in aortic dissection-imaging and pathologic correlation. Radiology 1994;190:167–74.

33. Kapoor V, Ferris JV, Fuhrman CR, et al. Intimomedial rupture: a new CT finding to distinguish true from false lumen in aortic dissection. AJR Am J Roentgenol 2004;183:109–12.

34. Park KH, Lim C, Choi JH, et al. Prevalence of aortic intimal defect in surgically treated acute type A intramural hematoma. Ann Thorac Surg 2008;86: 1494–500.

35. Beauchesne LM, Veinot JP, Brais MP, et al. Acute aortic intimal tear without a mobile flap mimicking an intramural hematoma. J Am Soc Echocardiogr 2003;16:285–8.

36. Berdat PA, Carrel T. Aortic dissection limited to the ascending aorta mimicking intramural hematoma. Eur J Cardiothorac Surg 1999;15:108–9.

37. Neri E, Capannini G, Carone E, et al. Evolution toward dissection of an intramural hematoma of the ascending aorta. Ann Thorac Surg 1999;68: 1855–6.

38. Vilacosta I, Román JA. Acute aortic syndrome. Heart 2001;85:365–8.

39. Sueyoshi E, Matsuoka Y, Imada T, et al. New development of an ulcerlike projection in aortic intramural hematoma: CT evaluation. Radiology 2002;224: 536–41.

40. Jang YM, Seo JB, Lee YK, et al. Newly developed ulcer-like projection (ULP) in aortic intramural haematoma on follow-up CT: is it different from the ULP seen on the initial CT? Clin Radiol 2008;63: 201–6.

41. Eyler WR, Clark MD. Dissecting aneurysms of the aorta: roentgen manifestations including a comparison with other types of aneurysms. Radiology 1965;85: 1047–57.

42. Nienaber CA, von Kodolitsch Y, Petersen B, et al. Intramural hemorrhage of the thoracic aorta. Diagnostic and therapeutic implications. Circulation 1995;92:1465–72.

43. Krinsky GA, Rofsky NM, DeCorato DR, et al. Thoracic aorta: comparison of gadolinium-enhanced three-dimensional MR angiography with conventional MR imaging. Radiology 1997;202:183–93.

44. Coady MA, Rizzo JA, Elefteriades JA. Pathologic variants of thoracic aortic dissections: penetrating atherosclerotic ulcers and intramural hematomas. Cardiol Clin 1999;17:637–57.

45. Shon DW, Jung JW, Oh BH, et al. Should ascending aortic intramural hematoma be treated surgically? Am J Cardiol 2001;87:1024–6.

46. Song JM, Kim HS, Song JK, et al. Usefulness of the initial noninvasive imaging study to predict the adverse outcomes in the medical treatment of acute type A aortic intramural hematoma. Circulation 2003; 108(Suppl II):II324–8.

47. Evangelista A, Dominguez R, Sebastia C, et al. Long-term follow-up of aortic intramural hematoma: predictors of outcome. Circulation 2003;108:583–9.

48. Sueyoshi E, Matsuoka Y, Sakamoto I, et al. Fate of intramural hematoma of the aorta: CT evaluation. J Comput Assist Tomogr 1997;21:931–8.

49. Hayashi H, Matsuoka Y, Sakamoto I, et al. Penetrating atherosclerotic ulcer of the aorta: imaging features and disease concept. Radiographics 2000;20:995–1005.

50. Quint LE, William DM, Francis IR, et al. Ulcerlike lesions of the aorta: imaging features and natural history. Radiology 2001;218:719–23.

51. Hirris JA, Bis KG, Glover JL, et al. Penetrating atherosclerotic ulcers of the aorta. J Vasc Surg 1994;19:90–8.

52. Ganaha F, Miller DC, Sugimoto K, et al. Prognosis of aortic intramural hematoma with or without penetrating atherosclerotic ulcer: a clinical and radiological analysis. Circulation 2002;106:342–8.

53. Cho KR, Stanson AW, Potter DD, et al. Penetrating atherosclerotic ulcer of the descending thoracic aorta and arch. J Thorac Cardiovasc Surg 2004; 127:1393–401.

54. Coady MA, Rizzo JA, Hammond GL, et al. Penetrating ulcer of the thoracic aorta: what is it? How do we recognize it? How do we manage it? J Vasc Surg 1998;27:1006–15.

55. Jean J, Waite S, White CS. Nontraumatic thoracic emergencies. Radiol Clin North Am 2006;44: 273–93.

56. Takakuwa KM, Halpern EJ. Evaluation of a "triple rule-out" coronary CT angiography protocol: use of 64-section CT in low-to-moderate risk emergency department patients suspected of having acute coronary syndrome. Radiology 2008;248: 438–46.

57. Lee HY, Yoo SM, White CS. Coronary CT angiography in emergency department patients with acute chest pain: triple rule-out protocol versus dedicated coronary CT angiography. Int J Cardiovasc Imaging 2009;25:319–26.

58. Picano E. Sustainability of medical imaging. BMJ 2004;328:578–80.

59. Coady MA, Rizzo JA, Elefteriades JA. Developing surgical intervention criteria for thoracic aortic aneurysms. Cardiol Clin 1999;17:827–39.

60. Scott RA, Tisi PV, Ashton HA, et al. Abdominal aortic aneurysm rupture rates: a 7-year follow-up of the entire abdominal aortic aneurysm population detected by screening. J Vasc Surg 1998;28:124–8.

61. Gonsalves CF. The hyperattenuating crescent sign. Radiology 1999;211:37–8.

62. Thurnher SA, Grabenwoger M. Endovascular treatment of thoracic aortic aneurysms: a review. Eur Radiol 2002;12:1370–87.

Congenital Thoracic Vascular Anomalies

José A. Maldonado, MD[a], Travis Henry, MD[b],
Fernando R. Gutiérrez, MD[c],*

KEYWORDS

- Multidetector computed tomography • Congenital
- Vascular • Anomalies

Congenital vascular anomalies of the thorax represent an important group of entities that can occur either in isolation or in association with different forms of congenital heart disease. From a clinical viewpoint, they can be totally silent or, because of associated cardiac anomalies or compression of the airway and esophagus, result in cardiovascular, respiratory, or feeding problems that result in morbidity and mortality. It is extremely important that radiologists have a clear understanding of these entities, their imaging characteristics, and their clinical relevance.

The imaging armamentarium available to diagnose these diverse conditions is ample, and has evolved from such traditional methods as chest radiography, barium esophagography, and angiography to new modalities that include echocardiography, multidetector row CT (MDCT), and MR imaging. These imaging modalities have added safety, speed, and superb resolution in diagnosis and, as in the case of MDCT, provide additional information about the airway and lung parenchyma, resulting in a more comprehensive examination with greater anatomic coverage.[1,2] This article reviews the most important congenital thoracic vascular anomalies, their embryologic foundation, clinical presentation, and imaging characteristics, especially those of MDCT.

TECHNIQUE

Although infants and children are the most frequently affected by congenital vascular

anomalies of the thorax, such anomalies can also be seen in adults, sometimes incidentally and as part of an examination for a totally unrelated indication. Therefore, examinations should be tailored to take into account radiation issues, need for sedation, and other indications so that that diagnosis is safe, comprehensive, and efficient. To accomplish this, those indications, along with available clinical and imaging data, should be systematically and carefully reviewed in consultation with referring physicians before the examination is prescribed according to the patient's individual needs.

Radiation exposure, particularly in infants and children, must be carefully considered when deciding whether MDCT or MR imaging is more appropriate. This risk should be weighed against the longer imaging time required for MR imaging, which necessitates expanded sedation or anesthesia with their inherent risks.

Due to the fast scanning times of MDCT, sedation is seldom required for older children and adults. For infants and children younger than 5 years of age, however, sedation may be necessary. The American College of Radiology has issued helpful guidelines to assist radiologists in the safe and effective use of conscious sedation for pediatric patients undergoing imaging and therapeutic procedures.[3] At our institution, we induce conscious sedation with chloral hydrate (50–100 mg per kilogram body weight, maximum dose of 2000 mg) in patients younger than 18 months and with intravenous pentobarbital sodium (up to 6 mg per kilogram body weight, maximum dose of

[a] Cardiothoracic Imaging Section, Department of Diagnostic Radiology, University of Puerto Rico School of Medicine, San Juan, Puerto Rico
[b] Mallinckrodt Institute of Radiology, Washington University School of Medicine, 660 South Euclid Avenue, Campus Box 8131, St Louis, MO 63110, USA
[c] Cardiothoracic Section, Mallinckrodt Institute of Radiology, Washington University, St Louis, MO, USA
* Corresponding author.
E-mail address: gutierrezf@mir.wustl.edu (F.R. Gutiérrez).

Radiol Clin N Am 48 (2010) 85–115
doi:10.1016/j.rcl.2009.09.004
0033-8389/09/$ – see front matter © 2010 Published by Elsevier Inc.

200 mg) in those older than 18 months. Scans are obtained during a single breath-hold. In sedated and uncooperative patients, images are obtained during quiet respiration. In general, anatomic coverage extends from the thoracic inlet to below the level of the diaphragm. In a 64-row MDCT, scanning of the entire thorax can be accomplished in a single breath-hold of less than 5 seconds.

For vascular opacification, a nonionic low-osmolarity contrast agent that contains 300 mg of iodine per milliliter or greater is injected via an antecubital vein using a mechanical injector. A saline bolus chase is applied. In adult patients, a contrast material dose of 1.5 mL/kg body weight and a flow rate of 3 to 4 mL/s through an 18-gauge catheter are prescribed. In pediatric patients, the flow rate varies with the size of the intravenous catheter. Suggested rates are 1.5 to 2.0 mL/s for a 22-gauge catheter and 2 to 3 mL/s for a 20-gauge catheter. For catheters smaller than 22 gauge, the contrast medium should be administered by hand. An automated bolus tracking system is used to determine the scanning delay time. A cursor is placed in the region of interest and the attenuation threshold set at 120 Hounsfield units. In pediatric patients, an empiric delay of 12 to 15 seconds after the start of intravenous contrast injection can be used for patients who weigh less than 10 kg. A delay of 20 to 25 seconds is used in larger patients.[4]

We use a 64-section CT scanner (Sensation 64; Siemens Medical Solutions, Forchheim, Germany) with a detector collimation of 64 × 0.6 mm, pitch of 1.4, and gantry rotation time of 330 ms. In adult patients, tube current is set to 220 mA and tube voltage to 120 kV. In pediatric patients, low radiation dose techniques are used. Tube current is adjusted by weight in the following manner: 25 mAs in patients weighing less than 15 kg, 30 mAs in patients weighing between 15 and 24 kg, 45 mAs in patients weighing between 25 and 34 kg, 75 mAs in patients weighing between 35 and 44 kg, 100 mAs in patients weighing between 45 and 54 kg, and 120 to 140 mAs in patients weighing more than 54 kg. Tube voltage dosages of 80 kV are used for patients weighing less than 50 kg. For patients weighing more than 50 kg, tube voltage dosages of 100 to 120 kV are used.

For the evaluation of congenital thoracic vascular anomalies, we do not routinely synchronize the CT data acquisition with the ECG tracing. An ECG-gated CT of the thorax increases scanning time and, more importantly, the radiation dose. In some cases, however, ECG-gating may be necessary to evaluate concomitant complex cardiac abnormalities, to assess ventricular and valvular function, or to reduce motion artifacts that obscure the anatomy. Scanning parameters then include a detector collimation of 32 × 0.6 mm, section collimation of 64 × 0.6 mm by means of a z-flying focal spot, gantry rotation time of 330 ms, pitch of 0.2, and tube potential of 100 to 120 kilovolt (peak) (kv[p]). We routinely use ECG-controlled tube current modulation. The supervising physician must determine on a patient-by-patient basis if the benefit of the additional information to be obtained by ECG-gating outweighs the risks of the increased radiation dose.

With the advent of MDCT, postprocessing techniques have become routine. They are helpful in conveying relevant imaging data to the referring physicians and can provide surgeons with detailed anatomic information for surgical planning. Although the source axial images are in most instances sufficient for diagnosis, two-dimensional reformatted and three-dimensional volume-rendered reconstructions can provide additional information about the nature and extent of the lesion in question. During thoracic CT angiography for the evaluation of congenital thoracic vascular anomalies, these postprocessed images are particularly useful in assessing stenoses and change of caliber of small structures that run obliquely to the imaging plane.[5] If concomitant airway narrowing is present, three-dimensional volume-rendered images from an external and internal perspective ("virtual bronchoscopy") readily show the extent.[6]

EMBRYOLOGY

Familiarity with the embryologic development of the thoracic vasculature is crucial in the proper understanding of the potential anomalies and anatomic variations. So, a brief review of this development follows, with an emphasis on the systemic and pulmonary circulations.

By the third week of embryonic development, paired angioblastic cords canalize to form endothelial tubes that quickly fuse into a single cardiac tube beginning at the cranial end. The cardiac tube elongates and develops alternate dilatations and constrictions that mark its several segments. Progressing caudally, these are truncus arteriosus, bulbus cordis, ventricle, atrium, and sinus venosus.

Separation of the aorta and pulmonary trunk is brought about by ingrowth of a spiral aorticopulmonary septum within the truncus arteriosus, which develops cephalad to caudad. The truncus arteriosus at the cranial end is continuous with the aortic sac from which symmetric aortic arches arise. Six paired aortic arches develop. These terminate in the dorsal aortas of the corresponding side. Portions of these arches regress and disappear, but several remnants normally persist.

The first and second aortic arches regress, except for small portions that form parts of the maxillary and stapedial arteries, respectively. In humans, the fifth aortic arches are rarely or only transiently present.[7] The third, fourth, and sixth aortic arches are the most important for final vascular development. The third pair of aortic arches forms the common carotid arteries and part of the internal carotid arteries. The left fourth aortic arch forms part of the definitive left aortic arch. The aortic sac contributes to the proximal part of the aortic arch, and the left dorsal aorta contributes to the distal part of the aortic arch. The right fourth aortic arch forms the proximal subclavian artery; the distal subclavian artery forms from the dorsal aorta and right seventh intersegmental artery. The left subclavian artery is formed from the left seventh intersegmental artery. The left and right pulmonary arteries are derivatives of the sixth aortic arches. The left sixth aortic arch also forms the ductus arteriosus.[8–10] The embryologic double aortic arch has on each side an aortic arch and a potential ductus arteriosus. The normal configuration of a left aortic arch with a left descending aorta and left ligamentum arteriosus occurs when the embryologic right arch regresses between the right subclavian artery and the descending aorta. The right subclavian artery fuses superiorly with the right common carotid artery and inferiorly with the brachiocephalic artery.[11] Fusion of the two dorsal aortas begins in the abdomen and progresses toward the thorax. The right thoracic dorsal aorta gradually regresses, leaving only the left dorsal aorta as the single descending thoracic aorta.

In the early developing embryo, the systemic venous system is bilateral and symmetric with both sides emptying into the caudal end of the cardiac tube via left and right horns of the sinus venosus. The left-sided venous system, mostly the left anterior and posterior cardinal veins, eventually regresses, leaving the coronary sinus as its only major remnant. At the same time, the left horn of the sinus venosus regresses and the right horn dilates to receive the entire systemic venous return via the inferior and superior vena cavae. The right horn of the sinus venosus becomes incorporated into the posterior wall of the right atrium. The pulmonary venous system is at first connected to the systemic venous system. With time, individual pulmonary veins form a confluence behind the primitive left atrium. An outpouching from the dorsal wall of the primitive left atrium—the common pulmonary vein—joins this confluence. As this communication between the left atrium and the pulmonary veins develops, the primitive pulmonary connections with the systemic venous system regress and disappear. Incorporation of the pulmonary veins into the left atrium typically gives rise to four separate pulmonary veins, one superior and one inferior in each side.[12]

AORTOPULMONARY ANOMALIES
Truncus Arteriosus

Truncus arteriosus, also known as truncus arteriosus communis or common arterial trunk, is an uncommon congenital vascular anomaly accounting for 2% of all congenital cardiac disease.[13] It is caused by failed septation of the embryologic truncus. As a result, a single vessel (the persistent truncus) receives the output of both ventricles and gives rise to the systemic, pulmonary, and coronary circulations (Fig. 1). There is a single truncal valve, usually dysplastic with a variable number of leaflets (up to six). This may cause regurgitation, stenosis, or both. A ventricular septal defect results from the absence of the right ventricular infundibular septum. A single coronary artery can be present. Patients present with cyanosis and cardiac failure in infancy. Truncus arteriosus invariably requires operative repair, which consists of patch-closure of the ventricular septal defect, and committing the truncus arteriosus and valve to the left ventricle. The pulmonary arteries are excised from their truncal origins and anastomosed to a prosthetic or aortic homograft valved conduit used to reconstruct the right ventricular outflow tract.

Truncus arteriosus is usually an isolated finding, though it can occasionally be associated with other anomalies, including DiGeorge syndrome, right aortic arch with mirror image branching, and CATCH-22 deletion. It has been classified in four anatomic types according to the origin of the pulmonary arteries (Collett and Edwards classification). In type I, a short pulmonary trunk arising from the truncus arteriosus gives rise to both pulmonary arteries. This is the most common type. In type II, each pulmonary artery arises directly from the posterior aspect of the truncus arteriosus. In type III, each pulmonary artery arises from the lateral aspect of the truncus arteriosus. In type IV, the pulmonary arteries arise from the descending aorta. Currently, this latter type is considered a severe form of tetralogy of Fallot with pulmonary atresia, rather than a true type of truncus arteriosus ("pseudotruncus"). The blood vessels from the descending aorta represent aortopulmonary collaterals rather than pulmonary arteries. More recently, a modified Van Praagh classification has been proposed involving three

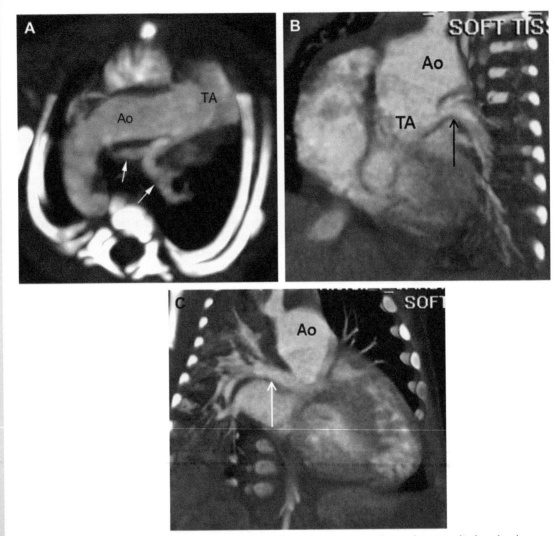

Fig. 1. Truncus arteriosus. (*A*) Oblique axial maximum intensity projection shows the aorta (Ao) and pulmonary arteries (*arrows*) arising from a type I truncus arteriosus (TA). (*B* and *C*) Sagittal oblique maximum intensity projection images show the left pulmonary artery (*arrow* in *B*) and right pulmonary artery (*arrow* in *C*) each arising from the short main pulmonary artery.

main categories: (1) truncus arteriosus with confluent or near confluent pulmonary arteries, (2) truncus arteriosus with absence of one pulmonary artery, and (3) truncus arteriosus with interrupted aortic arch or coarctation.[14]

Hemitruncus Arteriosus

In hemitruncus arteriosus, a pulmonary artery (more commonly the right) arises anomalously from the ascending aorta, and the opposite pulmonary artery originates from the main pulmonary artery (Fig. 2).[15] This anomaly is likely due to failure of migration of the sixth aortic arch to join its contralateral counterpart before the truncus arteriosus is divided. As a result, the right pulmonary

artery remains in continuity with the divided truncus arteriosus. MDCT readily shows the origin and course of the anomalous vessel and allows differentiation from comparable conditions, such as absence of the ipsilateral pulmonary artery.

Aorticopulmonary Window

An aorticopulmonary window is a communication, usually large, between the ascending aorta and main pulmonary artery, in the presence of two semilunar valves. This latter finding is key in distinguishing this condition from truncus arteriosus. In addition, the ventricular septum is usually intact in this anomaly, while it is invariably present in truncus arteriosus. An aorticopulmonary window

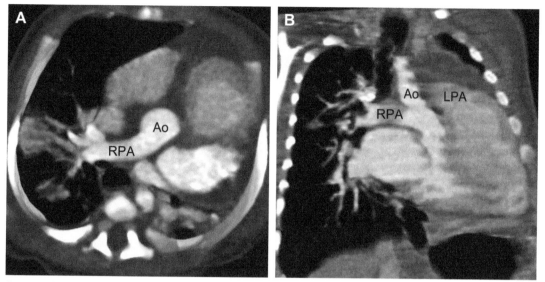

Fig. 2. Right hemitruncus. (*A*) Axial maximum intensity projection image shows the right pulmonary artery (RPA) arising from the aorta (Ao). (*B*) Oblique sagittal maximum intensity projection redemonstrates the continuity of the right pulmonary artery (RPA) and ascending aorta (Ao). The left pulmonary artery (LPA) arises from the right ventricle and contains dilute contrast in comparison to the left heart chambers. The right ventricle is shifted into the left hemithorax because of left lower lobe collapse.

results from partial failure of partitioning of the truncus arteriosus. As the term *windows* implies, there is little if any length to the communication; a ductus-type of communication is rare. The lower margin of the window is usually at or only a few millimeters above the aortic valvular ring. Clinically and hemodynamically, findings resemble a large patent ductus arteriosus and patients are diagnosed in infancy.[16] Treatment is with patch closure with a prosthetic or pericardial patch.

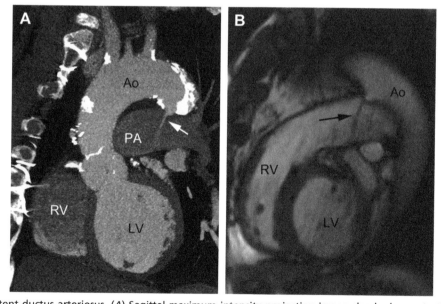

Fig. 3. Patent ductus arteriosus. (*A*) Sagittal maximum intensity projection image clearly demonstrates a jet of opacified blood (*arrow*) flowing from the aorta (Ao) into the pulmonary artery via a patent ductus arteriosus. This jet would be almost impossible to recognize on standard axial images. Median sternotomy wires and surgical clips along the ascending aorta are related to coronary artery bypass grafting. (*B*) Static frame of a steady-state free-precession magnetic resonance cine shows a dephasing jet (*arrow*) directed toward the pulmonary artery, correlating with the CT findings. LV, left ventricle; RV, right ventricle; PA, pulmonary artery.

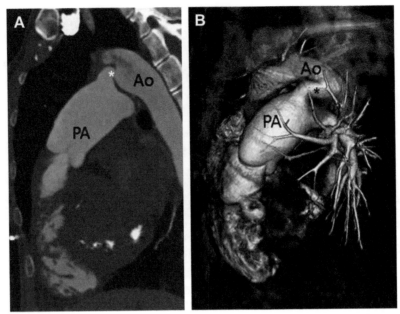

Fig. 4. Patent ductus arteriosus. (*A*) Sagittal maximum intensity projection image and (*B*) three-dimensional volume-rendered reconstruction demonstrate a patent ductus (*asterisk*) between the main pulmonary artery (PA) and proximal descending aorta (Ao). This patient has Eisenmenger syndrome with a right-to-left shunt as the descending aorta is opacified with contrast (through the patent ductus) but no contrast is present in the left heart. Calcifications in the left ventricle are due to underlying endocardial fibroelastosis.

Patent Ductus Arteriosus

The ductus arteriosus is derived from the left sixth aortic arch and connects the distal main or proximal left pulmonary artery to the descending aorta. It is a normal pathway of the fetal circulation, carrying deoxygenated blood from the right ventricle to the placenta via the descending aorta. Normally, the

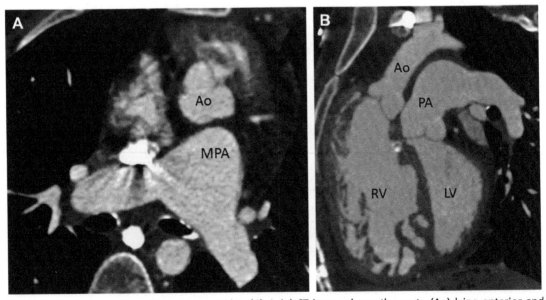

Fig. 5. Dextro-transposition of the great arteries. (*A*) Axial CT image shows the aorta (Ao) lying anterior and slightly to the right of the main pulmonary artery (MPA). (*B*) Sagittal maximum intensity projection image depicts the aorta (Ao) arising from the right ventricle (RV) and the main pulmonary artery (PA) arising from the left ventricle (LV). The great arteries have a parallel orientation and do not cross.

ductus closes functionally by 48 hours of age and anatomically several weeks later. When the ductus fails to close, an extracardiac left-to-right shunting of blood occurs and pulmonary hypertension can develop (**Figs. 3** and **4**). While echocardiography is the modality of choice for diagnosis, CT may play an important role in preoperative treatment planning. It can accurately assess the size and shape of the ductus to determine if transcatheter embolotherapy is feasible.[17,18]

Transposition of the Great Arteries

Dextro-transposition of the great arteries, also known as complete transposition of the great vessels, is the most common cyanotic lesion found in neonates and accounts for approximately 2.5% to 5% of congenital cardiac malformations. It results from failed spiraling of the aorticopulmonary septum. There is a strong association with right aortic arch and mirror-image branching. The

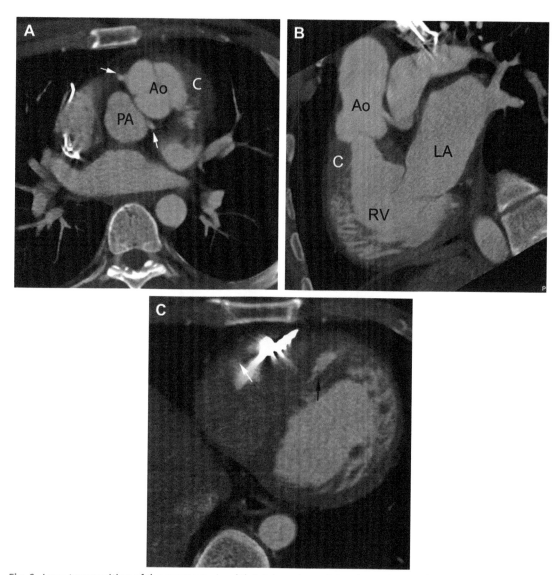

Fig. 6. Levo-transposition of the great arteries. (*A*) Axial maximum intensity projection shows the aorta (Ao) lying anterior and to the left of the main pulmonary artery (PA). The aorta gives rise to the coronary arteries (*arrows*), but is continuous with the muscular conus (C), a morphologic feature of the right ventricle. (*B*) Oblique coronal maximum intensity projection image along the axis of the right ventricle (RV) shows connection with the left atrium (LA) and aortic valve (atrioventricular and ventriculoarterial discordance). Note the muscular conus (C). (*C*) Axial maximum intensity projection image near the inferior wall of the heart shows the moderator band (*black arrow*), another morphologic feature of the right ventricle. Note the presence of a transvenous pacemaker lead (*white arrow*) in the left ventricle as these patients are prone to arrhythmia.

hallmark of this anomaly is ventriculoarterial discordance: The aorta arises from the right ventricle and receives systemic venous blood, and the main pulmonary artery arises from the left ventricle and receives pulmonary venous blood. In this manner, two independent parallel circulations are established. The majority of patients have an intact ventricular septum or a restrictive ventricular septal defect; the minority of patients have an unrestrictive ventricular septal defect with or without left ventricular (pulmonary outflow tract) obstruction. Regardless of the type of associated anomalies, most neonates present in the first few hours of life with cyanosis. Surgical repair is necessary for long-term survival and is nowadays accomplished by anatomic switching of the great vessels and coronary arteries (Jatene arterial switch procedure).[19–21]

Levo-transposition of the great arteries, also known as double discordance or congenitally corrected transposition, is an uncommon form of transposition that does not cause cyanosis in and of itself. It results from malrotation of the bulboventricular loop, which twist to the left in an opposite direction from normal. This anomaly is characterized by both atrioventricular and ventriculoarterial discordance (ie, "double discordance"): The morphologic right ventricle, from which the aorta arises, lies on the left and the morphologic left ventricle, from which the main pulmonary artery arises, lies on the right. Systemic venous return from the vena cavae flows into a normally positioned right atrium and then crosses a mitral valve into the morphologic left ventricle. The pulmonary venous return flows into a normally positioned left atrium and then

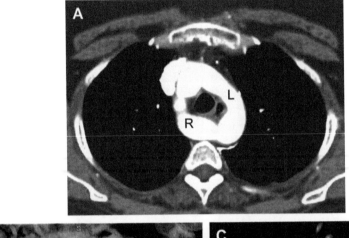

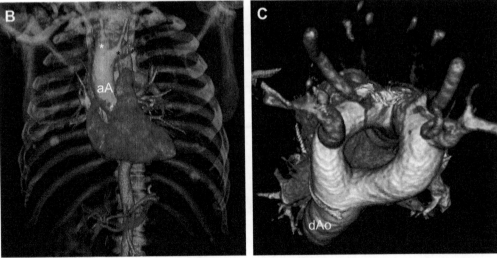

Fig. 7. Double aortic arch. (*A*) Axial CT image shows a complete ring around the esophagus and trachea formed by a double aortic arch. R, right arch; L, left arch. (*B*) Coronal and (*C*) superior three-dimensionally rendered reconstructions show two arches arising from the ascending aorta and joining posteriorly. The right-sided arch (*white asterisk in B*) is of larger caliber and more superior than the left-sided arch (*black asterisk in B*). Two epiaortic arteries arise from each arch. aAo, ascending aorta; dAo, descending aorta.

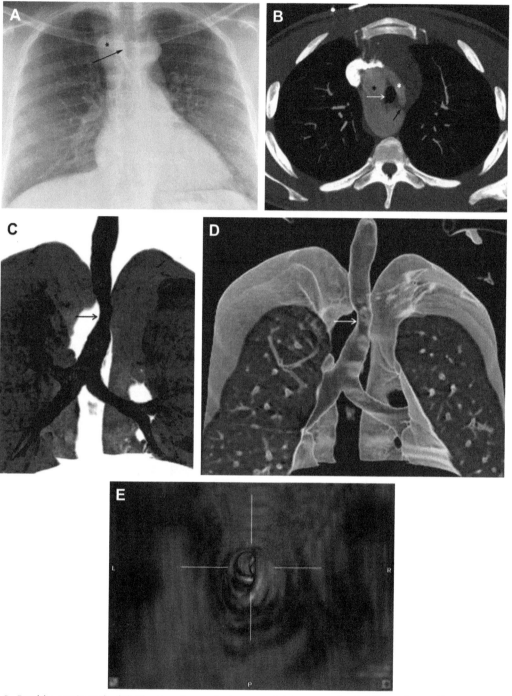

Fig. 8. Double aortic arch. (*A*) Chest radiograph shows a right paratracheal fullness (*asterisk*) indenting the trachea (*arrow*). (*B*) Axial maximum intensity projection image demonstrates a double aortic arch with right (*black asterisk*) and left (*white asterisk*) limbs encircling the airway. An atretic fibrous cord (*black arrow*) completes the arch on the left. Tracheal indentation is again noted (*white arrow*). (*C*) Minimum intensity projection image, (*D*) three-dimensional volume-rendered reconstruction, and (*E*) "virtual bronchoscopy" concomitant evaluations of the tracheal narrowing (*arrow* in *C* and *D*).

crosses a tricuspid valve into the morphologic right ventricle. Thus, "two anatomic wrongs make a physiologic right" and the circulatory pattern is in series and functionally correct: Systemic venous blood is delivered to the lungs and pulmonary venous blood is delivered to the body. Unfortunately, in the vast majority of cases, other cardiac anomalies coexist, including ventricular septal defects, conduction derangements, coronary artery anomalies, pulmonary stenosis, and systemic atrioventricular (tricuspid) valve deformities.[22,23] In the exceptional cases that lack additional cardiac abnormalities, this lesion may go undetected until adulthood.

In dextro-transposition of the great arteries, axial CT images at the level of the semilunar valves show the ascending aorta anterior and to the right of the main pulmonary artery (Fig. 5). In levo-transposition of the great arteries, the aorta is anterior and slightly to the left of the main pulmonary artery (Fig. 6). There may also be a rather horizontal interventricular septum with a relative superoinferior relationship of the ventricular chambers ("piggy-back configuration"). Dextrocardia is present in approximately one fourth of cases of levo-transposition of the great arteries.

SYSTEMIC ARTERIAL ANOMALIES
Left Aortic Arch with Aberrant Right Subclavian Artery

Embryologically, a left aortic arch with aberrant right subclavian artery results from interruption of the right

arch between the right common carotid artery and right subclavian artery. This is the most common congenital lesion of the aortic arch, occurring in 0.5% of the population,[24] and is usually asymptomatic, although dysphagia has been reported (dysphagia lusoria). The aberrant subclavian artery is the last main branch artery of the aortic arch, arising at the junction with the descending aorta. On an esophagogram, it may be noted to indent the posterior wall of the esophagus as it courses through the mediastinum to the right. The origin of the aberrant vessel may have a focal enlargement known as the diverticulum of Kommerell.

Double Aortic Arch

Double aortic arch is the most common cause of a vascular ring and is seldom associated with congenital heart disease. It results from persistence of both fourth aortic arches and is characterized by left and right aortic arches that arise from the ascending aorta, encircling the trachea and esophagus. Both arches join posteriorly after each one has given rise to a subclavian and common carotid artery. The single descending aorta formed is usually left sided. The right-sided limb in a double aortic arch is usually of larger caliber and more cephalad positioned than the left (Fig. 7). The left limb may have an atretic segment with a fibrous cord that completes the ring. In either case, such symptoms as severe stridor and dysphagia, which result from tracheal and esophageal compression, are common. CT readily shows the presence of the vascular ring from which four epiaortic arteries arise (ie, "four artery sign"). It can also help determine the surgical approach by depicting the

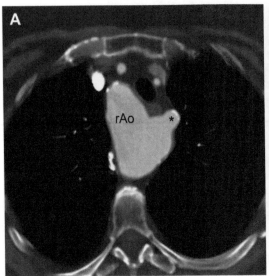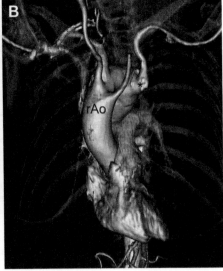

Fig. 9. Right aortic arch with aberrant left subclavian artery. (A) Axial CT image and (B) three-dimensional volume-rendered reconstruction demonstrate a right aortic arch (rAo). An aberrant retroesophageal left subclavian artery (asterisk) is the last artery to arise from the arch.

smaller limb, which is usually surgically ligated. The extent of tracheal narrowing can be demonstrated simultaneously (**Fig. 8**).[25]

Right Aortic Arch Anomalies

A right aortic arch occurs in approximately 0.1% of adults. The types of right arch anomalies depend on the point at which the left aortic arch is interrupted and include (1) right aortic arch with an aberrant left subclavian artery, (2) right aortic arch with mirror image branching, and (3) right aortic arch with isolated left subclavian artery. The latter is extremely rare.[11]

Right aortic arch with aberrant left subclavian artery is the most common right arch anomaly and the second most common cause of vascular ring after double aortic arch (**Fig. 9**). A left-sided ligamentum arteriosus completes the ring. Depending on the tightness of the ring and the extent to which the trachea and esophagus are encircled, the anomaly may or may not be symptomatic. This type of right arch anomaly is

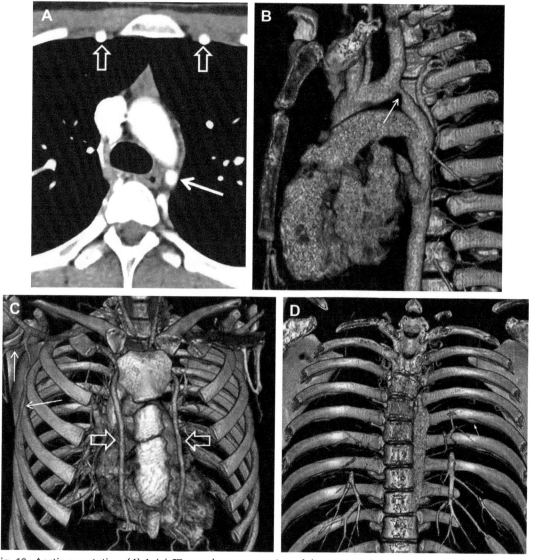

Fig. 10. Aortic coarctation. (*A*) Axial CT scan shows narrowing of the aortic arch lumen distal to the origin of the subclavian artery (*solid arrow*). The internal mammary arteries are enlarged (*open arrows*). (*B*) Three-dimensional volume-rendered reconstruction depicts the coarctation (*arrow*). (*C*) Frontal view shows enlarged internal mammary (*open arrows*) and right subscapular and lateral thoracic arteries (*white arrows*) that provide collateral circulation to the descending aorta. (*D*) Three-dimensional volume-rendered reconstruction (heart and anterior ribs removed) shows enlarged intercostals arteries but only mild rib notching of the left fifth rib (*arrow*) since most of the collateral flow is through the anterior arterial arcades.

associated with a low prevalence of congenital heart disease. Conversely, right aortic arch with mirror image branching is associated with a 98% prevalence of severe congenital heart disease, particularly tetralogy of Fallot, truncus arteriosus, and ventricular septal defect. In its usual configuration, in which the ligamentum arteriosus is on the right side, there is no formation of a vascular ring.[26]

Aortic Coarctation

In coarctation of the aorta, a congenital constriction of the lumen occurs at the junction of the aortic arch and the descending aorta (Fig. 10). Coarctation may be classified as preductal (infantile type) or postductal (adult type).[27] Both types are readily demonstrated by CT and MR imaging. With the latter

modality, important flow-sensitive hemodynamic measurements may be obtained noninvasively.

In the preductal type of coarctation, the obstruction occurs proximal to the ductus arteriosus, which often remains patent. A long segment of the transverse arch may show tubular hypoplasia, in addition to the focal constriction. A ventricular septal defect frequently coexists and resultant pulmonary arterial hypertension is common. This type usually presents in infancy with congestive heart failure.

In the postductal form, the obstruction occurs distal to the ductus arteriosus, which usually closes. The constriction consists of a shelflike indentatation in the posterolateral aortic wall. A bicuspid aortic valve occurs in over 70% of cases, but frank aortic

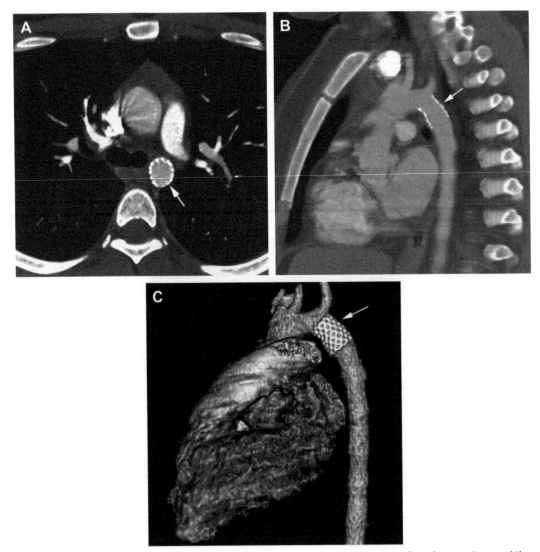

Fig. 11. Endovascular stent for aortic coarctation treatment. Using a combination of axial source images (A) and postprocessed images, including sagittal maximum intensity projection (B) and three-dimensional volume-rendered images (C), position, patency, and integrity of the stent (arrow) is accurately depicted with MDCT.

stenosis is rarely encountered during infancy. In fact, this form of coarctation is most commonly found in older (adult) patients. Physical examination may reveal a left sternal border systolic ejection murmur, differences in blood pressure between the upper and lower extremities, or decreased lower extremity pulses. A bicuspid aortic valve is usually present and may be complicated by aortic stenosis or regurgitation or both. Chronic hypertension, cerebrovascular accidents, left ventricular hypertrophy, mitral

valve disease, and subaortic stenosis are potential late problems.[28]

In coarctation, a high pressure gradient across the area of constriction provokes the formation of systemic collateral vessels to maintain blood flow to low-pressure regions. Collateral pathways include (1) internal thoracic (mammary) arteries arising from the subclavian arteries and connecting with the descending thoracic aorta via the intercostal arteries and with the external iliac

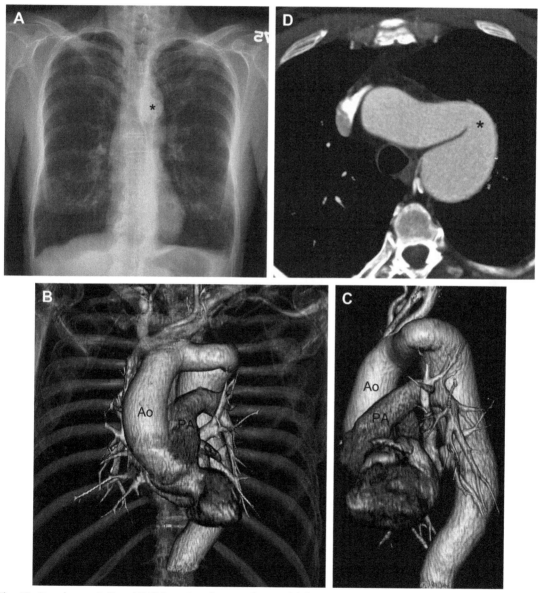

Fig. 12. Pseudocoarctation. (A) This patient has an abnormal left paratracheal density (asterisk) that represents the aorta buckling on itself. (B) Three-dimensional volume-rendered anteroposterior and (C) oblique sagittal reconstructions from a different patient with pseudocoarctation demonstrate a more pronounced buckling of a tortuous aortic arch. Ao, aorta; PA, pulmonary artery. (D) Axial maximum intensity projection image shows the buckling of the aortic arch (asterisk). Note that the internal mammary arteries are normal caliber.

arteries via the superior and inferior abdominal epigastric arteries, (2) thoracoacromial and descending scapular arteries arising from the subclavian arteries and connecting with the descending thoracic aorta via the intercostal arteries, and (3) vertebral arteries arising from the subclavian arteries and connecting with the descending thoracic aorta via the anterior spinal artery and intercostal arteries.[29] Inferior notching of the third to sixth ribs by dilated intercostal arteries is a classic radiographic finding.

Choice of treatment must take into account the patient's age and the site, extent, and hemodynamic severity of the coarctation. Intervention options include open surgery, balloon angioplasty,

stent implantation, and extra-anatomic bypass graft techniques. CT is well suited for the postoperative evaluation, including those for both adults and children.[30] Residual or recurrent stenosis, aneurysm formation, and other endovascular stent-related complications (eg, leaks, migration, fracture, infection, thrombosis, and dissection) are readily shown (**Fig. 11**).[29,31–33]

Aortic Pseudocoarctation

Aortic pseudocoarctation is an uncommon congenital anomaly that occurs when the third and seventh aortic dorsal segments fail to fuse properly.[11] It is characterized by buckling or kinking of a tortuous aortic arch at the level of the ligamentum arteriosus

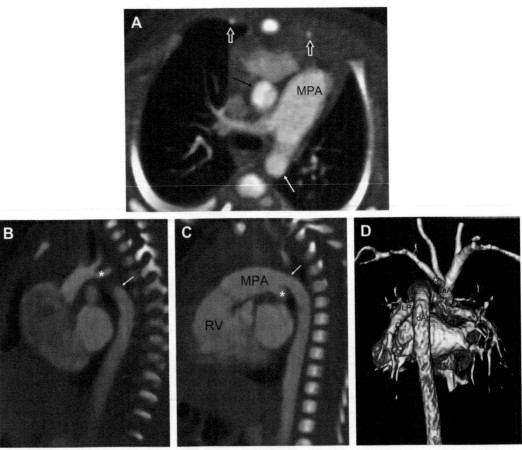

Fig. 13. Interrupted aortic arch. (*A*) Axial maximum intensity projection image shows the descending aorta (*white arrow*) communicating with the pulmonary artery through a large ductus arteriosus. Note the subtle difference in attenuation between the ascending aorta (*black arrow*) and the descending aorta. The internal mammary arteries (*open arrows*) are enlarged. MPA, main pulmonary artery. (*B*) Sagittal maximum intensity projection image demonstrates interruption of the aortic arch just beyond the left subclavian artery (*asterisk*). This is a type A interrupted aortic arch. Black arrow indicates ascending aorta. White arrow indicates descending aorta. (*C*) Sagittal maximum intensity projection image shows continuity of the descending aorta (*arrow*) with the main pulmonary artery (MPA) through a large ductus arteriosus. Asterisk indicates left pulmonary artery. RV, right ventricle. (*D*) Three-dimensional volume-rendered reconstruction from a posterior perspective shows an overview of this complex anatomy. Asterisk indicates left subclavian artery. aAo, ascending aorta; dAo, descending aorta; LPA, left pulmonary artery.

(Fig. 12). Although some degree of luminal narrowing and turbulence may be present, the hallmark of a pseudocoarctation is the absence of a significant pressure gradient. Therefore, systemic collateral vessels are not formed. This anomaly is usually asymptomatic and needs to be differentiated from true aortic coarctation, aneurysms, or mediastinal tumors.[34] Before cross-sectional imaging, clinicians occasionally found this distinction difficult to identify. Nowadays, however, both CT and MR imaging provide accurate morphologic information noninvasively. By demonstrating the absence of a pressure gradient, phase-contrast magnetic resonance can be diagnostic.

Interruption of the Aortic Arch

In an interrupted aortic arch, there is complete discontinuity of the aortic lumen between the ascending and descending aorta. An atretic fibrous cord may span the gap. Interrupted aortic arch is rare and accounts for less than 1.5% of congenital heart disease cases. Three basic types have been described, according to the site of interruption:

Type A: distal to the left subclavian artery
Type B: between the left common carotid and left subclavian artery
Type C: between the innominate and left common carotid artery

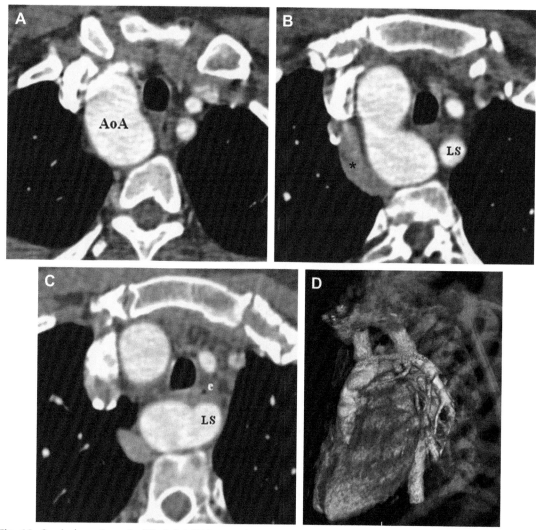

Fig. 14. Cervical aortic arch. (A) Axial CT image shows a right-sided aortic arch (AoA) extending above the sternum. (B and C) The distal arch crosses the mediastinum posterior to the esophagus (e) before descending in the left. The anomalous origin of the retroesophageal left subclavian (LS) artery is demonstrated. The azygous vein (asterisk) is just to the right of the aortic arch. (D) Oblique three-dimensional volume-rendered reconstruction shows the cervical arch rising above the sternum. The arch is partially obscured by patient motion.

A patent ductus arteriosus is invariably present and provides flow to the distal aorta. Associated anomalies include ventricular septal defect and some form of left ventricular outflow tract obstruction.[35] A right-sided descending aorta with interrupted arch is almost always associated with DiGeorge syndrome. In most cases, neonates nowadays undergo a single primary repair via a median sternotomy. The aortic arch is reconstructed, with a prosthetic patch if necessary, and the ventricular septal defect closed.[36] MDCT readily shows the abnormality and can be helpful in preoperative planning (Fig. 13). The distance between the discontinuous segments, the size of the patent ductus arteriosus, and the narrowest dimension of the left ventricular outflow tract are important anatomic features useful to the surgeon.[37]

Cervical Aortic Arch

A cervical aortic arch is characterized by an elongated aortic arch that runs upward above the sternum to the base of the neck, more often on the right side. It is frequently associated with a retroesophageal course of the descending aorta contralateral to the arch, and with an anomalous origin of the subclavian artery arising

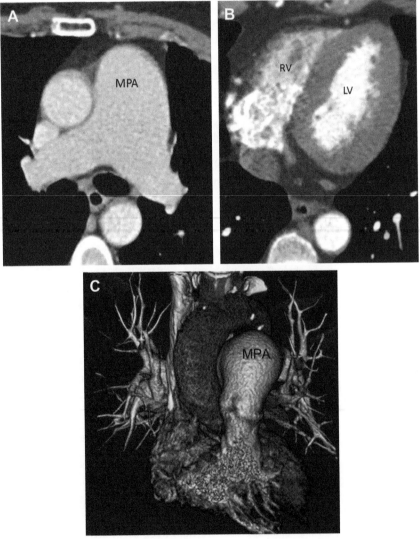

Fig. 15. Idiopathic dilatation of the pulmonary artery trunk. (A) Axial CT image demonstrates a dilated main pulmonary artery (MPA). (B) There is no associated right cardiac chamber dilatation or hypertrophy. LV, left ventricle; RV, right ventricle. There is no pulmonic stenosis (not shown). (C) Three-dimensional volume-rendered coronal reconstruction demonstrates the enlarged main pulmonary artery (MPA) in relation to a normal-caliber aortic arch. This patient had normal pulmonary artery pressures at cardiac catheterization.

from the descending aorta (**Fig. 14**). It may form a vascular ring if the ligamentum arteriosus is on the side opposite the arch. In the asymptomatic patient, this lesion is of little clinical significance. Patients may experience, however, swallowing or respiratory difficulties. Clinically, a pulsating mass in the supraclavicular area is a characteristic finding. This lesion results from persistence of the embryonic third aortic arch instead of the fourth.[38]

PULMONARY ARTERIAL ANOMALIES
Idiopathic Dilatation of the Pulmonary Artery Trunk

In idiopathic dilatation of the pulmonary artery trunk, there is enlargement of the pulmonary trunk without cardiac or pulmonary conditions that would otherwise account for the dilatation. This anomaly is asymptomatic and nonprogressive, and is usually detected incidentally. The idiopathic dilatation may involve the right and left pulmonary arteries (**Fig. 15**).[39]

Absence or Proximal Interruption of a Pulmonary Artery

In proximal interruption of the right or left main pulmonary artery, the intrapulmonary vascular network continues to develop independently and is supplied by aortopulmonary and transpleural collaterals. Right-sided involvement, which is much more common than left-sided involvement, is in most instances an isolated finding. Conversely, interruption of the left pulmonary artery is usually associated with a right aortic arch and other congenital cardiovascular anomalies, most commonly tetralogy of Fallot.[39–41] Most patients with this disorder are

symptomatic and present with recurrent pulmonary infections, mild dyspnea, and hemorrhage. Hemoptysis due to rupture of enlarged collateral vessels may occur. Pulmonary arterial hypertension develops in up to 25% of cases and is an important determinant of the prognosis.

Contrast-enhanced MDCT can be diagnostic, enabling concurrent evaluation of the major vascular structures, bronchial tree, and lung parenchyma. It will show absence of the main pulmonary artery or proximal interruption about the hilum, which is decreased in size. Hemithoracic volume loss with ipsilateral mediastinal shift and elevation of the hemidiaphragm is common (**Fig. 16**). There is hyperinflation and herniation of the contralateral lung into the smaller hemithorax. The bronchial branching pattern and pulmonary venous drainage are normal. The affected hemithorax may be hyperlucent. There is, however, no air trapping, and this is a distinguishing feature from Swyer-James syndrome. Lung windows may demonstrate peripheral parenchymal linear opacities perpendicular to the pleural surface. Transpleural systemic vessels cause these opacities. The latter may originate from the intercostal, internal thoracic (mammary), subclavian, and innominate arteries. Rib notching may also be present.

Pulmonary Arterial Stenosis

Pulmonary artery stenosis without ventricular septal defect accounts for approximately 8% of congenital heart disease cases. It is classified according to the level of the stenosis, which can be single or multiple, central or peripheral,

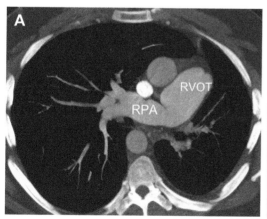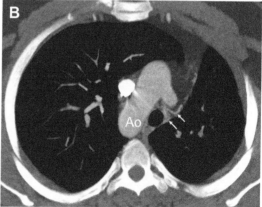

Fig. 16. Absence of the left main pulmonary artery. (*A*) Oblique axial maximum intensity projection image shows absence of the left main pulmonary artery. (*B*) Axial maximum intensity projection image at a higher level shows a right aortic arch (Ao) with mirror-image branching (not shown). There is left hemithoracic volume loss and leftward mediastinal shift. Enlarged collateral arteries to the left lung are abundant (*arrows*). RPA, right main pulmonary artery; RVOT, right ventricular outflow tract.

unilateral or bilateral. In type I, there is a single central stenosis (main, right, or left pulmonary artery) without peripheral branch involvement. In type II, a stenosis at the bifurcation of the pulmonary arterial trunk extends to the origins of the right and left pulmonary arteries, without peripheral branch involvement. In type III, there are peripheral but no central pulmonary artery stenoses. In type IV, there are both central and peripheral pulmonary artery stenoses. These lesions may be associated with well-characterized syndromes (Williams, Alagille, Noonan, Ehlers-Danlos, and Silver) and in

utero exposure to rubella virus. In general, patients are asymptomatic unless they have suprasystemic right ventricular pressures or associated cardiac disease. Treatment is with balloon pulmonary angioplasty (**Fig. 17**).[42–45]

Pulmonary Sling

A pulmonary sling is created by an anomalous origin of the left pulmonary artery that arises from the posterior aspect of the right pulmonary artery and crosses leftward between the trachea and

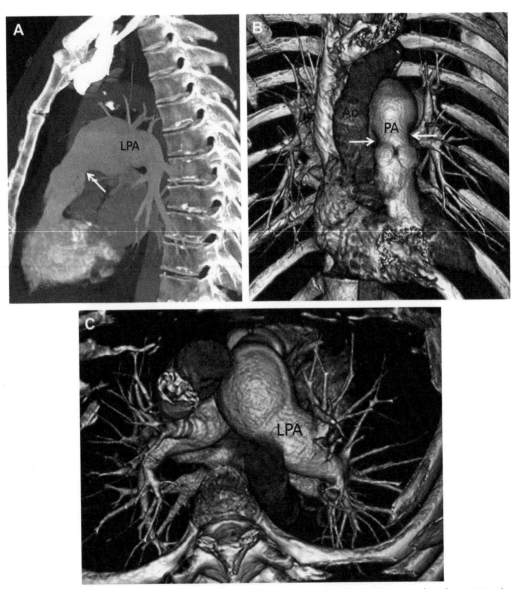

Fig. 17. Supravalvular pulmonic stenosis. Narrowing of the pulmonary trunk (*white arrows*) and poststenotic dilatation of the left main pulmonary artery (LPA) are shown clearly in this sagittal maximum intensity projection image (*A*) and in these three-dimensional volume-rendered reconstructions from a frontal (*B*) and superior (*C*) perspective. Ao, aorta; PA, pulmonary artery.

esophagus. The term *sling* refers to this vascular loop around the airway (**Fig. 18**). Along its proximal course, the anomalous vessel may compress the right main-stem bronchus or distal trachea. The esophagus may be indented anteriorly but is seldom functionally constricted. The ligamentum arteriosus completes a vascular ring that encircles the trachea but not the esophagus.[41,46]

Approximately 50% of patients with this anomaly have congenital tracheal stenosis due to complete cartilaginous rings, a condition in which the posterior membranous component of the trachea is absent and the tracheal cartilages are O-shaped

rather U-shaped. The result may be either a short- or long-segment tracheal stenosis. Additional concomitant malformations of the trachea include tracheomalacia, abnormal pulmonary lobulation, and bronchus suis. Congenital heart defects are present in 50% of patients with pulmonary artery sling, including ventricular septal defects, tetralogy of Fallot, and right ventricle with double outlet.[47,48]

Patients are usually symptomatic early in infancy, presenting with respiratory distress. Occasionally, this anomaly may be discovered incidentally in asymptomatic adults. When clinically indicated, treatment consists of reimplantation of the

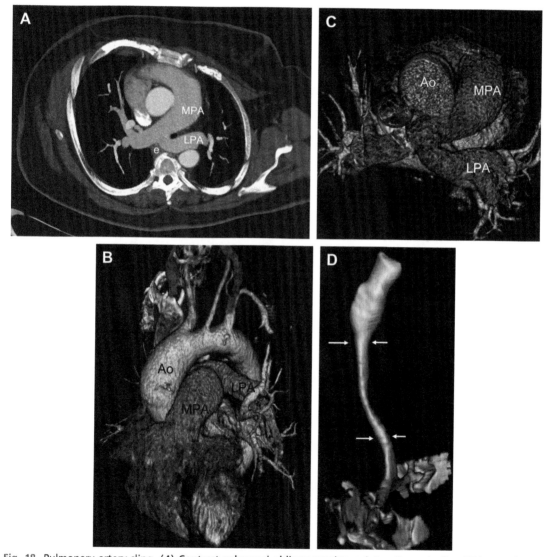

Fig. 18. Pulmonary artery sling. (*A*) Contrast-enhanced oblique maximum intensity projection CT image shows the left pulmonary artery (LPA) crossing between the trachea and esophagus (e) toward the left. (*B*) Sagittal oblique and (*C*) axial three-dimensional volume-rendered reconstructions show the anomalous origin and course of the left pulmonary artery and its relationship to the aorta. (*D*) Three-dimensional volume-rendered reconstruction of the trachea shows diffuse intrathoracic narrowing of the airway—tracheomalacia—a commonly associated finding (*arrows*). Ao, aorta; MPA, main pulmonary artery.

anomalous left pulmonary artery. If congenital tracheal stenosis is also present, tracheal reconstruction may be necessary. Resection with end-to-end anastomosis is the procedure of choice for short-segment tracheal stenosis. For long-segment stenosis, tracheoplasty may be performed.[49,50]

PULMONARY VENOUS ANOMALIES
Partial Anomalous Pulmonary Venous Return

In partial anomalous pulmonary venous return (PAPVR), one or more lobes drain into the right

atrium or into one of its tributaries (eg, vena cavae, azygous vein, coronary sinus, left vertical vein). The anomalous connection to the right heart or systemic venous circulation results in left-to-right shunting that may or may not be hemodynamically significant. In the second most common type of PAPVR, the right superior pulmonary vein drains to the low superior vena cava or to the superior cavoatrial junction.[51] In up to 90% of cases, a sinus venosus type of atrial septal defect is also present (Fig. 19). When both anomalies coexist, the resultant shunt may be hemodynamically significant and lead to cardiovascular symptoms.[52,53]

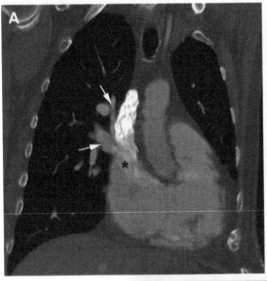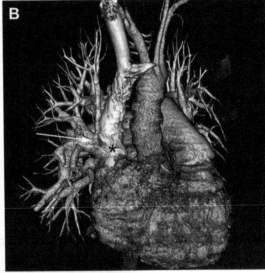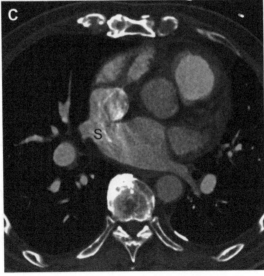

Fig. 19. Right upper lobe and middle lobe PAPVR. (A) Axial maximum intensity projection image and (B) three-dimensional volume-rendered reconstruction show the right upper lobe and right middle lobe pulmonary veins (arrows) draining into the superior vena cava (asterisk). Note the mixing of dense contrast from the superior vena cava with diluted contrast from the pulmonary veins. (C) Axial CT image shows a large sinus venosus atrial septal defect (S) with nondilute contrast passing into the left atrium.

In left upper lobe PAPVR, which is the most common PAPVR without heart disease, a vertical anomalous pulmonary vein courses lateral to the aortic arch and cephalad before joining the left brachiocephalic vein (**Fig. 20**). Because a left superior vena cava (LSVC) is similarly placed lateral to the aortic arch, it is important to determine whether a connection to the coronary sinus exists to distinguish the two anomalies (an LSVC can be followed inferiorly to the coronary sinus, which is usually dilated). In addition, two vessels anterior to the left main bronchus are present with an LSVC: the normal left superior pulmonary vein and the LSVC. With PAPVR, there is no vessel anterior to the bronchus.[51,54,55]

A right-sided anomalous venous drainage to the inferior vena cava (IVC), portal, hepatic, or other systemic vein usually involves the middle and lower lobes. It has been termed the *scimitar*, *venolobar* or *hypogenetic lung syndrome* when it is associated with right lung and pulmonary artery hypoplasia, systemic arterial supply, and mediastinal shift. The spectrum of associated anomalies, including congenital heart disease, horseshoe lung, and pulmonary arteriovenous malformations (PAVMs), is variable and determines the need for surgical correction.[56] The term *scimitar* refers to the appearance of the anomalous pulmonary vein, often resembling a scimitar, a curved Turkish saber (Fig. 21).

Total Anomalous Pulmonary Venous Return

When all pulmonary veins fail to drain directly to the left atrium, total anomalous pulmonary venous

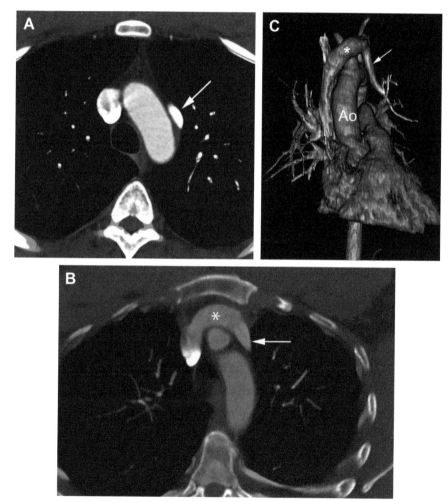

Fig. 20. Left upper lobe PAPVR. (*A*) Axial maximum intensity projection image shows an abnormal vessel to the left of the aortic arch—the vertical vein (*arrow*). (*B*) An oblique axial maximum intensity projection image shows the vertical vein (*arrow*) draining into the left brachiocephalic vein (*asterisk*). (*C*) Three-dimensional volume-rendered reconstruction depicts the left upper lobe pulmonary veins draining into the vertical vein (*arrow*) and depicts the entire course of the vertical vein. Asterisk indicates left brachiocephalic vein. Ao, aorta.

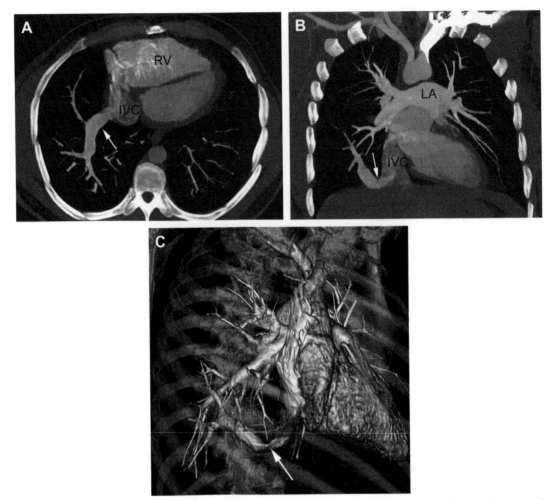

Fig. 21. Right lower lobe PAPVR. (*A*) Axial maximum intensity projection shows an anomalous pulmonary vein (*arrow*) draining into the IVC. The right ventricle (RV) is enlarged from the left-to-right shunt. (*B*) Coronal maximum intensity projection and (*C*) three-dimensional volume-rendered reconstruction from a right perspective demonstrate the full course of the anomalous right lower lobe vein (*arrow*) as it drains into the IVC. LA, left atrium.

return (TAPVR) is present. The embryologic defect occurs when the common pulmonary vein does not incorporate into the left atrium. Pulmonary venous drainage returns to the right side of the heart via persistent primitive communications. An obligatory atrial septal defect allows blood to reach the left cardiac chambers (Fig. 22).

TAPVR is an admixture lesion classified into supracardiac, cardiac, infracardiac, and mixed types, depending on the routes of venous drainage. The clinical picture is determined by the size of the interatrial communication and the magnitude of the pulmonary vascular resistance. The latter is related to the site of anomalous connection. For instance, in the infracardiac type, drainage into a high-resistance channel (ie, portal system) causes pulmonary venous hypertension

and congestive heart failure. Most patients with TAPVR have symptoms during the first year of life and require corrective surgery, which consists of anastomosing the confluence of pulmonary veins to the left atrium.

PULMONARY ARTERIOVENOUS MALFORMATION

PAVMs consist of direct communications between a pulmonary artery and a pulmonary vein without an intervening capillary network. These lesions occur as isolated entities or, in more than 60% of cases, in association with hereditary hemorrhagic telangiectasia. Also known as Osler-Weber-Rendu disease, hemorrhagic telangiectasia is an autosomal-dominant

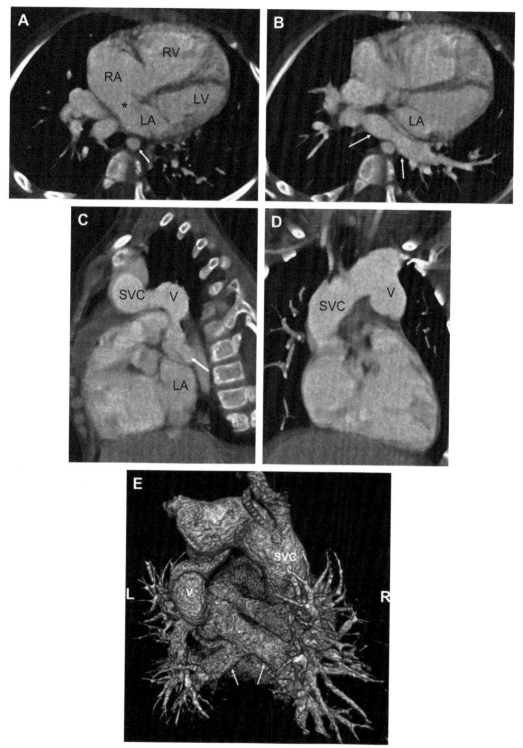

Fig. 22. TAPVR. (*A*) Oblique axial maximum intensity projection image through all four cardiac chambers shows a large atrial septal defect (*asterisk*) with marked enlargement of the right ventricle (RV) and right atrium (RA). The left ventricle (LV) and left atrium (LA) are normal size. The descending aorta (*arrow*) is small caliber and contains little intravenous contrast. (*B*) Oblique axial maximum intensity projection at a higher level shows that there is no communication between the left atrium (LA) and the pulmonary veins (*arrows*). (*C*) Sagittal maximum intensity projection shows that the pulmonary venous confluence (*arrow*) drains cephalad into an abnormal vein (V) that returns blood to the superior vena cava (SVC), a supracardiac type of TAPVR. (*D*) Coronal maximum intensity projection image shows marked increase in caliber of the superior vena cava and the large supracardiac vein (V). (*E*) Three-dimensional volume-rendered reconstruction from a posterior prospective shows the pulmonary veins (*arrows*) draining into the tortuous supracardiac vein (V) and superior vena cava (SVC).

condition with the clinical triad of epistaxis, mucocutaneous or visceral telangiectasia, and family history of disease.[57]

PAVMs cause right-to-left shunting of blood. Small malformations may be asymptomatic. If large and numerous, however, these lesions may cause hypoxemia, stroke, and paradoxic emboli. Although individual lesions were once treated by surgical resection, percutaneous transcatheter embolization is now considered the treatment of choice.[58,59] Most PAVMs (>70% cases) have a single feeding artery and a single draining vein. Up to 50% of patients with PAVMs have multiple lesions. By depicting the size, extent, and angioarchitecture of the malformations, MDCT plays an important role in the preinterventional planning and posttreatment follow-up (Fig. 23). Generally, arteriovenous malformations with feeding arteries greater than 3 mm require treatment. Because the size of the feeding artery determines management, this value should be included in any CT report in which a PAVM is described.

SYSTEMIC VENOUS ANOMALIES
Persistent Left Superior Vena Cava

A persistent LSVC has been reported to occur in 0.3 to 0.5% of the general population[60–62] and in 4.4% of patients with congenital heart disease. It results

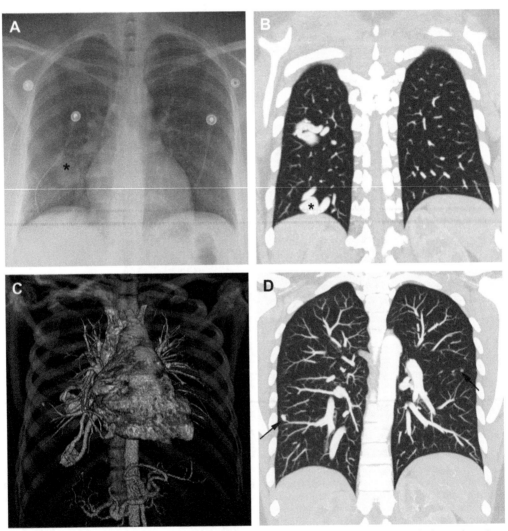

Fig. 23. Hereditary hemorrhagic telangiectasia with PAVMs. (A) A mass (asterisk) in the right lower lung is noted on the chest radiograph. (B) Oblique coronal maximum intensity projection image and (C) three-dimensional volume-rendered reconstruction demonstrate that the radiographic abnormality represents the nidus of a large PAVM (asterisk). Note the presence of a second large PAVM superiorly. (D) Sagittal maximum intensity projection image demonstrates additional small PAVMs (arrows).

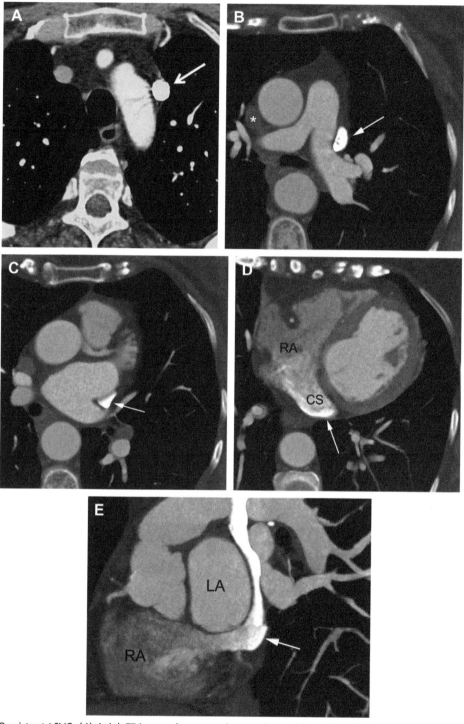

Fig. 24. Persistent LSVC. (*A*) Axial CT image shows an abnormal vessel lateral to the aortic arch that represents a persistent LSVC (*arrow*). (*B*) Axial maximum intensity projection image from a coronary CT angiogram in a different patient shows the LSVC (*arrow*) coursing lateral to the pulmonary artery. Note the presence of a right-sided superior vena cava that is not opacified with contrast (*asterisk*) since the injection was performed through the left upper extremity. (*C*) The LSVC (*arrow*) shown adjacent to the left atrium coursing inferiorly toward the coronary sinus. (*D*) The LSVC (*arrow*) drains into a dilated coronary sinus (CS). RA, right atrium. (*E*) Oblique coronal maximum intensity projection image depicts the course of the LSVC (*arrow*) as it drains into the right atrium (RA). Note the relationship to the left atrium (LA).

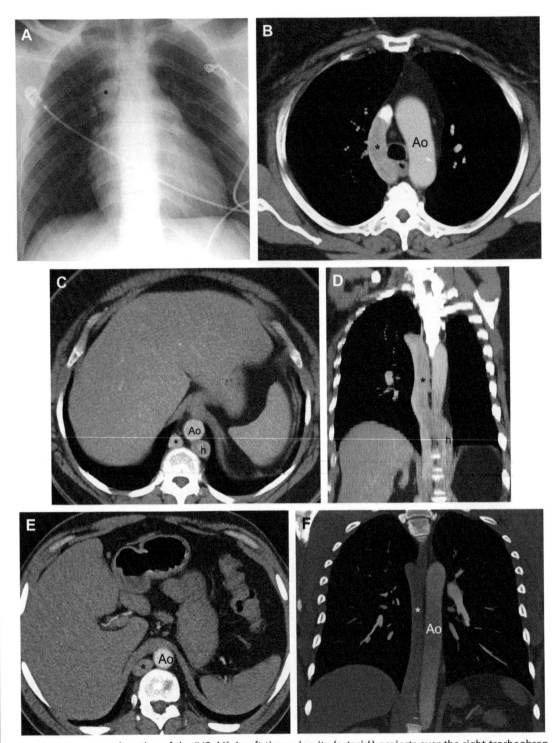

Fig. 25. Azygous continuation of the IVC. (*A*) A soft tissue density (*asterisk*) projects over the right tracheobronchial angle on the chest radiograph. (*B*) Axial maximum intensity projection image shows that a dilated azygous arch (*asterisk*) accounts for the radiographic density. Ao, aorta. (*C*) Axial CT image and (*D*) coronal maximum intensity projection image in a patient with azygous vein (*asterisk*) continuation of the IVC shows associated enlargement of the hemiazygous vein (h). (*E*) Axial CT image and (*F*) coronal maximum intensity projection image show that not all patients with azygous vein (*asterisk*) continuation of the IVC will have an enlarged hemiazygous vein. Ao, aorta.

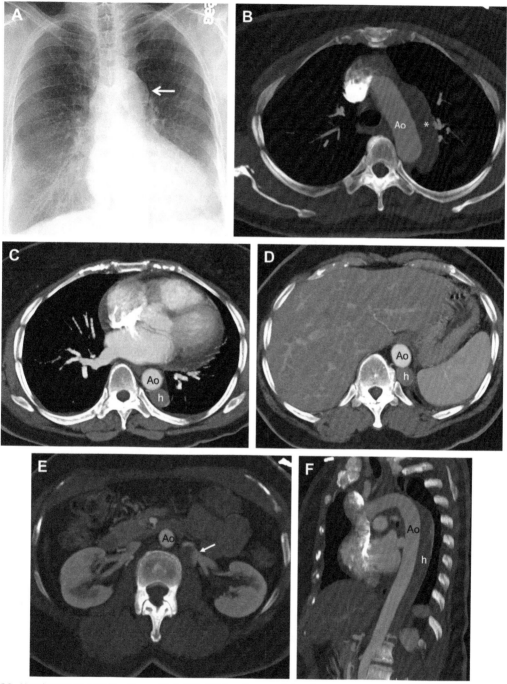

Fig. 26. Hemiazygous continuation of left IVC. (*A*) An abnormal density is present adjacent to the aortic knob on the chest radiograph (*arrow*). (*B*) Axial maximum intensity projection image reveals that the abnormal density corresponds to a dilated left superior intercostal vein (*asterisk*) alongside the aortic arch (Ao). (*C*) Axial maximum intensity projection image at the level of the left atrium shows the dilated hemiazygous vein (h) to the left and posterior of the aorta (Ao). (*D*) Axial maximum intensity projection image through the liver shows the hemiazygous vein (h) to the left of the aorta (Ao). A right-sided IVC is absent. (*E*) Axial maximum intensity projection image at a lower level in the abdomen shows the left renal vein draining into a left-sided IVC (*arrow*). Ao, aorta. (*F*) Oblique sagittal maximum intensity projection image through the chest shows why the dilated hemiazygous vein (h) could be mistaken for a thoracic aortic dissection. Ao, aorta.

from persistence of the left anterior cardinal vein. In the majority of cases, a right superior vena cava is also present. An anastomosis between the right and LSVC (bridging vein) is present in only 35% of cases. In 92% of individuals, the LSVC arises from the left brachiocephalic vein and travels inferiorly, lateral to the aortic arch and anterior to the left hilum, and drains into the coronary sinus through the vein of Marshal (Fig. 24). Blood therefore flows craniocaudally. As a vessel coursing lateral to the aortic arch, the LSVC must be differentiated from a vertical vein related to left upper lobe PAPVR (see PAPVR section). In the remaining cases, the persistent LSVC terminates in the left atrium, resulting in a right- to left-sided shunt.[63] Raghib complex denotes a developmental anomaly in which termination of the LSVC in the left atrium, an atrial septal defect, and absence of the coronary sinus coexist.[64]

The presence of an LSVC is usually an incidental finding during cardiovascular imaging, often detected after observing an unusual course of a central venous catheter. In most cases, a persistent LSVC is an isolated finding. Almost 40% of patients with a persistent LSVC, however, have associated cardiac anomalies, such as atrial septal defects, bicuspid aortic valve, coarctation of aorta, coronary sinus atresia, and cor triatrum. These associated cardiac anomalies are more common when the right superior vena cava is absent.

Azygous/Hemiazygous Continuation of the Inferior Vena Cava

Another common thoracic venous anomaly is azygous continuation of the IVC (prevalence of 0.6%). Also termed *absence of the hepatic segment of the IVC with azygous continuation*, this anomaly results from interruption of the intrahepatic IVC with atrophy of the right subcardinal vein. Blood is directed to the azygous vein, which courses superiorly along the spine to drain into the superior vena cava (Fig. 25). Hemiazygous continuation of a left-sided IVC is less common and presents with three possible routes for blood to reach the right heart. The hemiazygous vein can drain to the azygous vein or into a persistent LSVC. Also, it can drain to the accessory hemiazygous vein, left superior intercostal vein, and left brachiocephalic vein into a normal right superior vena cava (Fig. 26).[52,65]

SEQUESTRATION

Bronchopulmonary sequestration consists of a portion of nonfunctioning lung parenchyma that has no communication with the tracheobronchial tree and receives its blood supply from a systemic artery. The anomaly is commonly classified as intralobar or extralobar. While some intralobar sequestrations may be congenital, most are acquired secondary to chronic inflammation and bronchial obstruction. Affected patients present during adolescence or adulthood with recurrent pneumonias. This form is the most common, accounting for up to 75% of cases. It is seldom associated with other anomalies and is characterized by contiguity with the normal lung parenchyma and investment within the same visceral pleura.[66] Conversely, extralobar sequestration is always congenital, has a separate pleural investment, and is often associated with other anomalies,

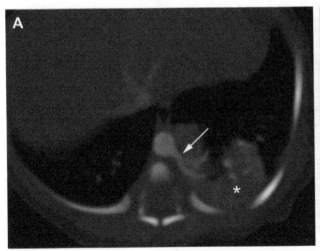
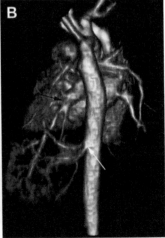

Fig. 27. Intralobar sequestration. (*A*) Axial maximum intensity projection image in a 1-day-old patient shows an enhancing mass in the left lower lobe (*asterisk*) with a feeding vessel arising directly from the descending thoracic aorta (*arrow*). (*B*) Posterior oblique three-dimensional volume-rendered reconstruction shows the feeding vessel arising from the aorta (*white arrow*) and drainage of the sequestration via pulmonary veins (*black arrow*).

including congenital diaphragmatic hernia, congenital cystic adenomatoid malformation, and fistulous connection to the esophagus or stomach. It presents during the neonatal period. In intralobar sequestration, venous drainage is typically through a pulmonary vein. Extralobar sequestrations drain to systemic veins, usually via the azygous/hemiazygous vein or IVC. All forms of bronchopulmonary sequestrations are more common on the left side and in the lower lobes (Fig. 27). Treatment is by surgical excision.[67,68]

The appearance of bronchopulmonary sequestration in MDCT is variable, ranging from a heterogeneous solid mass, a conglomeration of cystic lesions, or a cavitary lesion with air-fluid levels. Adjacent emphysematous lung caused by collateral air drift at the margins of the sequestration is usually seen. The use of multiplanar reconstructions may facilitate the depiction of both the aberrant arterial feeding vessel and draining vein. When prescribing the anatomic coverage, the scan must include the upper abdomen, as the anomalous artery may arise from the upper abdominal aorta. The preoperative depiction of the involved angioarchitecture can be pivotal to avoid accidental incision and hemorrhage.[69]

SUMMARY

The ability to diagnose congenital vascular thoracic anomalies has evolved tremendously in the past 20 years. Traditional methods of plain radiographs and barium swallow studies as well as invasive angiography have now been supplanted with MR imaging and MDCT, minimally invasive methods that provide superb resolution and a large field of view. Physicians involved in the performance of these studies must have a clear understanding of the large variety of arterial and venous anomalies included in this diverse group of entities. Specific imaging strategies must be prescribed to better delineate the relevant anatomy so that proper care can be instituted.

REFERENCES

1. Baron RL, Gutierrez FR, Sagel SS, et al. CT of anomalies of the mediastinal vessels. AJR Am J Roentgenol 1981;137:571–6.
2. Haramati LB, Glickstein JS, Issenberg HJ, et al. MR Imaging and CT of vascular anomalies and connections in patients with congenital heart disease: significance in surgical planning. Radiographics 2002;22:337–49.
3. American College of Radiology. 2005. ACR practice guideline for pediatric sedation/analgesia, Retrieved February 2009 from American College of Radiology: Available at: http://www.acr.org/SecondaryMain MenuCategories/quality_safety/guidelines/pediatric/pediatric_sedation.aspx. Accessed February 12, 2009.
4. Siegel MJ. Multiplanar and three-dimensional multi-detector row CT of thoracic vessels and airways in the pediatric population. Radiology 2003;229:641–50.
5. Lee EY, Siegel MJ, Hildebolt CF, et al. MDCT evaluation of thoracic aortic anomalies in pediatric patients and young adults: comparison of axial, multiplanar and 3D images. AJR Am J Roentgenol 2004;182:777–84.
6. Ravenel JG, McAdams HP. Multiplanar and three-dimensional imaging of the thorax. Radiol Clin North Am 2003;41(3):475–89.
7. Effmann EL, Whitman SA, Smith BR. Aortic arch development. Radiographics 1986;6(6):1065–89.
8. Moore KL, Persaud TV. The developing human. Philadelphia: W B Saunders; 1993.
9. Arey JB. Embryology of the heart and great vessels. In: Arey JB, editor. Cardiovascular pathology in infants and children. Philadelphia: W B Saunders; 1984. p. 9–54.
10. Gedgaudas E, Moller JH, Casteñeda-Zúñiga W, et al. Embryology and anatomy of the heart. In: Gedgaudas E, Moller JH, Casteñeda-Zúñiga W, et al, editors. Cardiovascular radiology. 1st edition. Philadelphia: W B Saunders; 1985. p. 1–15.
11. Soler R, Rodriguez E, Requejo I, et al. Magnetic resonance imaging of congenital abnormalities of the thoracic aorta. Eur Radiol 1998;8:540–6.
12. Dillman JR, Yarram SG, Hernandez RJ. Imaging of pulmonary venous developmental anomalies. AJR Am J Roentgenol 2009;192:1272–85.
13. Gedgaudas E, Moller JH, Casteñeda-Zúñiga W, et al. Congenital heart disease: cyanosis and increased pulmonary arterial vascularity. In: Gedgaudas E, Moller JH, Casteñeda-Zúñiga W, et al, editors. Cardiovascular radiology. 1st edition. Philadelphia: W B Saunders; 1985. p. 101–25.
14. Jacobs ML. Congenital heart surgery nomenclature and database project: truncus arteriosus. Ann Thorac Surg 2000;69:50–5.
15. Choe YH, Kim YM, Han BK, et al. MR imaging in the morphologic diagnosis of congenital heart disease. Radiographics 1997;17:403–22.
16. Arey JB. Malformations of the conus and troncus arteriosus. In: Arey JB, editor. Cardiovascular pathology in infants and children. Philadelphia: W B Saunders; 1984. p. 136–8.
17. Leschka S, Oechslin E, Husmann L, et al. Pre- and postoperative evaluation of congenital heart disease in children and adults with 64-section CT. Radiographics 2007;27(3):829–46.
18. Goitein O, Fuhman CR, Lacomis JM. Incidental finding on MDCT of patent ductus arteriosus: use

of CT and MRI to assess clinical importance. AJR Am J Roentgenol 2005;184:1924–31.

19. Gaca AM, Jaggers JJ, Dudley LT, et al. Repair of congenital heart disease: a primer—Part 1. Radiology 2008;247(3):617–31.

20. Donnelly LF, Higgins CB. MR imaging of conotruncal abnormalities. AJR Am J Roentgenol 1996;166:925–8.

21. Barboza JM, Dajani NK, Glenn LG, et al. Prenatal diagnosis of congenital cardiac anomalies: a practical approach using two basic views. Radiographics 2002;22(5):1125–38.

22. Reddy GP, Caputo GR. Congenitally corrected transposition of the great arteries. Radiology 1999; 213(1):102–6.

23. Chang DS, Barack BM, Lee MH, et al. Congenitally corrected transposition of the great arteries: imaging with 16-MDCT. AJR Am J Roentgenol 2007;188: W428–30.

24. Cole TJ, Henry DA, Jolles H, et al. Vascular structures that simulate neoplasms on chest radiographs: clues to the diagnosis. Radiographics 1995;15(4): 867–91.

25. Schlesinger AE, Krishnamurthy R, Sena LM, et al. Incomplete double aortic arch with atresia of the distal left arch: distinctive imaging appearance. AJR Am J Roentgenol 2005;184:1634–9.

26. Shuford WH, Sybers RG, Edwards FK. The three types of right aortic arch. Am J Roentgenol 1970; 109(1):67–74.

27. Gutierrez FR, Ho M-L, Siegel MJ. Practical applications of magnetic resonance In congenital heart disease. Magn Reson Imaging Clin N Am 2008;16:403–35.

28. Gersony WM, Rosenbaum MS. Congenital heart disease in the adult. New York: McGraw-Hill; 2002.

29. Sebastia C, Quiroga S, Boye R, et al. Aortic stenosis: spectrum of diseases depicted at multisection CT. Radiographics 2003;23:S79–91.

30. Fidler JL, Cheatham JP, Fletcher SE, et al. CT angiography of complications in pediatric patients treated with intravascular stents. AJR Am J Roentgenol 2000;174:355–9.

31. Shih MC, Tholpady A, Kramer CM, et al. Surgical and endovascular repair of aortic coarctation: normal findings and appearance of complications on CT angiography and MR angiography. AJR Am J Roentgenol 2006;187:W302–12.

32. Libby P, Bonow RO, Mann DL, et al. 8th editionIn: Braunwald's heart disease: a textbook of cardiovascular medicine, vol. 2. Philadelphia: Saunders; 2008.

33. Corno AF, Festa P. Congenital heart defects: decision making for surgery. Heidelberg, Germany: Steinkopff Verlag; 2009.

34. Steinberg I, Engle MA, Holswade GR, et al. Pseudocoarctation of the aorta associated with congenital heart disease: report of ten cases. AJR Am J Roentgenol 1969;106(1):1–20.

35. Dillman JR, Yarram SG, D'Amico AR, et al. Interrupted aortic arch: spectrum of MRI findings. Am J Roentgenol 2008;190:1467–74.

36. Gaca AM, Jaggers JJ, Dudley LT, et al. Repair of congenital heart disease: a primer—Part 2. Radiology 2008;248(1):44–60.

37. Goo HW, Park I-S, Ko JK, et al. CT of congenital heart disease: normal anatomy and typical pathologic conditions. Radiographics 2003;23:S147–65.

38. Bisset GS, Towbin RB, Strife JL, et al. Pediatric case of the day: cervical aortic arch. Radiographics 1987; 7(1):186–9.

39. Castañer E, Gallardo X, Rimola J, et al. Congenital and acquired pulmonary artery anomalies in the adult: radiologic overview. Radiographics 2006;26: 349–71.

40. Davis SD. Proximal interruption of the right pulmonary artery. Radiology 2000;217(2):437–40.

41. Zylak CJ, Eyler WR, Spizarny DL, et al. Developmental lung anomalies in the adult: radiologic-pathologic correlation. Radiographics 2002;22:S25–43.

42. Kreutzer J, Landzberg MJ, Preminger TJ, et al. Isolated peripheral pulmonary artery stenoses in the adult. Circulation 1996;93:1417–23.

43. Gupta H, Mayo-Smith WW, Mainiero MB, et al. Helical CT of pulmonary vascular abnormalities. AJR Am J Roentgenol 2002;178:487–92.

44. Shah R, Cestone P, Mueller C. Congenital multiple peripheral pulmonary artery stenosis (pulmonary branch stenosis or supravalvular pulmonary stenosis). Am J Roentgenol 2000;175:856–7.

45. Baum D, Khoury GH, Ongley PA, et al. Congenital stenosis of the pulmonary artery branches. Circulation 1964;29:680–7.

46. Kussman BD, Geva T, McGowan FX. Cardiovascular causes of airway compression. Paediatr Anaesth 2004;14:60–74.

47. Berdon WE. Rings, slings, and other things: vascular compression of the infant trachea updated from the mid-century to the millenium. Radiology 2000;216(3):624–32.

48. Berdon WE, Baker DH, Wung J-T, et al. Complete cartilage-ring tracheal stenosis associated with anomalous left pulmonary artery: the ring-sling complex. Radiology 1984;152(1):57–64.

49. McLaren CA, Elliot MJ, Roebuck DJ. Vascular compression of the airway in children. Paediatr Respir Rev 2008;9:85–94.

50. Oshima Y, Yamaguchi M, Yoshimura N, et al. Management of pulmonary artery sling associated with tracheal stenosis. Ann Thorac Surg 2008;86:1334–8.

51. Ho M-L, Bhalla S, Bierhals A, et al. MDCT of partial anomalous pulmonary venous return (PAPVR) in adults. J Thorac Imaging 2009;24(2):89–95.

52. Demos TC, Posniak HV, Pierce KL, et al. Venous anomalies of the thorax. Am J Roentgenol 2004;182:1139–50.

53. Gustafson RA, Warden HE, Murray GF, et al. Partial anomalous pulmonary venous connection to the

right side of the heart. J Thorac Cardiovasc Surg 1980;98:861–8.

54. Dillon EH, Camputaro C. Partial anomalous drainage of the left upper lobe vs duplication of the superior vena cava: distinction based on CT findings. Am J Roentgenol 1993;160:375–9.

55. Pennes DR, Ellis JH. Anomalous pulmonary venous drainage of the left upper lobe shown by CT scans. Radiology 1986;159:23.

56. Woodring JH, Howard TA, Kanga JF. Congenital pulmonary venolobar syndrome revisited. Radiographics 1994;14(2):349–69.

57. Jaskolka J, Wu L, Chan RP, et al. Imaging of hereditary hemorrhagic telangiectasia. AJR Am J Roentgenol 2004;183:307–14.

58. Abdel-Aal AK, Hamed MF, Biosca F, et al. Occlusion time for Amplatzer vascular plug in the management of pulmonary arteriovenous malformations. Am J Roentgenol 2009;192(3):793–9.

59. Gupta P, Mordin C, Curtis J, et al. Pulmonary arteriovenous malformations: effect of embolization on right-to-left shunt, hypoxemia, and excercise tolerance in 66 patients. AJR Am J Roentgenol 2002;179:347–55.

60. Cha EM, Khoury GH. Persistent left superior vena cava. Radiologic and clinical significance. Radiology 1972;103(2):375–81.

61. Goyal SK, Punnam SR, Verma G, et al. Persistent left superior vena cava: a case report and review of literature. Cardiovasc Ultrasound 2008;50:50.

62. Kellman GM, Alpern MB, Sandler MA, et al. Computed tomography of vena caval anomalies with embryologic correlation. Radiographics 1988; 8(3):533–56.

63. Pretorius PM, Gleeson FV. Right-sided superior vena cava draining into left atrium in a patient with persistent left-sided superior vena cava. Radiology 2004; 232:730–4.

64. Raghib G, Ruttenberg HD, Anderson RC, et al. Termination of left superior vena cava in left atrium, atrial septal defect, and absence of coronary sinus: a developmental complex. Circulation 1965;31:906–18.

65. Bass JE, Redwine MD, Kramer LA, et al. Spectrum of congenital anomalies of the inferior vena cava: cross-sectional imaging findings. Radiographics 2000;20:639–52.

66. Frazier AA, Rosado de Christenson ML, Stocker JT, et al. Intralobar sequestration: radiologic-pathologic correlation. Radiographics 1997; 17:725–45.

67. Rosado de Christenson ML, Frazier AA, Stocker JT, et al. Extralobar sequestration: radiologic-pathologic correlation. Radiographics 1993;13:425–41.

68. Ellis K. Developmental abnormalities in the systemic blood supply to the lungs. AJR Am J Roentgenol 1991;156:669–79.

69. Ko S-F, Ng S-H, Lee T-Y, et al. Noninvasive imaging of bronchopulmonary sequestration. AJR Am J Roentgenol 2000;175:1005–12.

Multidetector Computed Tomography in the Preoperative Assessment of Cardiac Surgery Patients

Nila J. Akhtar, MD[a], Alan H. Markowitz, MD[b], Robert C. Gilkeson, MD[a,b,*]

KEYWORDS

• Multidetector CT • Preoperative • Cardiac • Surgery

Over the last 50 years, the volume of cardiac surgery has increased and associated operative morbidity and mortality has decreased secondary to advances in surgical technique, cardiopulmonary bypass, imaging, and perioperative care. There has been an increase in complex cardiac disease due to the aging population, who often present with severe coronary artery and degenerative valvular disease. These patients often require reoperative valvular surgery and coronary artery bypass grafting (CABG), and are frequently candidates for cardiac surgery. A recent study has shown that aortic valve replacement can be performed in octogenarians with acceptable surgical outcomes.[1]

Chest radiography, echocardiography (echo), and catheter angiography traditionally have been the primary modalities in the preoperative imaging evaluation of cardiac surgical patients. Improvements in multidetector computed tomography (MDCT) technology allow MDCT to play an increasing role in noninvasive cardiac imaging.[2,3] Increased numbers of detector rows with MDCT enhance the depiction of small structures such as coronary arteries with ever improving spatial resolution and anatomic coverage. Significant reduction in cardiac motion artifacts is possible with the improved temporal resolution enabled by faster gantry rotation times and the development of dual-source computed tomography (DSCT).

MDCT image acquisition yields large 3-dimensional (3D) volume datasets from which multiplanar reconstruction (MPR), maximum-intensity projection (MIP), and volume-rendered (VR) images are created using advanced computer graphics algorithms. Reconstructions can be performed in any plane as well as in any phase of the cardiac cycle if retrospective electrocardiographic (ECG) gating is used.

Whereas the MDCT source axial images are diagnostic, MPR, MIP, and VR are powerful tools that provide additional information regarding the nature and extent of disease and accurately illustrate pertinent anatomic relationships. Image postprocessing greatly aids in conveying the imaging findings to the referring surgeon. Hemminger and colleagues[4] demonstrated that surgeons benefited from real-time 3D imaging in the preoperative assessment of 23 complex cardiothoracic MDCT cases. The addition of 3D images changed the surgical plan in 65% of cases, increased the surgeon's confidence on average 40% per case, and correlated with the anatomy found at surgery in 95% of cases.

[a] Department of Radiology, University Hospitals, Case Medical Center, 11100 Euclid Avenue, Cleveland, OH 44106, USA
[b] Heart Valve Center, Harrington-McLaughlin Heart & Vascular Institute, University Hospitals, Case Medical Center, 11100 Euclid Avenue, Cleveland, OH 44106, USA
* Corresponding author.
E-mail address: robert.gilkeson@uhhospitals.org (R.C. Gilkeson).

Radiol Clin N Am 48 (2010) 117–139
doi:10.1016/j.rcl.2009.09.002
0033-8389/09/$ – see front matter © 2010 Elsevier Inc. All rights reserved.

The purpose of this article is to illustrate and discuss the importance of preoperative MDCT imaging in the preoperative evaluation of cardiac surgical patients. The questions posed by the surgeon in planning both native and reoperative surgery, and key points of the operative technique are outlined. Aortic, valvular, coronary, pericardial, and congenital heart disease requiring surgery are addressed. The imaging protocol is tailored to each patient and an imaging protocol guide is provided, which includes techniques to minimize radiation dose.

PROTOCOL

Preoperative cardiac imaging at the authors' institution is mainly performed on a dual-source MDCT scanner (Siemens SOMATOM Definition, Siemens Medical Solutions, Forchheim, Germany). One of 4 general protocols is applied to answer the surgeon's specific questions before surgery (Table 1). The key points of each protocol are briefly highlighted; however, ECG gating, contrast administration, delay time to scan, and radiation dose reduction mechanisms are discussed separately here as they are integrated into the majority of protocols.

The first protocol is assessment of the thoracic aorta (see Table 1). A major protocol consideration is the use of intravenous contrast. If the assessment is for aortic caliber or the presence and distribution of atherosclerotic plaque in the aorta and major branches, a noncontrast study is performed. The remainder of studies, including those for aneurysm, aortic dissection, and ulcerative atherosclerotic plaque, are performed with contrast. It should be noted that an initial noncontrast MDCT is included in the aortic dissection protocol for evaluation of intramural hematoma, a dissection equivalent, and dissection complicated by mediastinal hemorrhage, hemothorax, and hemorrhagic pericardial effusion. The second major protocol consideration is the use of ECG gating. If aortic pathology involves the aortic root, ascending aorta, arch, or arch vessels, ECG gating is used to minimize pulsation artifact. Finally, a right-sided arm injection is used for all contrast-enhanced aortic studies. The contrast bolus from a left arm injection can cause significant beam hardening artifact in innominate vein, which often limits evaluation of the proximal arch vessels.

The second protocol is assessment of the coronary arteries (see Table 1), which is performed to exclude significant coronary artery disease in patients with surgical noncoronary cardiac disease and a low pretest predictive value of coronary artery disease. This study is also indicated to delineate the course of anomalous coronary arteries suspected by echo or catheter angiography.

The third protocol is general cardiac evaluation (see Table 1), which is requested in patients with valvular pathology, congenital heart disease, cardiac mass, or pericardial disease. These 3D acquisitions complement findings obtained with echo and magnetic resonance (MR) imaging. When particular cardiac chamber anatomy is of clinical interest, the major protocol consideration is delay time to scan. If the clinical question involves the left-sided chambers or valves, the delay time to scan is based on opacification of the aortic root. If right-sided chambers or valves are of interest, the delay time to scan is based on opacification of the main pulmonary artery.

The fourth protocol is for assessment of coronary artery graft position and patency when reoperative cardiac surgery is considered. The major protocol consideration is the range of the scan. If there is a known or questionable left or right internal mammary artery graft (LIMA or RIMA), the image acquisition should begin more superiorly at the base of the neck to include the origins of the internal mammary arteries from the anterior subclavian arteries. If CABG history does not include LIMA or RIMA bypass grafts, image acquisition should begin at the superior level of the aortic arch to include saphenous vein grafts arising from the anterior mid ascending aorta.[5]

PROTOCOL: ECG GATING

ECG gating can be performed retrospectively or prospectively. Retrospective ECG gating acquires images throughout the cardiac cycle or R-R interval, which is usually divided into 5% or 10% phases. Each phase can be reviewed separately, and the entire dataset can be run in a cine mode for myocardial and valvular functional evaluation. Prospective ECG gating acquires images in a preselected diastolic phase of the cardiac cycle, and thus no functional evaluation can be performed. Although the 2 techniques have similar image quality, prospective ECG gating radiation dose is 77% less than that of retrospective ECG gating.[6] The decreased temporal resolution in prospective ECG-gating techniques requires heart rates less than 70 beats per minute. In addition, if there is 10% heart rate variability during preimaging monitoring, prospective ECG gating should be performed with phase padding. Phase padding widens the preselected phase by 5% to 10% on each side of the preselected phase, improving imaging flexibility in imaging the coronary arteries. However, the radiation dose reduction drops to approximately 68% when 5% phase padding is used and 56% when 10% phase padding is used.[7]

PROTOCOL: β BLOCKADE

Although it has been shown that coronary artery image quality on dual-source computed tomographic angiography (CTA) is independent of heart rate when retrospective ECG gating is used,[8] prospective ECG gating requires a heart rate less than 70 beats per minute. In the absence of contraindications, such as severe aortic stenosis and obstructive lung disease, a β-blocker is prescribed by referring clinicians to be taken by the patient the night before and on the morning of the examination, to enable heart rates of less than 70 beats per minute.

PROTOCOL: CONTRAST

Contrast-enhanced studies use nonionic, low osmolar Isovue (Isovue 370). The volume of contrast is calculated by multiplying the estimated scan length in seconds (s) by the rate of contrast injection in cubic centimeters per second (cc/s); however, this calculation will vary with different scanners. A minimum of 80 cc is used in cardiac CTA and a minimum of 100 cc is used in aortic CTA. The rate of injection is 5 cc/s for both cardiac and aortic CTA. The delay time to scan following the injection of contrast is determined by the timing bolus method. A 20-cc test bolus of contrast followed by a 40-cc saline flush is administered, and sequential images measuring peak attenuation are acquired at the same slice position through the region of interest. The delay time to scan is equal to time in seconds to maximum enhancement in the region of interest plus 5 seconds. All contrast-enhanced studies are performed with a biphasic injection of contrast followed by a 40-cc saline flush. Some physicians use a triphasic contrast injection when right cardiac chamber enhancement is of interest.[9]

PROTOCOL: RADIATION DOSE REDUCTION

The principle of "as low as reasonably achievable" (ALARA) should be followed in all imaging modalities that expose the patient to ionizing radiation, including cardiac CTA. Decreasing the voltage from the 120 to 100 kV can decrease radiation dose by approximately 46%, depending on scanner type and specific protocol.[10] Given the overall decrease in image quality with reduced voltage,[11] a body mass index (BMI; calculated as the weight in kilograms divided by height in meters squared) of less than 25 to 30 is required. Prospective ECG gating should be used when possible, as discussed earlier. Retrospective ECG-gated studies should be performed with automated exposures control (AEC), Caredose (Siemens Medical Solutions, Forchheim, Germany) and ECG-gated tube current modulation (ECGTM), Mindose (Siemens Medical Solutions, Forchheim, Germany).

PROTOCOL: RECONSTRUCTIONS

MPR, MIP, and VR are performed on a Siemens Leonardo workstation (Siemens Medical Solutions, Forchheim, Germany), Philips Extended Brilliance Workstation (Philips Medical Systems, Eindhoven, the Netherlands), and Voxar 3D Workstation (Barco Medical Systems, Brussels, Belgium). Although the number of reconstructions is essentially limitless, standard aortic reconstructions include oblique coronal MPR of the aortic root and sagittal oblique/"candy cane" MPR of the aortic arch. Standard cardiac reconstructions include 4-chamber/horizontal long axis, 2-chamber/vertical long axis, 3-chamber/left ventricular outflow tract, and short-axis views of the heart. Standard coronary reconstructions include curved and straight centerline MIP and VR reconstructions.

IMAGING CONSIDERATIONS: CHEST WALL

Preoperative imaging should address anterior vascular structures in close proximity to the inner table of the sternum, which have been shown to be at greatest risk for injury during prebypass dissection followed by sternotomy.[12] Venous structures at risk for injury include the innominate vein and right ventricle. Imaging evaluation should document the presence or absence of an intact fat plane between right ventricle and right ventricular outflow tract and the inner table of the sternum, which may be significantly decreased or obliterated because of adhesions (**Fig. 1**), right-sided chamber enlargement secondary to right heart failure, and pectus excavatum deformity. Arterial structures at risk include ascending aortic aneurysms or pseudoaneurysms, which may also be in close proximity to the sternum secondary to size. Coronary artery bypass grafts, including internal mammary artery and saphenous vein grafts, may have a retrosternal course and are at risk for injury. Coronary artery bypass grafts are discussed separately in this article. Risk is increased for increasing number of reoperations and in patients with prior chest radiation secondary to adhesions, which may immobilize vascular structures and fix them to the chest wall (**Fig. 2**A and B). Imaging allows the surgeon to plan for more difficult prebypass dissection, which

Table 1
MDCT protocols

	Thoracic Aorta		Heart		
Indication	Caliber and calcification	Dissection and aneurysm	Coronary	Valve, pericardium, congenital heart disease, or mass	Reoperative CABG
Range	Entire thorax	Entire thorax	Carina to cardiac apex	Carina to cardiac apex	Inferior neck and entire thorax
ECG gating	No	Yes	Yes	Yes	Yes
Radiation dose reduction: use prospective ECG gating	—	If heart rate <70 beats/min	If heart rate <70 beats/min and no functional assessment needed	Valvular assessment requires retrospective ECG gating	If heart rate <70 beats/min
Radiation dose reduction: if retrospective ECG gating required	—	Use EGTCM	Use EGTCM	Use EGTCM	Use EGTCM
Contrast	No	Yes	Yes	Yes	Yes
Contrast volume (cc)	—	[Estimated scan time(s) × rate of injection (cc/s)] Minimum 100 cc	[Estimated scan time(s) × rate of injection (cc/s)] Minimum 80 cc	[Estimated scan time(s) × rate of injection (cc/s)] Minimum 80 cc	[Estimated scan time(s) × rate of injection (cc/s)] Minimum 100 cc
Rate of injection of contrast	—	5 cc/s	5 cc/s	5 cc/s	5 cc/s

Contrast phasicity	—	Biphasic	Biphasic	Biphasic or triphasic	Biphasic
Determination of scan delay	—	Timing bolus on proximal descending aorta	Timing bolus on aortic root	Left: timing bolus on aortic root Right: timing bolus on main pulmonary artery	Timing bolus on proximal descending aorta
Slice thickness	2 mm	Noncontrast: 5 mm Contrast: 2 mm	0.75 mm	0.75 mm	0.75 mm
Increment	1 mm	Noncontrast: 5 mm Contrast: 1 mm	0.4 mm	0.4 mm	0.4 mm
kV	120	120	120	120	120
Radiation dose reduction: use 100 kV	If BMI <30	If BMI <30	If BMI <30	If BMI <30	If BMI <30
mA	250	500	800	800	800
Radiation dose reduction: use AEC	Yes	Yes	Yes	Yes	Yes
Filter	B25f	B25f	B25f	B25f	B25f

Abbreviations: AEC, automated exposure control; BMI, body mass index; CABG, coronary artery bypass grafting; EGTCM, ECG-gated tube current modulation.

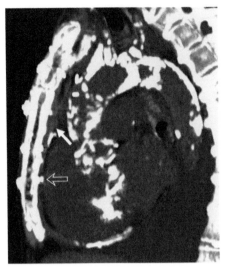

Fig. 1. A 74-year-old woman with history of critical aortic stenosis, CABG × 3, and Hodgkin lymphoma treated with radiation therapy. Noncontrast chest CT obtained before aortic valve replacement. Sagittal MPR demonstrates linear soft tissue density compatible with adhesions between the inner table of the sternal body and right ventricular outflow tract (*arrow*). A sternal wire abuts the anterior free wall of the right ventricle (*open arrow*). Note the diffuse and dense atherosclerotic calcification of the thoracic aorta.

may involve a more superior extensive initial dissection before sternotomy or the initiation of cardiopulmonary bypass before dissection or sternotomy.

IMAGING CONSIDERATIONS: INTRAOPERATIVE PERFUSION

Direct ascending aortic cannulation has been the traditional route of continuous antegrade cerebral perfusion during cardiopulmonary bypass (CPB) in cardiac surgery. Ascending aortic aneurysm and atherosclerotic disease can preclude its cannulation. The presence of atherosclerotic disease in the ascending aorta is the most important risk factor for postoperative stroke,[13] being the major cause of postoperative morbidity and mortality in cardiac surgery.[14] Atheroemboli from ascending aortic cannulation are believed to be responsible for stroke.[15] Axillary artery cannulation is now the favored alternative cannulation site, as the axillary artery rarely contains atherosclerotic plaque. Axillary artery cannulation has been shown to decrease the risk of microemboli during CPB.[16,17]

Preoperative noncontrast MDCT is the preferred imaging modality to identify calcified atherosclerotic plaque in the thoracic aorta and risk stratify patients with respect to CPB, especially "no-touch aortas" with diffuse atherosclerotic disease requiring axillary artery cannulation (see **Fig. 1**).[18] CPB via axillary artery cannulation is achieved by clamping the base of the innominate artery with antegrade cerebral perfusion via the right common carotid artery. Perfusion of the contralateral cerebral hemisphere relies on an intact circle of Willis. Arch anomalies are easily identified on MDCT. Favorable variant arch anatomy for axillary cannulation is a common origin of the innominate artery and left common carotid artery, which results

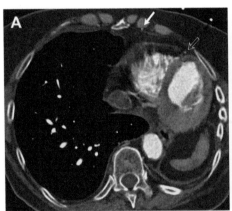
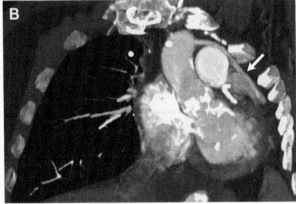

Fig. 2. (*A, B*) A 70-year-old woman presented with unstable angina, history of CABG × 2, severe aortic stenosis, and lung cancer treated with left pneumonectomy and radiation therapy. Cardiac catheterization demonstrated 2 tandem high-grade stenoses in the left anterior descending artery. Retrospective ECG-gated CT obtained before reoperative CABG. (*A*) Axial image shows significant leftward mediastinal shift and increased distance between the proposed left internal mammary artery bypass graft (*arrow*) and the distal left anterior descending artery (LAD) (*open arrow*). (*B*) Coronal oblique slab-MIP shows leftward mediastinal shift and saphenous vein graft (*arrow*) abutting the chest wall likely due to adhesions. Due to extensive postsurgical and postradiation changes, reoperative CABG and aortic valve replacement were not technically feasible. Medical management was elected.

antegrade cerebral perfusion via bilateral common carotid artery flow (**Fig. 3**A and B). MDCT evaluation should also identify important contraindications to right axillary cannulation. Important congenital variants to identify are a left-sided aortic arch with an aberrant right subclavian artery (**Fig. 4**A and B) and a right-sided aortic arch. If right axillary artery cannulation is performed in the presence of an aberrant right subclavian, the cerebral circulation is bypassed with perfusion of only the descending thoracic aorta. In the setting of a right-sided aortic arch, the separate origins of the right subclavian artery and right carotid common carotid artery preclude cerebral perfusion via right axillary cannulation. The second contraindication is flow-limiting atherosclerotic disease in the innominate, right axillary, or subclavian arteries (**Fig. 5**A and B).

IMAGING CONSIDERATIONS: AORTA

Preoperative imaging of the thoracic aorta is most frequently performed with MDCT due to its widespread availability, speed, high spatial resolution, and relatively motion-free assessment of the proximal aorta with ECG gating. An accurate description of the extent of aortic disease and measurements are needed by the surgeon for aortic repair, which involves resection of the diseased aorta followed by synthetic graft replacement. Image postprocessing with MPR, MIP, and VR aids in conveying these findings to the surgeon.[19] When ECG gating is used, information regarding cardiac structures, including the aortic valve and coronary arteries, can be obtained concurrently.

The advantages of preoperative MDCT imaging are best exemplified by evaluation of a Stanford type A aortic dissection, which warrants immediate surgical management when patients present acutely. MDCT is the modality of choice for evaluation of aortic dissection because it has a sensitivity and specificity of 100% for the detection of aortic dissection, and is superior to both transesophageal echocardiography and MR imaging for arch vessel involvement.[20] MDCT evaluation of aortic dissection should include the proximal and distal extent of the intimal flap, presence of extension into aortic branch vessels and coronary arteries, presence of intimal flap fenestrations, and size and patency of the true and false lumens (**Fig. 6**A–C).

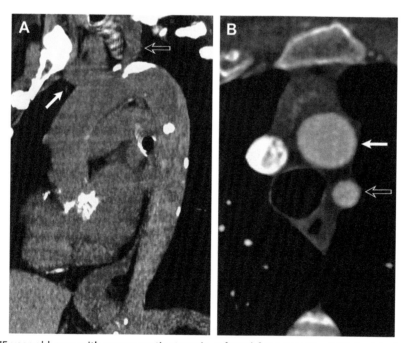

Fig. 3. (*A*) A 75-year-old man with severe aortic stenosis, referred for noncontrast CT chest before aortic valve replacement. Sagittal slab image demonstrates a common origin of the right innominate artery and left common carotid artery (*arrow*). Left subclavian artery (*open arrow*) arises separately from the aortic arch. (*B*) A 75-year-old woman with mixed stenosis and regurgitation of the aortic and mitral valves secondary to rheumatic heart disease, referred for cardiac CT before mitral and aortic valve replacement for more detailed valvular assessment. Axial CT image demonstrates a common origin of the right innominate artery and left common carotid artery (*arrow*). Left subclavian artery (*open arrow*) arises separately from the aortic arch.

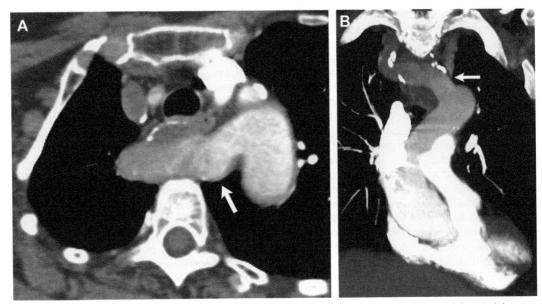

Fig. 4. (A, B) An 83-year-old woman with hypoxia. Axial MIP CT (A) and coronal oblique slab-MIP (B) images demonstrate an aneurysmal and aberrant right subclavian artery (arrows), which courses posterior to the trachea and esophagus.

Thoracic aortic aneurysm is the most common indication for aortic surgery, and therefore a frequent indication for preoperative MDCT imaging. Surgical replacement is generally performed when the caliber is greater than or equal to 5 cm. The authors routinely include a standardized report of thoracic aortic caliber, which includes the aortic root, sinotubular junction, mid ascending aorta, arch, and mid descending aorta. More accurate aortic caliber measurements are

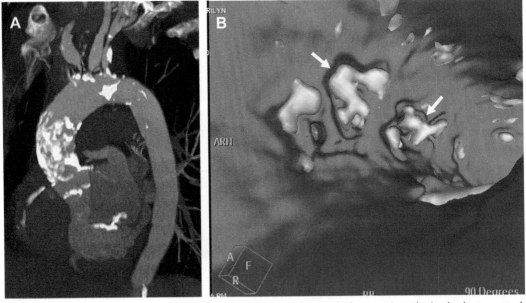

Fig. 5. (A, B) A 79-year-old woman referred for preoperative evaluation before aortic and mitral valve surgery. (A) Sagittal oblique volume rendered images demonstrate extensive atherosclerotic disease of the aortic arch and arch vessels. Note significant narrowing of the proximal arch vessels. (B) Virtual endoscopic image of the aortic arch demonstrates extensive calcified plaque obstructing the origins of the left carotid and left subclavian arteries (arrows).

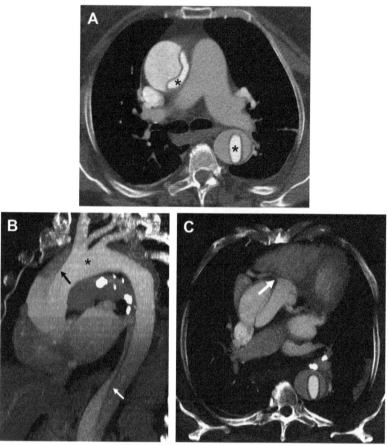

Fig. 6. (A–C) A 66-year-old woman with history of hypertension presented with acute chest pain, and was referred for CT for evaluation of aortic dissection. (A) Axial CT image demonstrates type A dissection and delineates the true lumen (*asterisks*), which is compressed and more brightly enhanced than the laterally displaced false lumen. (B) Sagittal oblique slab MIP view shows the type A aortic dissection flap (*arrows*) extending from the aortic root to the visualized superior abdominal aorta. (C) Sagittal oblique MIP demonstrates dissection flap (*arrow*) extending to the origin of the right coronary artery.

achieved with the use of MPR, which is most useful for the proximal aorta (Fig. 7). The type, location, maximal dimension of the aneurysm, and the relationship of the branch vessels to the aneurysm should be given.

Special surgical considerations include connective tissue disease, and the presence or absence of coexisting aortic valvular disease. The threshold for aortic repair often decreases to greater than or equal to 4 cm in patients with connective tissue disorders, such as Marfan or Loeys-Dietz syndrome.[21] If there is coexisting aortic valvular disease, patients with aneurysmal dilatation of the aortic root and ascending aorta will undergo composite aortic valve-graft replacement (Fig. 8). If the aortic valve is competent, valve-sparing root replacement is performed, which involves telescoping the graft over the aortic annulus and subcentimeter residual rim of aortic root,

resuspension of the aortic valvular commissures within the graft, and coronary artery reimplantation.[21]

The high sensitivity of MDCT for the presence and distribution of aortic atherosclerotic calcification is essential when coronary reimplantation or complex aortic arch repair is planned. The Bentall button procedure is the technique of choice for coronary artery reimplantation.[22] The Bentall button procedure involves dissection of the coronary artery ostia along with a cuff of native adjacent aorta. The Bentall button procedure is feasible when there is ample atherosclerotic disease-free aortic tissue adjacent to the coronary artery ostia. At the authors' institution the surgeon requires at least 2 mm of disease-free aortic tissue adjacent to the coronary ostia. Knowledge of the density and distribution of atherosclerotic calcification of the arch vessels is also needed by the

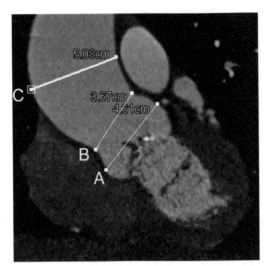

Fig. 7. A 69-year-old man with bicuspid aortic valve and worsening aortic stenosis and aneurysmal dilatation of the ascending aorta. Coronary CT obtained for coronary clearance before aortic valve replacement. Coronal oblique slab MIP of the proximal thoracic aorta demonstrates standard measurements of the aortic root (A), sinotubular junction (B), and mid ascending aorta (C). Patient underwent successful aortic valve replacement, aortic root replacement with reimplantation of the coronary arteries, and ascending aorta and hemiarch replacement.

surgeon to plan graft repair of the aortic arch (see Fig. 6).

IMAGING CONSIDERATIONS: CARDIAC VALVES

Echo is the gold standard imaging modality for the assessment of cardiac valves. The advantages of echo include its widespread availability, real-time image acquisition, lack of ionizing radiation, and ability to provide transvalvular peak velocity and pressure gradients. The disadvantages of echo are operator dependence, poor acoustic windows, and low spatial resolution.

Cardiac MR imaging routinely provides useful information regarding cardiac valve morphology and function, which complements echo. MR imaging has adequate spatial and temporal resolution, can acquire transvalvular peak velocity and pressure gradients with phase contrast imaging, and does not require contrast because of the inherent T2 weighting of blood on steady-state free precession (SSFP) cine images. However, MR imaging is not widely available, is time consuming and costly, and is contraindicated in patients with indwelling devices such as pacemakers.

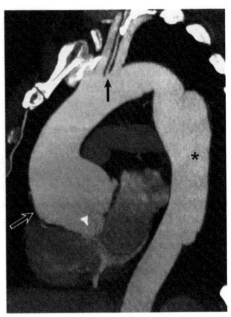

Fig. 8. An 80-year-old man with severe aortic regurgitation and enlarging aortic root aneurysm. Coronary CT obtained for coronary clearance before aortic valve replacement and evaluation of aortic arch anatomy. Sagittal oblique slab MIP of the thoracic aorta demonstrates an aortic root aneurysm measuring 8 cm in greatest dimension (open arrow), localized type B aortic dissection (asterisk) extending 10 cm in craniocaudal dimension, and a direct origin of the left vertebral artery (arrow). There was normal coronary artery anatomy and no significant coronary artery stenosis (not shown). Patient underwent successful aortic valve replacement and aortic root replacement, with reimplantation of the coronary arteries. Recognition of the direct origin of the vertebral artery was important in the planning of ascending aorta and hemiarch replacement.

There is a growing body of literature supporting the role of MDCT in cardiac valvular imaging due to the rapid advancement in MDCT technology that meets or approximates the requirements of high temporal and spatial resolution.[23–29] MDCT offers superior spatial resolution of 0.4 to 0.6 mm which, coupled with intravenous contrast, allows excellent visualization of the valvular apparatus, including the annulus, valve leaflets, chordae tendinae, and papillary muscles (Fig. 9).[24] Retrospective ECG gated cine images allow functional valvular assessment of leaflet excursion and coaptation (Fig. 10).[25] Mitral regurgitation is the most common valvular disease. The most common cause of mitral regurgitation is congenital mitral valve prolapse (Fig. 11). The key findings of mitral valve prolapse are lengthening and rupture of the chordae tendinae with

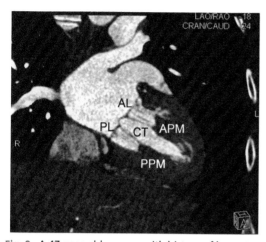

Fig. 9. A 47-year-old woman with history of hypertension presenting with recurrent atypical chest pain, and normal echo and nuclear stress test, referred for coronary CTA to exclude coronary artery disease, which was negative. The components of the mitral valve are well delineated on vertical long axis image of the heart. The mitral valve is composed of the annulus, which is located in the atrioventricular groove and serves as the insertion site for the anterior valve leaflet (AL) and posterior valve leaflet (PL). The anterolateral (APM) and posteromedial (PPM) papillary muscles arise from the lateral wall of the left ventricle, and provide chordae tendinae (CT) to each leaflet, which are responsible for end-systolic positioning of the leaflets.

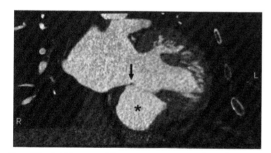

Fig. 10. A 77-year-old-woman presented with syncopal episode, and was found to have ST-elevation myocardial infarction. Urgent cardiac catheterization revealed 100% occluded right coronary artery, high-grade circumflex artery stenosis, and left ventricular inferior wall aneurysm. Patient referred for cardiac CT evaluation of left ventricular aneurysm morphology before Dorr repair and coronary artery bypass grafting. Vertical long-axis view of the heart clearly depicts a large, broad-based basal posterolateral wall aneurysm (*asterisk*), which spares the posterior mitral valve leaflet (*arrow*), chordae tendinae, and posteromedial papillary muscle. There was normal mitral valvular function on cine images (not shown).

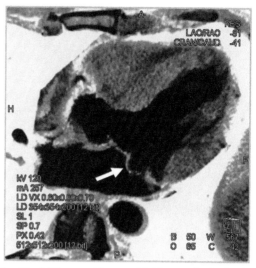

Fig. 11. A 50-year-old man with history of mitral valve prolapse and severe mitral regurgitation complained of progressive exertional dyspnea. Coronary CT obtained for coronary clearance before mitral valve repair. Four-chamber reverse-ramp view shows thickening and prolapse of the mitral valve leaflets (*arrow*). There was normal coronary artery anatomy and no significant coronary artery stenosis (not shown).

more frequent rupture of the chordae to the posterior leaflets. Acquired causes include infective endocarditis (**Fig. 12**), myocardial infarction, and annular dilatation secondary to left ventricular dilatation. MDCT can assess for annular calcification, leaflet thickening, thickened chordae, leaflet prolapse, and incomplete leaflet apposition and excursion.[27] Secondary signs of mitral regurgitation include left atrial and ventricular enlargement and right heart dilatation in long-standing cases.

However, whereas the temporal resolution of MDCT has improved to 83 milliseconds with DSCT and 83 to 250 milliseconds on MDCT depending on scanner type and reconstruction method, echo has superior temporal resolution of approximately 50 milliseconds.[24] Other disadvantages of MDCT are the inability to determine peak velocity and pressure gradient, ionizing radiation, and contrast.

The most common valvular pathology encountered on preoperative MDCT at the authors' institution is aortic stenosis (AS); the most common valvular disease treated with valve replacement. Patients are referred for noncontrast MDCT for CPB planning and coronary CTA for preoperative coronary clearance before aortic valve replacement. Surgical indications for aortic valvular replacement are dependent on the severity of

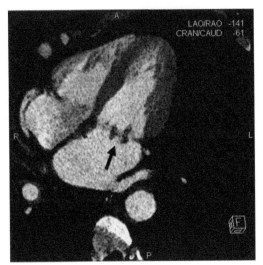

Fig. 12. A 61-year-old man with no significant medical history presented with fever, cough, and mental status changes. Echo shows a vegetation on the anterior leaflet of the mitral valve, which was perforated with severe mitral regurgitation. Patient ultimately diagnosed with Austrian syndrome, *Streptococcus pneumoniae* endocarditis, meningitis, and pneumonia. Coronary CT for coronary clearance before mitral valve replacement complements echo findings of nodular vegetations of the mitral valve (*arrow*).

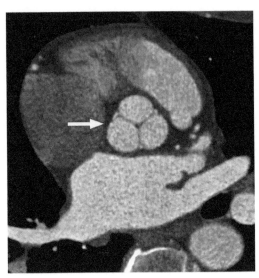

Fig. 13. A 54-year-old asymptomatic man with equivocal stress echo and family history of coronary artery disease, referred for coronary CT to exclude significant coronary artery disease. There was normal coronary artery anatomy and no significant coronary artery stenosis (not shown). Short-axis MPR of the aortic valve in diastole illustrates a normal tricuspid aortic valve (*arrow*).

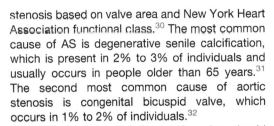

stenosis based on valve area and New York Heart Association functional class.[30] The most common cause of AS is degenerative senile calcification, which is present in 2% to 3% of individuals and usually occurs in people older than 65 years.[31] The second most common cause of aortic stenosis is congenital bicuspid valve, which occurs in 1% to 2% of individuals.[32]

MDCT evaluation of the aortic valve should include the number of leaflets, and identification of morphologic abnormalities such as leaflet thickening and calcification. The normal aortic valve is tricuspid, with uniform and thin valve leaflets that coapt completely in diastole (Fig. 13). The left and right cusps are most commonly fused in congenital bicuspid aortic valve (Fig. 14). MDCT findings of AS are leaflet thickening, valvular calcification, decreased valvular excursion, left ventricular hypertrophy, and poststenotic dilatation of the aortic root and ascending aorta. MDCT is the best imaging modality to assess aortic valve calcification,[33–37] and the degree of aortic valvular calcification is the greatest independent risk factor for disease progression and adverse clinical outcome.[38] Whereas calcification is usually scattered on the commissures and annulus of a bicuspid aortic valve (Fig. 15), calcification in acquired degenerative AS is greater and

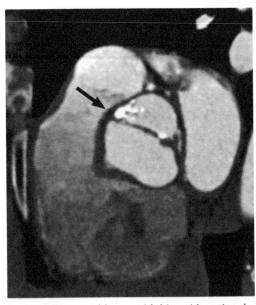

Fig. 14. A 69-year-old man with bicuspid aortic valve, and worsening aortic stenosis and aneurysmal dilatation of the ascending aorta. Coronary CT obtained for coronary clearance before aortic valve replacement. Diastolic aortic valve short-axis MPR clearly shows the bicuspid aortic valve with fusion of the left and right leaflets, and leaflet thickening and calcification (*arrow*). There was normal coronary artery anatomy and no significant coronary artery stenosis (not shown).

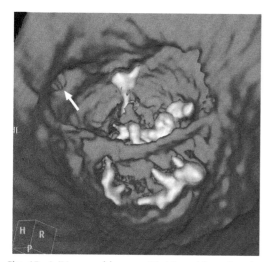

Fig. 15. A 74-year-old man with bicuspid aortic valve and progressive aortic stenosis, referred for coronary CT for coronary clearance before aortic valve replacement. Endoluminal view of the aortic valve demonstrates fusion of the left and right cusps, and diffuse valvular calcification of the aortic valve. Note relationship of the right coronary artery ostium (*arrow*). There was normal coronary artery anatomy and no significant coronary artery stenosis (not shown).

predominantly located on the valve leaflets. Quantification of aortic valvular calcification by electron beam CT and MDCT has been reported, and the severity of calcification correlates with increased pressure gradients on echo.[39,40] MDCT planimetry

can also assess maximal leaflet excursion in systole and estimate aortic valve area.[41]

Another congenital cause of aortic valve disease is quadricuspid aortic valve, which most commonly causes aortic insufficiency that may require aortic valve replacement (**Fig. 16**A and B). Quadricuspid aortic valve is very rare, with prevalence between 0.008% and 0.033%.[42,43] The primary diagnosis of quadricuspid aortic valve on MDCT has been reported, and requires an accurate short-axis MPR view of the aortic valve to assess the number or aortic valve leaflets.[44] An off-axis view of a normal tricuspid valve can make the left ventricular outflow tract appear as a false fourth cusp.[44] Coronary artery anomalies are the most frequently associated cardiac congenital anomaly with quadricuspid aortic valve, and should be excluded on preoperative cardiac MDCT to avoid coronary injury during aortic valve replacement.[45]

The normal tricuspid right-sided heart valves are not usually visualized on conventional MDCT. Abnormal tricuspid and pulmonic leaflet thickening can be detected on MDCT in disease states such as carcinoid heart disease. Carcinoid heart disease occurs in 50% of patients with hepatic metastases secondary to vasoactive substances released by tumor that reach and predominantly affect the right side of the heart.[46] Tricuspid regurgitation and pulmonic regurgitation or stenosis with right atrial and ventricular dilatation are most characteristic (**Fig. 17**A). Left-sided valvular involvement occurs in less than 10% of patients,

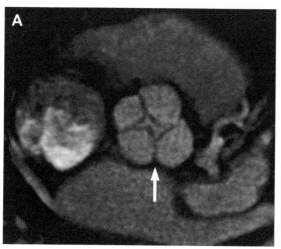

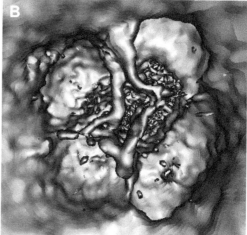

Fig. 16. (*A, B*) A 43-year-old woman with history of abnormal heart murmur since childhood, hypertension, and asthma presented with progressive exertional dyspnea and orthopnea. Severe aortic regurgitation and dilated aortic root were discovered on echo. Patient was referred for aortic valve replacement. Preoperative cardiac CT requested for more detailed aortic valve assessment. Diastolic aortic valve short-axis MPR (*A*) and endoluminal view (*B*) clearly depict a quadricuspid aortic valve (*arrow*) with incomplete coaptation of the valve leaflets, compatible with aortic insufficiency. There was normal coronary artery anatomy and no significant coronary artery stenosis (not shown).

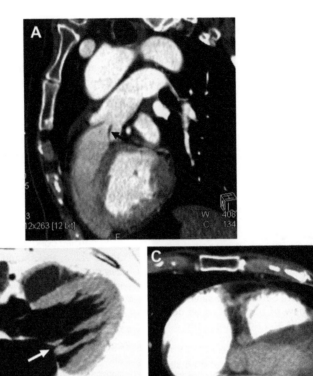

Fig. 17. A 59-year-old woman with metastatic carcinoid tumor presented with progressive shortness for breath. Echo demonstrated carcinoid heart disease involving all 4 heart valves secondary to patent foramen ovale with right-to-left shunting. (*A*) Sagittal image of the pulmonic valve demonstrates marked thickening of the valve leaflets (*arrow*). (*B*) Four-chamber reverse-ramp view demonstrates extensive thickening of the mitral valve and chordal attachments (*arrow*). (*C*) Four-chamber view demonstrates aneurysm of the fossa ovalis (*arrow*). Patent foramen ovale aneurysm was surgically resected during valve replacement.

and is usually associated with a patent foramen ovale (PFO) (**Fig. 17**C).[47]

IMAGING CONSIDERATIONS: CORONARY ARTERIES

Coronary artery disease is the leading cause of mortality in the United States.[48] Conventional coronary catheter angiography is the gold standard for the diagnosis of coronary artery disease. Although the major benefit of conventional coronary catheter angiography is the ability to perform procedures such as balloon angioplasty and coronary stent placement, most procedures are diagnostic for the detection and determination of the degree of coronary artery disease.

Coronary CTA is an evolving noninvasive imaging modality for direct visualization of the coronary arteries due to advances in ECG gating, improved spatial and temporal resolution, and image reconstruction techniques. In a meta-analysis comparing 16-slice and 64-slice coronary CTA with coronary catheter angiography, the per-patient analysis yielded excellent negative predictive value of 92% for 16-slice CTA and 96% for 64-slice CTA. The positive predictive value was lower, 79% for 16-slice CTA and 93% for 64-slice CTA, indicating that CTA can overestimate the degree of stenosis because of lower special resolution compared with coronary catheter angiography.[49] Image quality with 16- and 64-slice coronary CTA is also degraded by high heart rate and irregularity, as well as calcification. Newer dual-source coronary CTA has heart rate–independent image quality, with NPV 100% and PPV 93.6% by patient; however, image quality

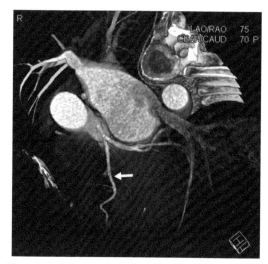

Fig. 18. A 54-year-old man with progressive mitral regurgitation, left ventricular enlargement, and declining ejection fraction. Coronary CT requested before mitral valve repair for coronary clearance. VR images demonstrate normal coronary artery anatomy without coronary artery stenosis (*arrow*).

exclusion of coronary artery disease in these patients (**Fig. 18**). In many patients imaged for this purpose, there is simultaneous evaluation of the primary surgical noncoronary artery disease.

Coronary artery anomalies are rare, occurring in 0.3% to 5.6% of the population, and are frequently an incidental finding in asymptomatic patients.[50] Life-threatening presentations include arrhythmia, myocardial infarction, and sudden death, and can occur in approximately 20% of patients.[51] Coronary arteries are divided into malignant and benign types. The malignant type occurs when the left main, left anterior descending, or right coronary artery arises from the opposite coronary sinus, and has an interarterial course between the aortic root and right ventricular outflow tract/pulmonary artery. Malignant coronary anomalies are most often associated with an adverse outcome, and are an indication for surgical correction. Coronary artery bypass is most frequently performed in adult patients (**Fig. 19**A and B). Benign types of coronary artery anomalies include those with a retroaortic or prepulmonic course. A common benign anomalous coronary artery is origin of the left circumflex artery from the right sinus of Valsalva or right coronary artery with a retroaortic course to the left atrioventricular groove, which can be injured by sutures or prosthetic ring during aortic or mitral surgery if the surgeon is unaware of the anomalous course. Knowledge of this anomalous artery allows the surgeon to prevent injury by first

remains prone to heart rate variability and calcification.[8] Given the high negative predictive value of coronary CTA, the use of coronary CTA for the exclusion of significant coronary artery disease in patients undergoing noncoronary cardiac surgery provides a noninvasive alternative for the

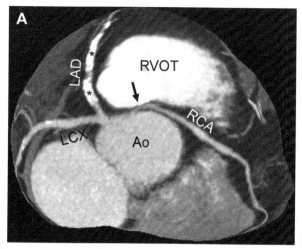
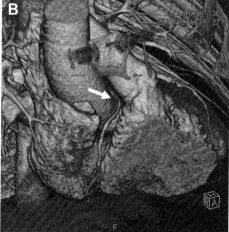

Fig. 19. A 78-year-old man with history of coronary artery disease and 2 LAD stents presented with unstable angina. Cardiac catheterization documented an anomalous origin of the right coronary artery (RCA) from the left coronary cusp. Coronary CT was recommended to preoperatively define the course of the anomalous RCA. (A) Coronary CT slab MIP globe reconstruction confirms an anomalous RCA origin from the left coronary sinus, which is separate from the left main coronary origin, and has interarterial course between the aorta (Ao) and right ventricular outflow tract (RVOT). A short segment of the RCA interarterial course is intramural within the anterior aortic wall (*arrow*). (B) VR images redemonstrate the interarterial course of the anomalous RCA (*arrow*). Patient underwent successful single CABG with a saphenous vein graft to the RCA.

dissecting the artery away from the valve during surgery.[52]

In the past, coronary artery anomalies were identified primarily by catheter angiography and autopsy. The limitation of catheter angiography is difficulty in determining the course of anomalous coronaries on a 2-dimensional view. Whereas the proximal course of anomalous coronaries may be assessed by echo and MR imaging, coronary CTA has become the imaging modality of choice to define the course of a coronary anomaly.[53] CT evaluation of the coronary arteries should be a systematic review of the ostia, course, and termination on the source axial images. MIP and VR images are useful in evaluating the ostia and course. Endoluminal views may be used to further assess the ostia.[54]

IMAGING CONSIDERATIONS: CORONARY ARTERY BYPASS GRAFTS

Catheter angiography traditionally has been the modality of choice for the evaluation of coronary artery bypass grafts in symptomatic patients after CABG and in reoperative cardiac surgical planning. Improvements in the temporal and spatial resolution of MDCT coupled with ECG-gated imaging support its use in defining graft anatomy and evaluating graft patency, especially in cases where catheter angiography fails to access bypass grafts.

Coronary artery bypass grafts include both left and right internal mammary artery grafts and saphenous vein grafts. The LIMA graft and, less frequently, the RIMA graft are primarily used to revascularize the left anterior descending artery (LAD). LIMA and RIMA grafts have better long-term, 10-year patency rates of 85% to 90% compared with saphenous vein grafts.[55] Internal mammary artery grafts course inferiorly and anteriorly from their origin in the anterior subclavian artery to their distal anastomosis with the LAD. Whereas care is taken to prevent the LIMA from becoming adherent to the posterior sternal table by routing it through a left pericardial slit,[56] the course of the RIMA graft to the left coronary distribution is always retrosternal, which is at risk for injury during reoperation. Saphenous vein grafts are used for the right coronary artery distribution as well as the left coronary artery distribution, including diagonal and obtuse marginal arteries. Saphenous vein grafts have an end-to-side proximal anastomosis from the anterior aspect of the ascending aorta, and have a variable course depending on the coronary distribution they supply.

CTA evaluation of coronary artery bypass grafts should include the number, type, course, and patency of grafts used by the surgeon. The evaluation of bypass graft course and patency is first reviewed on axial images and is aided by associated surgical clips, which are readily identified on MDCT. Multiplanar MIP and VR images accurately demonstrate the relationship between these grafts and the chest wall (Fig. 20A and B).[5] It is crucial that grafts that closely appose the inner table of the sternum or cross midline be documented (Fig. 21). Medially displaced LIMA grafts secondary to adhesions, RIMA grafts crossing midline, which may be adherent to the chest wall secondary to adhesions (Fig. 22A and B), and saphenous vein grafts anteriorly displaced or adherent to the chest wall secondary to adhesions (Fig. 23A and B) are at risk for injury during reoperative cardiac surgery. Gillinov and colleagues[56] reported a 5.3% frequency of internal mammary artery injury during reoperation and an associated mortality of 9% to 50%. Roselli and colleagues[12] reported a reduced frequency of internal mammary artery injury during reoperation of 3% with preoperative imaging, and recommended preoperative MDCT or MR imaging with 3D reconstructions optimized by contrast and ECG gating for evaluation of coronary artery grafts.

IMAGING CONSIDERATIONS: CONGENITAL HEART DISEASE

Although echocardiography is the primary imaging modality used both preoperatively and postoperatively in patients with congenital heart disease, cross-sectional imaging with MDCT and MR imaging is often obtained for complementary information. It is also important to note that undiagnosed adult congenital heart disease is not infrequently diagnosed by MDCT in symptomatic and asymptomatic adult patients obtained for unrelated reasons. Both MDCT and MR imaging offer a greater field of view to assess cardiovascular structures, such as the thoracic aorta and pulmonary vasculature. The greatest strengths of MR imaging are the ability to provide physiologic information, such as pulmonary to systemic perfusion ratio in patients with shunts and lack of ionizing radiation, whereas MDCT heralds superior spatial resolution, speed, and simultaneous evaluation of the extracardiac structures. MDCT provides primarily morphologic information on cardiac anatomy, but can also provide some functional information regarding wall motion and valvular function when retrospective ECG gating is used. MDCT imaging also provides simultaneous evaluation of related coronary artery anomalies and

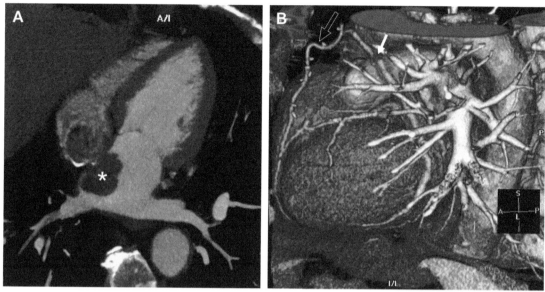

Fig. 20. A 76-year-old man with history of redo CABG × 3. A left atrial mass was seen on follow-up echo and surgical excision advised. Preoperative assessment included coronary catheterization and cardiac CT, which were concordant. (*A*) Horizontal long-axis MPR image of the heart delineates heterogeneous enhancement of a hypodense, lobulated, soft tissue mass (*asterisk*) at the level of the fossa ovalis. (*B*) VR image demonstrates significant stenosis in a saphenous vein graft to the left circumflex distribution (*arrow*) and patent LIMA graft to the LAD (*open arrow*). Patient underwent successful atrial myxoma resection and redo CABG, including a sequential radial artery graft to the second and third obtuse marginal arteries.

possible coexisting coronary artery disease in adult patients before surgery. Here, 2 case examples of congenital heart disease encountered on MDCT before surgical repair are discussed.

The most common congenital cardiac defect to present in adults is atrial septal defect (ASD).[57] There are 3 subtypes. Ostium secundum ASD is the most common, and is located in the superior septum bordered by the fossa ovalis. The ostium primum ASD is located in the inferior septum, and is associated with atrioventricular canal defects. The sinus venosus ASD, which is located in the posterior and superior septum near the superior vena cava (SVC), is associated with partial anomalous pulmonary venous return (PAPVR). Surgical repair of ASD or preferred percutaneous closure of qualifying isolated secundum subtype should be offered at any age in adults unless the ASD associated with significant pulmonary vascular disease.[58] In patients with an unrepaired sinus venosus ASD, pulmonary hypertension occurs 3 times more often and at an earlier age in comparison with patients with secundum ASD.[59] In addition, the surgical repair of a sinus venosus ASD in adults is associated with increased risk of late mortality, adverse cardiac events, and worse functional outcome when performed at an older age.[60]

MDCT findings in ASD include a defect in the interatrial septum best visualized on horizontal long-axis view of the heart (**Fig. 24**A). Important secondary findings include right-sided chamber

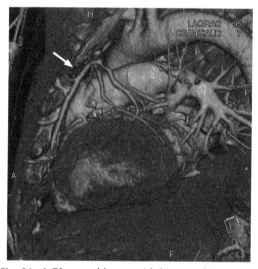

Fig. 21. A 70-year-old man with history of CABG × 5 presented with chest pain. CT aortic dissection protocol obtained and negative for aortic dissection. Sagittal reconstruction demonstrates close apposition of the saphenous vein graft to the inner table of the sternum.

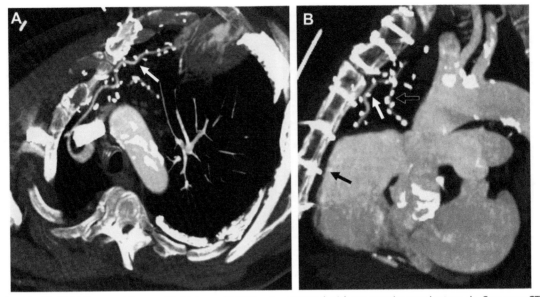

Fig. 22. (*A, B*) A 72-year-old man with history of CABG × 4 presented with progressive aortic stenosis. Coronary CT and coronary catheterization of the bypass grafts were performed before aortic valve replacement, which were concordant and did not reveal disease requiring redo CABG. Axial MIP (*A*) images show important anatomic relationships in preoperative planning. A patent RIMA graft (*white arrow*) is in very close proximity to the inner table of the sternum as it crosses midline to anastomose with the LAD. Sagittal slab MIP (*B*) demonstrates a patent LIMA graft (*open white arrow*), well separated from the sternum and terminating in the circumflex distribution. Also note the close apposition of the right ventricular free wall and RVOT to the inner table of the sternum and sternal wires (*black arrow*).

enlargement and right ventricular hypertrophy. When a sinus venosus ASD is identified or suspected, an imaging study for associated anomalous pulmonary venous anatomy is indicated. In

a recent large retrospective review of PAPVR diagnosed by contrast-enhanced MDCT of the chest, left upper lobe PAPVR was most common, followed by right upper lobe PAPVR.[61] In the

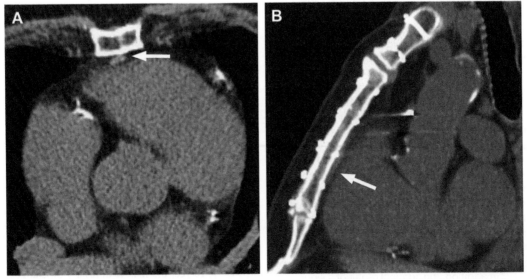

Fig. 23. (*A, B*) An 80-year-old man with history CABG × 2 presented with left arm pain, shortness of breath, and diaphoresis. Coronary catheterization revealed occlusion of the RCA and 80% stenosis of the saphenous vein graft to the LAD. Noncontrast CT chest was requested before redo CABG. Axial (*A*) and axial oblique MPR (*B*) images demonstrate adherence of a saphenous vein graft to the inner table of the sternum, and loss of the fat plane between the right ventricle and RVOT and the posterior aspect of the saphenous vein graft (*arrow*).

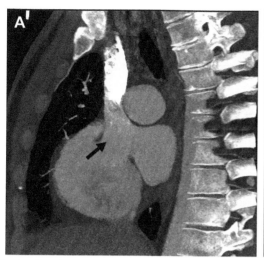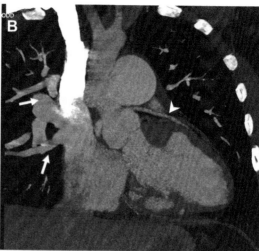

Fig. 24. (*A, B*) A 38-year-old asymptomatic man underwent echo after right bundle branch block discovered on routine physical ECG. Echo revealed dilated right atrium and right ventricle with mild right ventricular dysfunction. Sagittal oblique MPR from coronary CT obtained for preoperative coronary clearance clearly shows the relationship of the superior vena cava to the large sinus venosus ASD (*black arrow*) (*A*). Coronal oblique MPR (*B*) demonstrates anomalous right upper lobe and middle lobe pulmonary vein (*white arrows*) draining to the SVC. There was normal coronary artery anatomy and no significant coronary artery stenosis (*arrowhead*).

same study, right upper lobe PAPVR was associated with sinus venosus ASD in 42% of cases.[61] Although an anomalous pulmonary vein can be detected on echo, MDCT and MR imaging are commonly performed at the authors' institution (**Fig. 24B**).

A rare but surgically correctable congenital abnormality of the left atrium is cor triatriatum sinister. Cor triatriatum sinister is a fibromuscular membrane dividing the left atrium into a posterior chamber, which receives pulmonary venous drainage, and an anterior chamber, which gives rise to the left atrial appendage and mitral valve. Although the abnormality may be asymptomatic and discovered incidentally, patients may present with pulmonary venous hypertension that mimics mitral stenosis secondary to a gradient across the membrane.[62] A similar abnormality can occur in the right atrium and is called cor triatriatum dextra. Treatment of cor triatriatum is surgical resection.

Cor triatriatum sinister and dextra are best diagnosed on ECG-gated cardiac MDCT (**Fig. 25**).[63] The membrane is of variable size with variable fenestration. MPR is helpful in visualizing the membrane attachment sites. The vertical long-axis view is the best to visualize the attachment between the pulmonary vein ostium and left atrial appendage.

IMAGING CONSIDERATIONS: PERICARDIUM

The initial assessment of pericardial disease, most commonly pericardial effusion, is generally

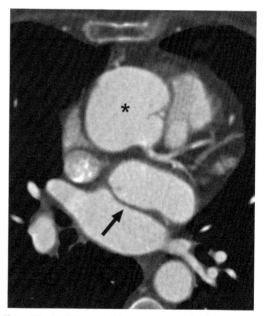

Fig. 25. A 50-year-old woman with history of membranous ventricular septal defect repair during childhood presented with cough and dyspnea. Preoperative cardiac CT requested, given history of congenital heart disease. Axial contrast CT image shows noncoronary sinus of Valsalva aneurysm (*asterisk*). A left atrial membrane compatible with cor triatriatum sinister (*arrow*) is identified. There was normal coronary artery anatomy and no significant coronary artery stenosis (not shown). Patient underwent successful aortic valve replacement as well as cor triatriatum membrane resection.

performed with echocardiography. Advantages of imaging the pericardium with MDCT or MR imaging include a larger field of view allowing visualization of the entire pericardium and extracardiac structures, better detection of pericardial thickening and loculated effusions, superior soft tissue contrast especially with MR imaging, and accurate localization of pericardial masses.[64] Advantages of MDCT over other imaging modalities include excellent detection of pericardial calcification and multiplanar reconstruction. The disadvantages of MDCT again include ionizing radiation and the administration of contrast.

MDCT is an excellent tool for the evaluation of constrictive pericarditis. Causes of pericarditis include cardiac surgery, radiation therapy, myocardial infarction, trauma, infection, collagen vascular disease, and uremia. The MDCT features of constrictive pericarditis include pericardial effusion, thickening and calcification of the pericardium, and pericardial enhancement. The most common cause of constrictive pericarditis in the United States is as a consequence of cardiac surgery and radiation therapy.[65] Constrictive pericarditis can mimic restrictive cardiomyopathy clinically. The diagnosis of constrictive pericarditis is important, as it is an indication for surgical pericardial decortication.

The MDCT findings suggestive of constrictive pericarditis are pericardial thickness greater than or equal to 4 mm, pericardial calcification, and secondary signs of constrictive physiology (**Figs. 26** and **27**).[66,67] Secondary signs include biatrial enlargement, tubular ventricular configuration, and leftward bowing of the interventricular

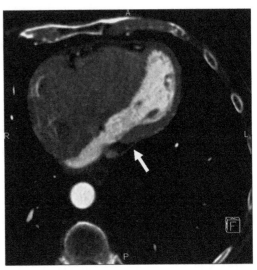

Fig. 27. A 69-year-old man with history of ankylosing spondylitis presented with dyspnea and persistent lower extremity edema. Cardiac catheterization revealed right ventricular pressure tracing, characteristic of constrictive physiology. Four-chamber view demonstrates marked limitation of diastolic relaxation of the ventricles due to constrictive pericardial band (*arrow*). Patient underwent successful pericardial decortication.

septum. Additional secondary findings include pleural effusions, enlargement of the inferior vena cava (IVC) and hepatic veins, reflux of contrast into the IVC and hepatic veins on contrast studies,

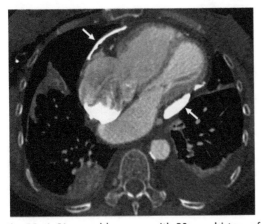

Fig. 26. A 61-year-old woman with 30-year history of constrictive pericarditis presented with respiratory failure. Preoperative cardiac CT obtained for evaluation of the pericardium. Axial image shows extensive pericardial calcification, which is most severe along the right and left atrioventricular grooves (*arrows*).

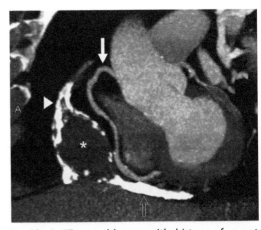

Fig. 28. A 47-year-old man with history of remote motorcycle accident presented with dyspnea. A pericardial collection (*asterisk*) with thick peripheral calcification (*arrowhead, open arrow*) exerts mass effect on the right ventricle and RCA (*white arrow*). The RCA is deviated posteriorly and to the left, but is patent with an intact surrounding fat plane. Patient underwent successful excision, with pathologic diagnosis of chronic pericardial hematoma.

and ascites. Of note, the diagnosis of constrictive pericarditis is clinical and the patient must be symptomatic in the setting of these imaging findings. When surgical treatment is planned for pericardial disease, ECG gating and 3D reconstruction delineate the relationship of the pericardial disease to the adjacent coronary artery (Fig. 28).

SUMMARY

The expanding imaging capabilities of MDCT have made it an important part of the preoperative assessment of the cardiac surgery patient. Ever decreasing imaging times, superior spatial resolution, and the 3D capabilities of MDCT improve diagnosis and enhance surgical planning. Understanding the imaging advantages of MDCT enable improved outcomes in this important patient population.

REFERENCES

1. Leontyev S, Walther T, Borger MA, et al. Aortic valve replacement in octogenarians: utility of risk stratification with EuroSCORE. Ann Thorac Surg 2009;87: 1440–5.
2. Flohr TG, Schoepf J, Ohnesorge BM. Chasing the heart: new developments for cardiac CT. J Thorac Imaging 2007;22:4–16.
3. Gilkeson RC, Markowitz A, Sachs P. Evaluation of the cardiac surgery patient with MSCT. J Thorac Imaging 2005;20:265–72.
4. Hemminger BM, Molina PL, Egan TM, et al. Assessment of real-time 3D visualization for cardiothoracic diagnostic evaluation and surgery planning. J Digit Imaging 2005;18(2):145–53.
5. Gilkeson RC, Markowitz AH. Multislice CT evaluation of coronary artery bypass graft patients. J Thorac Imaging 2007;22:56–62.
6. Shuman WP, Branch KR, May JM, et al. Prospective versus retrospective ECG gating for 64-detector CT of the coronary arteries: comparison of image quality and patient radiation dose radiology. Radiology 2008;248:431–7.
7. Shreter U, Londt J, Vass M, et al. Prospective ECG gating in cardiovascular CTA imaging delivers up to 5-fold dose reduction while maintaining image quality. Presented at: Cardiovascular Imaging 2006. NASCI 34th Annual Meeting and Scientific Sessions. Las Vegas (NV), October, 2006.
8. Brodoefel H, Burgstahler C, Tsiflikas I, et al. Dual-source CT: effect of heart rate, heart rate variability, and calcification on image quality and diagnostic accuracy. Radiology 2008;247:346–55.
9. Juergens KU, Fischbach R. Left ventricular function studied with MDCT. Eur Radiol 2006;16:342–57.
10. Hausleiter J, Meyer T, Franziska H, et al. Estimated radiation dose associated with cardiac CT angiography. JAMA 2009;301:500–7.
11. Abada HT, Larchez C, Daoud B, et al. MDCT of the coronary arteries: feasibility of low-dose CT with ECG-pulsed tube current modulation to reduce radiation dose. AJR Am J Roentgenol 2006;186(6 Supp 2):S387–90.
12. Roselli EE, Pettersson GB, Blackstone EH, et al. Adverse events during reoperative cardiac surgery: frequency, characterization, and rescue. J Thorac Cardiovasc Surg 2008;135:316–23.
13. Van der Linden J, Hadjinikolaou L, Bergman P, et al. Postoperative stroke in cardiac surgery is related to the location and extent of atherosclerotic disease in the ascending aorta. J Am Coll Cardiol 2001;38: 131–5.
14. Roach GW, Kanchuger M, Mangano M, et al. Adverse cerebral outcomes after coronary bypass surgery. N Engl J Med 1996;335:1857–63.
15. Fearn SJ, Pole R, Burgess M, et al. Cerebral embolism during modern cardiopulmonary bypass. Eur J Cardiothorac Surg 2001;20:1163–7.
16. Neri E, Massetti M, Capannini G, et al. Axillary artery cannulation in type A aortic dissection operations. J Thorac Cardiovasc Surg 1999;118:324–9.
17. Hedayati N, Sherwood JT, Schomisch SJ, et al. Axillary artery cannulation for cardiopulmonary bypass reduces cerebral microemboli. J Thorac Cardiovasc Surg 2004;128:389–90.
18. Morino Y, Hara K, Tanabe K, et al. Retrospective analysis of cerebral complications after coronary artery bypass grafting in elderly patients. Jpn Circ J 2000;64:46–50.
19. Bradshaw KA, Pagano D, Bonser RS, et al. Multiplanar reformatting and three-dimensional reconstruction: for pre-operative assessment of the thoracic aorta by computed tomography. Clin Radiol 1998; 53:198–202.
20. Sommer T, Fehske W, Holzknecht N, et al. Aortic dissection: a comparative study of diagnosis with spiral CT, multiplanar transesophageal echocardiography, and MRI imaging. Radiology 1996;199:347–52.
21. Parsa CJ, Hughes GC. Surgical options to contend with thoracic aortic pathology. Semin Roentgenol 2009;44(1):29–51.
22. Gelsomino S, Morocutti G, Frassani R, et al. Long-term results of Bentall composite aortic root replacement for ascending aortic aneurysms and dissections. Chest 2003;124:984–8.
23. Gilkeson RC, Markowitz AH, Balgude A, et al. MDCT evaluation of aortic valvular disease. AJR Am J Roentgenol 2006;186:350–60.
24. Vogel-Claussen J, Pannu H, Spevak PJ, et al. Cardiac valve assessment with MR imaging and 64-section multi-detector row CT. Radiographics 2006;26:1769–84.

25. Abbara S, Soni AV, Cury RC. Evaluation of cardiac function and valves by multidetector row computed tomography. Semin Roentgenol 2008;43(2):145–53.

26. Boxt LM. CT of valvular heart disease. Int J Cardiovasc Imaging 2005;21(1):105–13.

27. Manghat NE, Rachapalli V, Van Lingen R, et al. Imaging the heart valves using ECT-gated 64-detector row cardiac CT. Br J Radiol 2008;81(964):275–90.

28. Ryan R, Abbara S, Colen RR, et al. Cardiac valve disease: spectrum of findings on cardiac 64-MDCT. Am J Roentgenol 2008;190:W294–303.

29. Chen JJ, Jeudy J, Thorn E, et al. Computed tomography assessment of valvular morphology, function, and disease. J Cardiovasc Comput Tomogr 2009;3(Suppl 1):S47–56.

30. Bonow RO, Carabello BA, Kanu C, et al. ACC/AHA 2006 guidelines for the management of patients with valvular heart disease: a report of the American College of Cardiology/American Heart Association Task Force on Practice Guidelines (writing committee to revise the 1998 Guidelines for the Management of Patients With Valvular Heart Disease): developed in collaboration with the Society of Cardiovascular Anesthesiologists: endorsed by the Society for Cardiovascular Angiography and Interventions and the Society of Thoracic Surgeons. Circulation 2006;114(5):e84–231.

31. Lindroos M, Kupari M, Heikkila J, et al. Prevalence of aortic valve abnormalities in the elderly: an echocardiographic study of a random population sample. J Am Coll Cardiol 1993;21:1220–5.

32. Basso C, Boschello M, Perrone C, et al. An echocardiographic survey of primary school children for bicuspid aortic valve. Am J Cardiol 2004;93:661–3.

33. Koos R, Mahnken AH, Sinha AM, et al. Aortic valve calcification as a marker for aortic stenosis severity: assessment on 16-MDCT. Am J Roentgenol 2004;183:1813–8.

34. Morgan-Hughes GJ, Owens PE, Roobottom CA, et al. Three dimensional volume quantification of aortic valve calcification using multi-slice computed tomography. Heart 2003;89:1191–4.

35. Cowell SJ, Newby DE, Burton J, et al. Aortic valve calcification on computed tomography predicts the severity of aortic stenosis. Clin Radiol 2003;58:712–6.

36. Wagner S, Selzer A. Patterns of progression of aortic stenosis: a longitudinal hemodynamic study. Circulation 1982;65:709–12.

37. Stewart BF, Siscovick D, Lind BK, et al. Clinical factors associated with calcific aortic valve disease. J Am Coll Cardiol 1997;29:630–4.

38. Otto CM, Lind BK, Kitzman DW, et al. Association of aortic-valve sclerosis with cardiovascular mortality and morbidity in the elderly. N Engl J Med 1999;341:142–7.

39. Shavelle DM, Budoff MJ, Buljubasic N, et al. Usefulness of aortic valve calcium scores by electron beam computed tomography as a marker of aortic stenosis. Am J Cardiol 2003;92:349–53.

40. Liu F, Coursey CA, Grahame-Clarke, et al. Aortic valve calcification as an incidental finding at CT of the elderly: severity and location as predictors of aortic stenosis. Am J Roentgenol 2006;186:342–9.

41. Abbara S, Pena AJ, Maurovich-Horvat P, et al. Feasibility and optimization of aortic valve planimetry with MDCT. Am J Roentgenol 2007;188:356–60.

42. Simonds JP. Congenital malformations of the aortic and pulmonary valves. Am J Med Sci 1923;166:584–95.

43. Feldman BJ, Khandheria BK, Warnes CA, et al. Incidence, description and functional assessment of isolated quadricuspid aortic valves. Am J Cardiol 1990;65:937–8.

44. Bettencourt N, Sampaio F, Carvalho M, et al. Primary diagnosis of quadricuspid aortic valve with multislice computed tomography. J Cardiovasc Comput Tomogr 2008;2:195–6.

45. Tutarel O. To the editor: quadricuspid aortic valves and anomalies of the coronary arteries. J Cardiovasc Comput Tomogr 2003;127(3):897.

46. Fox DJ, Khattar RS. Carcinoid heart disease: presentation, diagnosis, and management. Heart 2004;90:1224–8.

47. Pellikka PA, Tajik AL, Khandheria BK, et al. Carcinoid heart disease. Clinical and echocardiographic spectrum in 74 patients. Circulation 1993;87:1188–96.

48. Lloyd-Jones D, Adams R, Carnethon M, et al. American Heart Association Heart disease and stroke statistics: 2009 update. a report from the American Heart Association Statistics Committee and Stroke Statistics Subcommittee. Circulation 2009;119(3):e21–e181.

49. Hamon M, Biondi-Zoccai GG, Malagutti P, et al. Diagnostic performance of multislice spiral computed tomography of coronary arteries as compared with conventional invasive coronary angiography: a meta-analysis. J Am Coll Cardiol 2006;48:1896–910.

50. Angelini P, Velasco JA, Flamm S. Coronary anomalies: incidence, pathophysiology, and clinical relevance. Circulation 2002;105:2449–54.

51. Datta J, White CS, Gilkeson RC, et al. Anomalous coronary arteries in adults: depiction at multidetector row CT angiography. Radiology 2005;235:812–8.

52. O'Blenes SB, Feindel CM. Aortic root replacement with anomalous origin of the coronary arteries. Ann Thorac Surg 2002;73:647–9.

53. Hendel RC, Patel MR, Kramer CM, et al. ACCF/ACR/SCCT/SCMR/ASNC/NASCI/SCAI/SIR 2006 Appropriateness criteria for cardiac computed tomography and cardiac magnetic resonance

imaging: a report of the American College of Cardiology Foundation Quality Strategic Directions Committee Appropriateness Criteria Working Group, American College of Radiology, Society of Cardiovascular Computed Tomography, Society for Cardiovascular Magnetic Resonance, American Society of Nuclear Cardiology, North American Society for Cardiac Imaging, Society for Cardiovascular Angiography and Interventions, and Society of Interventional Radiology. J Am Coll Cardiol 2006;48:1475–97.

54. Patel S. Normal and anomalous anatomy of the coronary arteries. Semin Roentgenol 2008;43(2):100–12.

55. Loop FD, Lytle BW, Cosgrove DM, et al. Influence of the internal-mammary-artery graft on 10-year survival and other cardiac events. N Engl J Med 1986;314:1–6.

56. Gillinov AM, Casselman FP, Lytle BW, et al. Injury to a patent left internal thoracic artery graft at coronary reoperation. Ann Thorac Surg 1999;67:382–6.

57. Hoffman J, Kaplan S. The incidence of congenital heart disease. J Am Coll Cardiol 2002;39:1890–900.

58. Rigatelli G, Cardaioli P, Hijazi ZM. Contemporary clinical management of atrial septal defects in the adult. Expert Rev Cardiovasc Ther 2007;5(6):1135–46.

59. Vogel M, Berger F, Kramer A, et al. Incidence of secondary pulmonary hypertension in adults with atrial septal or sinus venosus defects. Heart 1999; 82:30–3.

60. Luciani GB, Viscardi F, Pilati M, et al. Age at repair affects the very long-term outcome of sinus venosus defect. Ann Thorac Surg 2008;86:153–60.

61. Ho ML, Bhalla S, Bierhals A, et al. MDCT of partial anomalous pulmonary venous return (PAPVR) in adults. J Thorac Imaging 2009;24(2):89–95.

62. Slight RD, Nzewi OC, Buell R, et al. Cor-triatriatum sinister presenting in the adult as mitral stenosis: an analysis of factors which may be relevant in late presentation. Heart Lung Circ 2005;14(1):8–12.

63. Saremi F, Gurudevan S, Narula J, et al. Multidetector computed tomography (MDCT) in diagnosis of "cor triatriatum sinister". J Cardiovasc Comput Tomogr 2007;1:172–4.

64. Wang JW, Reddy GP, Gotway MB, et al. CT and MR imaging of pericardial disease. Radiographics 2003; 23:S167–80.

65. Ling LH, Oh JK, Schaff HV, et al. Constrictive pericarditis in the modern era: evolving clinical spectrum and impact on outcome after pericardectomy. Circulation 1999;100:1380–6.

66. Rienmuller R, Groll R, Lipton MJ. CT and MR imaging of pericardial disease. Radiol Clin North Am 2004; 42:587–601.

67. Suh SY, Rha SW, Kim JW, et al. The usefulness of three-dimensional multidetector computed tomography to delineate pericardial calcification in constrictive pericarditis. Int J Cardiol 2006;113: 414–6.

Multidetector CT of Solitary Pulmonary Nodules

Mylene T. Truong, MD[a],*, Bradley S. Sabloff, MD[a],
Jane P. Ko, MD[b]

KEYWORDS

- Chest imaging • CT • Lung • PET/CT
- Pulmonary nodules

A solitary pulmonary nodule is defined as "a round opacity, at least moderately well-marginated and no greater than 3 cm in maximum diameter."[1] The adjective *small* is occasionally used to characterize a nodule with a maximum diameter of less than 1 cm.[1] With the increasing use of multidetector CT (MDCT), small nodules are being detected with increasing frequency. In one screening study, the majority of patients who were screened had at least one nodule.[2] Although most incidentally discovered nodules are benign (usually the sequelae of pulmonary infection), malignancy remains an important consideration in the differential diagnosis of solitary pulmonary nodules (Table 1). According to the American Cancer Society,[3–5] 1 in 13 men and 1 in 16 women will be diagnosed with lung cancer and it is estimated that 20% to 30% of these patients will present with a solitary pulmonary nodule. Because many patients with early-stage lung cancer can present with a solitary pulmonary nodule, one of the main goals of imaging is to accurately differentiate malignant from benign lesions. Techniques for noninvasive image-based assessment and management of these nodules have rapidly evolved recently in large part because of data from ongoing screening studies and from thin-slice helical MDCT studies examining nodule morphology.

MDCT has improved nodule detection and characterization by increasing spatial and temporal resolution and decreasing misregistration artifacts. Typical reconstructions comprise 3- to 5-mm slice collimation for a nontargeted field of view. Obtaining images through the region of interest using a slice collimation of 1 to 1.5 mm improves spatial resolution and is useful in reducing partial volume averaging. If a 1.25-mm slice collimation has been used, as is common in CT angiography protocols to evaluate for pulmonary emboli, differentiating a vessel from a small central nodule is difficult and can be addressed with postprocessing techniques, such as maximum intensity projection, volume rendering, and cine viewing.[6–8] This article reviews the role of imaging in the detection and characterization of solitary pulmonary nodules. Strategies for evaluating and managing solitary pulmonary nodules are also discussed.

CLINICAL ASSESSMENT

How a nodule is managed depends on the probability of malignancy. Clinical factors associated with an increased risk of developing lung cancer include older age, presenting symptoms, smoking, and exposure to asbestos, uranium, or radon. In terms of clinical presentation, patients with hemoptysis are at increased risk for malignancy.[9] Past medical history is important as there is an increased risk of lung cancer in patients with

[a] Department of Radiology, University of Texas MD Anderson Cancer Center, 1515 Holcombe Boulevard, Unit 371, Houston, TX 77030, USA
[b] Department of Radiology, New York University Langone Medical Center, 560 First Avenue, IRM 236, New York, NY 10016, USA
* Corresponding author.
E-mail address: mtruong@mdanderson.org (M.T. Truong).

Radiol Clin N Am 48 (2010) 141–155
doi:10.1016/j.rcl.2009.09.005

radiologic.theclinics.com

Table 1
Differential diagnosis of solitary pulmonary nodules

Type of Cause	Disease
Neoplastic malignant	Primary lung malignancies (non–small cell, small cell, carcinoid, lymphoma); solitary metastasis
Benign	Hamartoma; arteriovenous malformation
Infectious	Granuloma; round pneumonia; abscess; septic embolus
Noninfectious	Amyloidoma; subpleural lymph nodule; rheumatoid nodule; Wegener granulomatosis; focal scarring; infarct
Congenital	Sequestration; bronchogenic cyst; bronchial atresia with mucoid impaction

a history of a prior neoplasm and in patients with pulmonary fibrosis.[9,10] Family history also plays a role in determining the likelihood of malignancy. In this regard, a susceptibility gene to lung cancer has been reported and the risk of developing lung cancer increases in patients who have a first-degree relative with lung cancer.[11] The overall assessment of a patient's risk for malignancy is important in the decision analysis concerning management. For example, in a patient presenting with fever, cough, and a new focal pulmonary opacity, radiographic follow-up to resolution may be all that is necessary to exclude malignancy and confirm a diagnosis of round pneumonia. However, if a new nodule is detected in a patient with a prior history of pulmonary sarcoma, the probability that this is a metastasis is high and tissue should be obtained for diagnosis (Fig. 1). For patients with a prior history of cancer, Ginsberg and colleagues[12] showed that nodules 5 mm or smaller were malignant in 115 of 275

(42%) patients undergoing video-assisted thoracoscopic resection of nodules. To identify independent predictors of malignancy, quantitative models have been developed using multiple logistic regression analysis. Independent predictors of malignancy include older age, current or past smoking history, and history of extrathoracic cancer more than 5 years before nodule detection.[13]

RADIOLOGICAL EVALUATION

Although CT detects an increasing number of solitary pulmonary nodules either incidentally or as part of a lung cancer screening study, many nodules are still initially detected on chest radiographs. If the nodule is diffusely calcified or if a comparison with older radiographs shows stability in size for more than 2 years, the nodule is presumed to be benign and no further evaluation is recommended. However, many nodules require

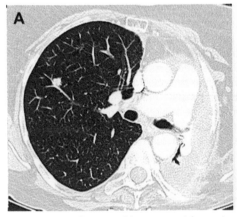
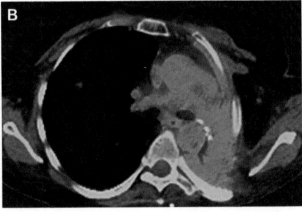

Fig. 1. Sixty-eight-year-old woman with a prior left pneumonectomy for a sarcoma. (*A*) Contrast-enhanced CT and (*B*) positron emission tomography/CT show a hypometabolic irregular right upper lobe nodule with standardized uptake value of 1.4. With advances in positron emission tomography technology, evaluation of nodules as small as 7 mm is possible. However, a negative positron emission tomography does not preclude malignancy. Because of the high clinical suspicion of malignancy with regards to the age of the patient and history of prior lung malignancy, transthoracic needle aspiration biopsy was performed and revealed an adenocarcinoma.

further imaging evaluation. MDCT optimally evaluates morphologic characteristics of the nodule and is useful in assessing for growth on serial studies. Nodules may be missed on MDCT because of a variety of factors, including central location, small size, low attenuation, and location in the lower lobes or adjacent to another abnormal pulmonary opacity, such as inflammatory change.[8] Difficulty with interpretation also occurs with CT as it may not be possible to determine whether a small opacity is a nodule, a vessel, or due to partial volume averaging of adjacent intrathoracic structures. However, the use of thin-section CT together with postprocessing techniques, such as maximum intensity projection, volume rendering, and cine viewing of images at a picture archiving and communication system workstation, has improved the ability to correctly determine whether a pulmonary opacity is a nodule.[8,14]

Nodule Morphology

Although there is considerable overlap in the morphology and appearance of benign and malignant solitary pulmonary nodules, several morphologic features are useful in assessing a nodule's malignant potential. These features include the size, margins, contour, internal morphology (attenuation, wall thickness in cavitary nodules, air bronchograms), presence of satellite nodules, halo sign, reverse halo sign, and growth rate.

The risk of malignancy correlates with nodule size. However, small nodule size does not exclude malignancy. In this regard, the widespread use of MDCT, coupled with the recent interest in CT screening for lung cancer, has resulted in the frequent and incidental detection of small nodules

(1–5 mm).[15–17] While the majority of these nodules are benign, studies of resected small nodules have shown that a considerable number are malignant—as high as 42% for patients with a known malignancy undergoing video-assisted thoracoscopic resection of nodules 5 mm or less.[12]

Typically, benign nodules have well-defined margins and a smooth contour while malignant nodules have ill-defined or spiculated margins and a lobular or irregular contour.[9,18,19] Lobulation is attributed to differential growth rates within nodules, while the irregular or spiculated margins are usually due to growth of malignant cells along the pulmonary interstitium.[20] However, there is considerable overlap between benign and malignant nodules regarding margins and contour. For example, although a spiculated margin with distortion of adjacent bronchovascular bundles (often described as a sunburst or corona radiata) is highly suggestive with a 90% predictive value of malignancy,[21] benign nodules due to infection/inflammation can also have this appearance (**Fig. 2**). Additionally, a smooth nodule margin does not exclude malignancy. Up to 20% of primary lung malignancies have smooth contours and well-defined margins and most metastatic nodules typically manifest as smooth margins.[9,19]

The halo sign is a poorly defined rim of ground-glass attenuation around the nodule (**Fig. 3**). This halo may represent hemorrhage, tumor infiltration, or perinodular inflammation. Originally described as a sign of invasive aspergillus infection, the CT halo sign may also be seen with bronchioloalveolar carcinoma.[22] Conversely, the reverse halo sign is a focal round area of ground-glass attenuation surrounded by a ring of consolidation (**Fig. 4**). Described in cryptogenic organizing pneumonia[23] and paracoccidioidomycosis, the reverse halo

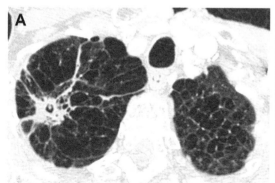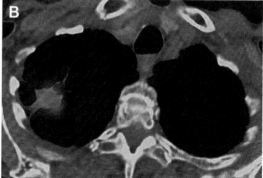

Fig. 2. Seventy-eight-year-old woman presenting with a chronic cough. (*A*) Contrast-enhanced CT and (*B*) positron emission tomography/CT show an irregular cavitary lesion in the right upper lobe with standardized uptake value of 4.1 suspicious for a primary lung cancer. Biopsy revealed acute and chronic inflammation with confluent colonies of fungiform bacteria consistent with actinomyces. Note that infectious and inflammatory conditions can accumulate ^{18}F-labeled 2-deoxy-D-glucose and be misinterpreted as malignant.

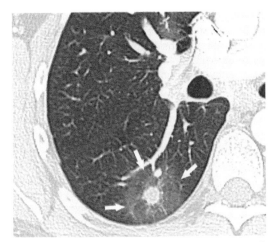

Fig. 3. Thirty-six-year-old man presenting with a cough. Contrast-enhanced CT shows a well-circumscribed right lower lobe nodule surrounded by a halo of ground-glass attenuation (*arrows*) and a satellite nodule anteriorly. Note that in patients with leukemia, the halo sign is highly suggestive of invasive aspergillus infection.

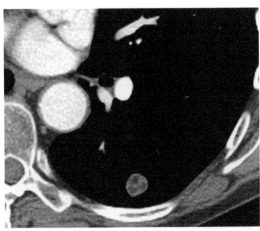

Fig. 5. Contrast-enhanced CT shows a well-circumscribed left lower lobe nodule. Low attenuation within the nodule (attenuation −46 Hounsfield units) is consistent with fat and is usually diagnostic of a hamartoma. Note that focal fat in a nodule can rarely be seen in liposarcoma metastases and lipoid pneumonia.

sign is histologically due to a greater amount of inflammatory cells in the periphery of the lesion than in the center. In invasive fungal pneumonias, the reverse halo sign is due to infarcted lung with a greater amount of hemorrhage in the peripheral solid ring than in the center ground-glass region.[24]

Fat within a nodule is a characteristic finding of a hamartoma and is detected by CT in up to 50% of these neoplasms (Fig. 5).[25] Rarely, lung metastases in patients with liposarcomas or renal cell cancers can manifest as fat-containing nodules.[26]

Calcification patterns can be useful in determining benignity of a nodule and CT is

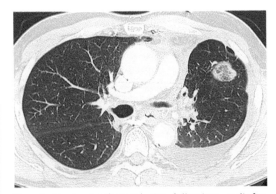

Fig. 4. Contrast-enhanced CT following radiofrequency ablation for a left upper lobe lung cancer shows a focal round area of ground-glass attenuation surrounded by a well-circumscribed region of consolidation (reverse halo sign). Note that the reverse halo sign is usually indicative of invasive fungal pneumonia in immunocompromised patients.

considerably more sensitive than radiography for detecting calcification in a nodule.[18,27,28] However, partial volume averaging can be problematic when thicker sections are obtained, making calcification within a small nodule visually undetectable. In these cases, thin sections (1–3 mm) to improve spatial resolution should be performed to detect calcification. With the introduction of dual-energy CT, simultaneous 80-kV and 140-kV images can be obtained. It has been shown that measurement of CT attenuation values obtained at different kilovolt peaks may be useful in identifying areas of fat, calcium, bone, soft tissue, and iodinated contrast[29] and in evaluating tumor perfusion. However, a multi-institutional trial has shown that dual-energy CT is unreliable for distinguishing benign from malignant nodules.[30–32]

Common benign patterns of calcification include diffuse, central, laminated, and "popcorn." However, lung metastases from chondrosarcomas or osteosarcomas can present with "benign" patterns of calcification (Fig. 6).[26,33] Calcification can be detected in up to 13% of all lung cancers on CT, although the incidence in patients with lung cancer manifesting as nodules less than 3 cm is only 2%.[34–36] Calcification patterns, such as stippled, eccentric, or amorphous, are indeterminate in etiology as they can be seen in both benign and malignant conditions (Fig. 7).[36]

The widespread use of MDCT images has increased the detection of "subsolid" nodules containing a component of ground-glass attenuation. The "subsolid" category comprises pure

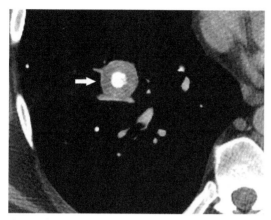

Fig. 6. Thirty-six-year-old man with a chondrosarcoma of the left proximal thigh. CT shows central calcification within the nodule in the right lower lobe (*arrow*). This appearance is highly suggestive of a benign calcified nodule secondary to granulomatous infection. However, knowledge of the clinical context must also be taken into account in establishing the diagnosis. Resection revealed metastatic chondrosarcoma.

ground-glass, as well as mixed solid and ground-glass (partly solid) lesions. In the ELCAP (Early Lung Cancer Action Project) study, 19% of positive results on the baseline screening were subsolid. Incidence of malignancy varies according to the degree of soft tissue attenuation. Henschke and colleagues[37] reported rates of malignancy for solid and subsolid nodules as 7% and 34%, respectively. Partly solid nodules had the highest incidence of malignancy (63%) (**Fig. 8**) while pure ground-glass nodules had an incidence of malignancy of 18%.

In terms of malignant potential, subsolid nodules have been associated with a spectrum of entities ranging from atypical adenomatous hyperplasia (a premalignant condition), to bronchioloalveolar carcinoma and invasive adenocarcinoma.[38] Atypical adenomatous hyperplasia (**Fig. 9**), a putative precursor to bronchioloalveolar carcinoma/adenocarcinoma, is defined by the World Health Organization as a

> ...*localized proliferation of mild to moderately atypical cells lining involved alveoli and sometimes respiratory bronchioles, resulting in focal lesions in peripheral alveolated lung, usually less than 5mm in diameter and generally in the absence of underlying interstitial inflammation and fibrosis.*[39]

Ground-glass nodules less than 1 cm may represent atypical adenomatous hyperplasia or bronchioloalveolar carcinoma. Subsolid nodules greater than 1 cm are more likely to represent

bronchioloalveolar carcinoma rather than atypical adenomatous hyperplasia. Noguchi and Shimosato[38] graded the spectrum of bronchioloalveolar carcinoma and invasive adenocarcinoma pathologically into types A through F, representing various degrees of aggressiveness. This grading system showed that the presence of solid component on CT in a ground-glass nodule is concerning for higher grades of adenocarcinoma.[40] In contradistinction, another study revealed that pure ground-glass opacities were less likely to have invasion and/or metastasis.[41]

Solid nodules have the lowest incidence of malignancy, as many infections, particularly mycoses and tuberculosis, have this appearance. However, despite the lower incidence of malignancy in solid nodules, most primary lung cancers and metastases present as solid nodules.[21]

Cavitation occurs in both infectious/inflammatory conditions as well as in primary and metastatic tumors. Up to 15% of primary lung malignancies cavitate and typically cavitation is seen in squamous cell histology (**Fig. 10**). Thick, irregular walls are typically seen in malignant cavitary nodules, whereas smooth, thin walls are seen in benign cavitary lesions.[19] It has been reported that 95% of cavitary nodules with a wall thickness greater than 16 mm are malignant and 92% with a wall thickness less than 4 mm are benign.[42,43] Although these measurements can add value in nodule evaluation, cavity wall thickness cannot be used to reliably differentiate benign and malignant nodules because of cavitary nodules with a wall thickness of 5 to 15 mm, 51% were found to be benign and 49% malignant.[43]

Additional morphologic imaging features that can be used in assessing the malignant or benign potential of solitary pulmonary nodules include the presence of internal lucencies, air bronchograms, and satellite nodules. Bronchioloalveolar carcinoma can also show small internal lucencies due to patent bronchi from lepidic growth of tumor cells (**Fig. 11**).[19] In one study, air bronchograms occurred more frequently in malignant nodules (30%) than in benign nodules (6%)[44]; and the differential diagnosis includes bronchioloalveolar carcinoma, lymphoma, and infection. Satellite nodules, small nodules adjacent to a dominant nodule, are more frequently associated with benign lesions. However, 6% to 16% of patients with lung cancer present with T4-satellite nodules.[45–47]

Nodule Growth

Nodule growth can be evaluated by reviewing prior films. Malignant nodules may double in volume

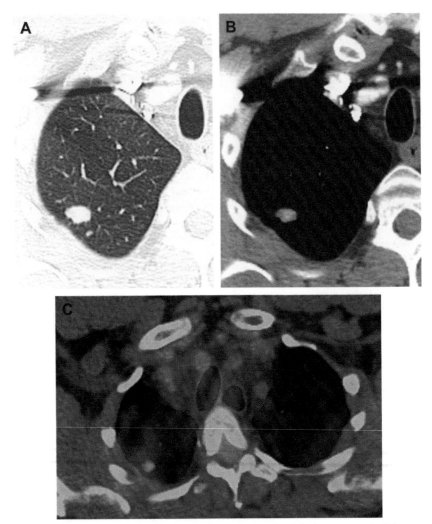

Fig. 7. Forty-seven-year-old man with a right upper lobe nodule with a lobular contour in (*A*) contrast-enhanced CT in lung windows, amorphous calcifications in (*B*) contrast-enhanced CT with mediastinal windows, and lack of ^{18}F-labeled 2-deoxy-D-glucose uptake in (*C*) positron emission tomography/CT. Despite the negative positron emission tomography, the lesion was biopsied because of the indeterminate calcification pattern and increase in size compared with 3 years earlier (not shown). Pathology revealed dense fibrosis, focal chronic inflammation, and no malignant cells.

between 30 and 400 days (**Fig. 12**).[48] Nodules that double in volume in less than 30 days are typically infectious or inflammatory in etiology but may also be seen in lymphoma or rapidly growing metastases (**Fig. 13**). Nodules that double in volume in greater than 400 days are usually benign neoplasms or sequelae of prior pulmonary infections. In general, the lack of growth over a 2-year period is reliable in determining benignity of a nodule.[49,50] This criterion does not apply to subsolid nodules because some well-differentiated adenocarcinoma and bronchioloalveolar carcinoma can have doubling times of up to 1346 days.[51] In a screening study analyzing the growth rates of small lung cancers, Hasegawa and

colleagues[52] found that approximately 20% (12 of 61) had volume-doubling time of greater than 2 years, typically seen with well-differentiated adenocarcinomas. Interestingly, the volume-doubling time was longer in nonsmokers than in smokers. Of small lung cancers, the longest doubling time was seen in nonsolid lesions, followed by partly solid lesions, and, finally, solid lesions.[52]

Because nodule growth is an important consideration when assessing lesions for malignant potential, the accuracy of growth assessment needs to be addressed. For a nodule to double in volume, the change in nodule diameter is approximately 26%. For a small nodule, this small

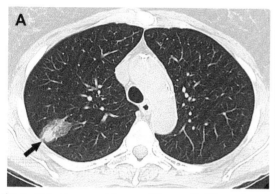
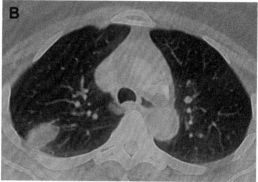

Fig. 8. Sixty-six-year-old man with a well-differentiated adenocarcinoma with bronchioloalveolar features manifesting as a partly solid right upper lobe nodule. (*A*) On CT, the nodule shows a solid component posteriorly (*arrow*). (*B*) Positron emission tomography/CT shows low metabolic activity with standardized uptake value of 3.3. Note that, compared with nonsolid and solid lesions, partly solid lesions have the highest likelihood of being malignant.

change in diameter may be difficult to detect. For example, a 4-mm nodule will increase to only 5 mm in diameter after doubling in volume. Additionally, it has recently been shown that significant inter- and intraobserver variability in lesion measurement, particularly in lesions with spiculated margins, are confounding factors in determining growth.[53,54] It has been suggested that, for evaluating nodule size and growth, the measurement of volume is a more accurate and reproducible than the measurement of diameters, and that automated volume techniques are potentially useful for assessing growth.[55,56]

Nodule Enhancement and Metabolism

There are qualitative and quantitative differences in nodule perfusion and metabolism when comparing benign and malignant lesions. Contrast-enhanced CT has been shown in a multi-institutional trial to be useful in determining the likelihood of malignancy of nodules between 5 mm and 3 cm.[57] The intensity of nodule enhancement is directly related to the vascularity of the nodule, which is increased in malignant lesions.[57–59] Malignant lesions greater than 3 cm may show necrosis and fail to enhance, leading to a false-negative study. In the CT-enhancement protocol, 3-mm collimation images of the nodule are obtained before and after the intravenous administration of contrast (2 mL/s; 300-mg iodine/mL; 420-mg iodine/kg of body weight). Serial 5-second spiral acquisitions (3-mm collimation scans with 2-mm reconstruction intervals; 120 kVp, 280 mA, pitch of 1:1; standard reconstruction algorithm; 15-cm field of view) are performed at 1,

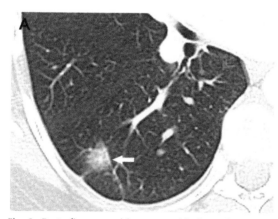
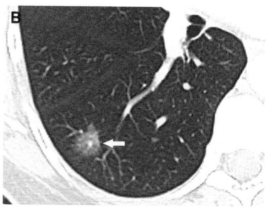

Fig. 9. Forty-five-year-old woman with thyroid cancer. (*A*) Contrast-enhanced CT shows a right lower lobe subsolid nodule (*arrow*) biopsy proven to be due to atypical adenomatous hyperplasia. (*B*) Contrast-enhanced CT 4 years later shows no change in nodule size and a decrease in nodule attenuation (*arrow*). Note that an exception to Fleischner's guidelines for evaluation of small pulmonary nodules is the nonsolid or partly solid nodule, for which reassessment may need to be continued beyond 2 years to exclude the risk of an indolent adenocarcinoma.

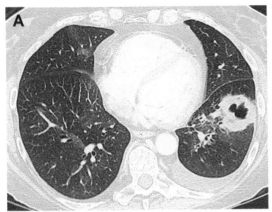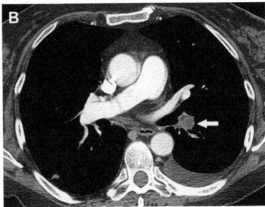

Fig. 10. Cavitary pulmonary infarction. (*A*) Contrast-enhanced CT shows a thick-walled cavitary nodule in left lower lobe suspicious for primary lung cancer. (*B*) Contrast-enhanced CT with mediastinal windows revealed clot in the left interlobar pulmonary artery consistent with pulmonary embolism (*arrow*).

2, 3, and 4 minutes after the onset of contrast injection. Enhancement is determined by subtracting the precontrast attenuation of the nodule from the peak nodule attenuation after contrast administration. To obtain measurements, the circular or oval region of interest is centered on the image closest to the nodule equator and should comprise roughly 70% of the diameter of a nodule. Region-of-interest measurements should be made on mediastinal window settings to minimize partial volume averaging. Careful inspection of the adjacent bronchovascular bundles to obtain region-of-interest measurements of the nodule at similar levels in the z-axis on serial scans is recommended. Typically, malignant nodules enhance more than 20 Hounsfield units (HU), while benign nodules enhance less than 15 HU.[57] When a cutoff

of 15 HU is used, the negative predictive value for malignancy is 96%.[57] There are, however, several potential limitations to clinical application of this technique. This technique should only be performed on nodules greater than 5 mm, relatively spherical in shape, and relatively homogeneous in attenuation (ie, without evidence of fat, calcification, cavitation, or necrosis). Because nodules that enhance less than 15 HU are almost certainly benign (sensitivity 98%, specificity 58%, accuracy 77%), the clinical utility of this technique, despite its limitations, does enable conservative management with serial imaging reassessment.

Recently, computer-aided diagnosis has been used to assist in differentiating benign from malignant nodules by examining vascular enhancement and nodule morphology. In a study by Shah and

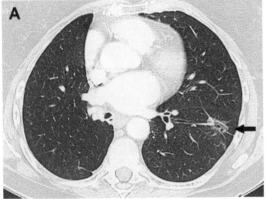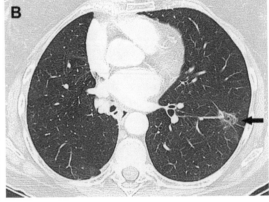

Fig. 11. Sixty-five-year-old woman with right lower lobectomy for lung cancer and left lower lobe subsolid nodule representing bronchioloalveolar carcinoma in (*A*) contrast-enhanced CT with small internal lucencies due to patent bronchi from lepidic growth of tumor cells (*arrow*). Comparison with a (*B*) contrast-enhanced CT 2 years earlier shows lack of growth (*arrow*). Note with small lung cancers, the longest doubling time is seen with nonsolid lesions, followed by partly solid lesions, and finally solid lesions.

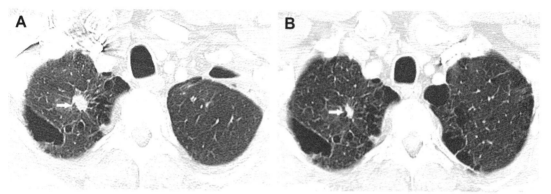

Fig. 12. Sixty-seven-year-old man with emphysema. (*A*) Contrast-enhanced CT shows a spiculated right apical lesion (*arrow*) has increased in size compared with (*B*) contrast-enhanced CT of 8 months earlier showing same lesion (*arrow*). Biopsy revealed a neuroendocrine carcinoma. Note that nodule growth is an important consideration when assessing lesions for malignant potential.

colleagues[60] a computer-aided diagnosis system used quantitative features to describe the nodule's size, shape, attenuation, and enhancement properties to differentiate benign from malignant nodules. This study showed that computer-aided diagnosis using volumetric and contrast-enhanced data from 35 CT data sets of solitary pulmonary nodules with a mean diameter of 25 mm (range 6–54 mm) is useful in assisting in the differentiation of benign and malignant solitary pulmonary opacities.

An alternative to CT enhancement to differentiate benign from malignant pulmonary nodules is functional imaging using ^{18}F-labeled 2-deoxy-D-glucose (FDG) positron emission tomography (PET). The most common semiquantitative method of evaluation of pulmonary lesions using PET is FDG standardized uptake value (SUV_{max}). Metabolism of glucose is typically increased in malignancies and an SUV_{max} cutoff of 2.5 has been used to differentiate benign from malignant nodules.[61] PET has a sensitivity and specificity of approximately 90% for detection of malignancy in nodules 10 mm or greater in diameter.[62] To properly tailor patient management, FDG PET evaluations of solitary pulmonary nodules must be considered alongside such clinical risk factors as patient age, smoking history, and history of malignancy (**Fig. 14**). For instance, in a patient with a low pretest likelihood of malignancy (20%) being considered for serial imaging reassessment, a negative PET will reduce the likelihood of

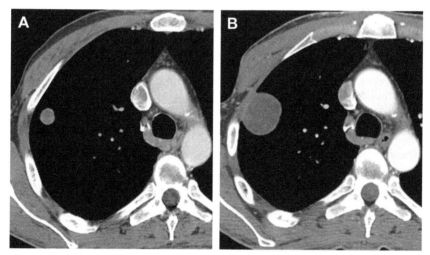

Fig. 13. Fifty-eight-year-old man with a pulmonary metastasis from a nasopharyngeal cancer. (*A*) Contrast-enhanced CT shows a small, well-circumscribed right upper lobe nodule. (*B*) Contrast-enhanced CT performed 28 days later shows a marked increase in size of right upper lobe lesion. Note that, although volume-doubling time of less than 30 days suggests infection, this can also be seen in lymphoma and rapidly growing metastases.

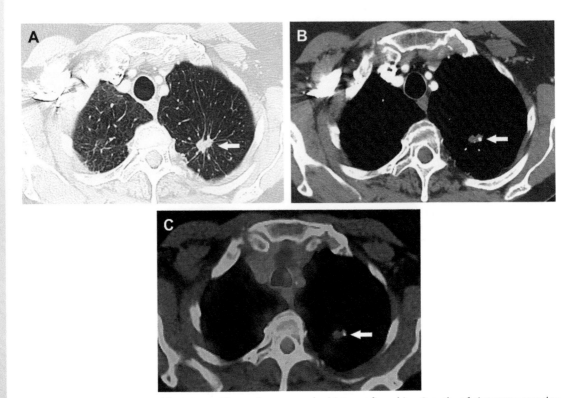

Fig. 14. Seventy-seven-year-old woman with emphysema and a history of smoking 3 packs of cigarettes per day for 40 years. (*A*) Contrast-enhanced CT with lung windows, (*B*) contrast-enhanced CT with mediastinal windows, and (*C*) PET/CT show a hypometabolic, spiculated left apical lung nodule with eccentric calcification (*arrow*). Despite the negative PET, further evaluation (biopsy or resection) is required because of the high clinical suspicion of malignancy owing to the age of the patient, smoking history, emphysema, and nodule characteristics of spiculation and eccentric calcification

malignancy to 1% and argues for conservative management.[62,63] However, in a patient with a high pretest likelihood of malignancy (80%), a negative PET will only reduce the likelihood of malignancy to 14%.[63,64] Accordingly, obtaining tissue for diagnosis with biopsy or resection would be recommended.

The high sensitivity and specificity of PET in the evaluation of solitary pulmonary nodules pertain to solid nodules of 10 mm or greater in diameter. However, FDG-uptake in malignant ground-glass and partly solid nodules is variable and cannot be used to differentiate benign from malignant lesions. In a recent study, 9 of 10 well-differentiated adenocarcinomas presenting as ground-glass nodular opacities were falsely negative on PET while 4 of 5 benign ground-glass nodular opacities were falsely positive.[65] The sensitivity (10%) and specificity (20%) for ground-glass opacities in this study were significantly lower than that for solid nodules (90% and 71%, respectively). Limitations in spatial resolution can also result in false-negative studies when lesions smaller than 10 mm in diameter are evaluated.[65,66] With

advances in PET technology, the evaluation of nodules of approximately 7 mm is possible.[67] Otherwise, false-negative PET results are uncommon, but may occur with carcinoid tumors and bronchioloalveolar carcinomas (Fig. 15).[68–70] The lower positive predictive value relates to the false-positive lesions due to infection and inflammation (Fig. 16).

The recent introduction of integrated PET/CT scanners has introduced the near-simultaneous acquisition of coregistered, spatially matched functional and anatomic data. The temporal and spatial fusion of these two data sets can be useful when used as the initial imaging modality in solitary pulmonary opacity characterization.[71] In a study comparing PET/CT and helical dynamic CT in the evaluation of solitary pulmonary nodules, PET/CT was more sensitive (96% vs. 81%) and accurate (93% vs. 85%) than helical dynamic CT.[71] However, the use of CT for attenuation correction of the PET images has introduced artifacts and quantitative errors that can affect the emission image and lead to misinterpretation.[72] For instance, imaging during different stages of

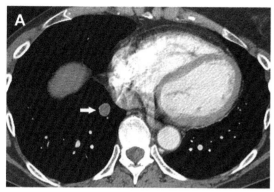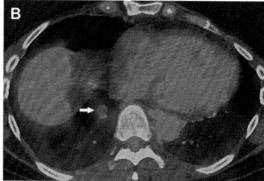

Fig. 15. Sixty-two-year-old woman with endometrial cancer and a right lung nodule detected on a preoperative chest radiograph. (A) Contrast-enhanced CT and (B) PET/CT show well-circumscribed hypometabolic nodule (arrow) in the right lower lobe. Transthoracic needle biopsy revealed a well-differentiated neuroendocrine tumor. Note that false-negative PET results may be seen with carcinoid and bronchioloalveolar carcinoma.

the patient's respiratory cycle may introduce a mismatch between the CT attenuation data obtained during breath-hold and the PET emission data obtained during quiet tidal breathing.[73,74] In addition to localization errors, this misregistration may also result in incorrect attenuation coefficients applied to the PET data that can affect the SUV_{max}, the most widely used parameter to quantify the intensity of FDG uptake.[73,75,76] Misregistration may lead to SUV_{max} being lower than expected and can potentially result in a false-negative study. Strategies to reduce the respiratory mismatch between the CT and PET images include obtaining the CT scan at end expiration, which most closely approximates the lung volumes during PET data acquisition at quiet tidal breathing. However, CT of the lungs at end expiration compromises anatomic detail and small nodules may be obscured. A more recent approach suggests the use of respiratory-averaged CT (CT cine images obtained over different portions of the respiratory cycle using four-dimensional CT techniques) to improve SUV_{max} quantification.[77] Respiratory-averaged CT used for attenuation correction of a PET scan has shown SUV_{max} differences of more than 50% in some lesions as compared with the standard method of CT attenuation using data obtained in the mid-expiratory phase.[77,78]

DECISION ANALYSIS

Management algorithms for solitary pulmonary nodules are determined by patients' clinical risk

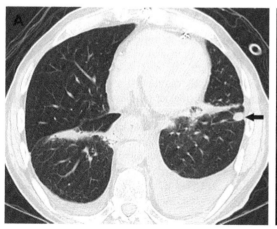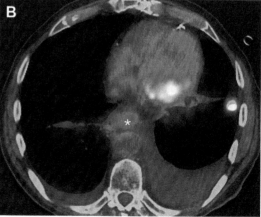

Fig. 16. Seventy-seven-year-old man with an esophageal cancer treated with chemoradiation. (A) CT and (B) PET/CT show a new well-circumscribed hypermetabolic left lower lobe nodule (arrow in A) with SUV_{max} of 9.3 suspicious for a metastasis. Asterisk in B shows esophageal cancer. Transthoracic needle aspiration biopsy revealed no malignant cells. Fungal elements morphologically consistent with Cryptococcus were identified. Note that infectious and inflammatory conditions with increased glucose metabolism can accumulate FDG and be misinterpreted as malignant.

factors as well as nodule characterization. Benign nodules, either because of their pattern of calcification or their stability over a long time, require no further evaluation. Nodules determined to be benign because of their pattern of calcification or their stability over a long time require no further evaluation. However, many nodules remain indeterminate in etiology after comprehensive noninvasive radiologic assessment. At this juncture in decision analysis, management options include observation with imaging reassessment, biopsy, or resection of the nodule. Detection of pulmonary nodules has increased with MDCT and many of these lesions are small (<7 mm) and benign. Multiple factors, including radiation exposure, cost, limited resources, patient anxiety, and the knowledge gleaned from the lung cancer CT screening trials have contributed to the recent release of guidelines for the management of pulmonary nodules discovered incidentally on routine and screening CT by the Fleischner Society[79] and more recently by the American College of Chest Physicians.[80] These guidelines take into consideration lesion size, morphology, and growth rate and patient age and smoking history.[79] In terms of size, small nodules (<4 mm) have a less than 1% chance of being a primary lung cancer, even in people who smoke, while the risk of malignancy increases to 10% to 20% in nodules in the 8-mm range.[79]

FLEISCHNER SOCIETY RECOMMENDATIONS

The following list gives the Fleischner Society's recommendations for an incidentally discovered nodule in an adult patient[79]:

A. Low-risk populations (little or no history of smoking, and no other risk factors)
  1. Nodule equal to or smaller than 4 mm: likelihood of malignancy very small and no reassessment is necessary.
  2. Nodule greater than 4 mm but less than or equal to 6 mm: reassessment CT at 12 months and, if stable, no further evaluation is required. The exception is the nonsolid or partly solid nodule, which may need to be reassessed to exclude the risk of an indolent adenocarcinoma.
  3. Nodule greater than 6 mm but less than or equal to 8 mm: reassessment CT at 6 to 12 months and, if stable, again at 18 to 24 months.
  4. Nodule greater than 8 mm: either reassessment CT scans at 3, 9, and 24 months to assess for stability in size or further evaluation with contrast-enhanced CT, PET/CT, or biopsy or resection.
B. High-risk populations (history of smoking, or other exposure or risk factor)
  1. Nodule equal to or smaller than 4 mm: reassessment at 12 months and, if stable, no further evaluation is required. The exception is the nonsolid or partly solid nodule, which may need to be reassessed to exclude the risk of an indolent adenocarcinoma.
  2. Nodule greater than 4 mm but less than or equal to 6 mm: Reassessment CT at 6 to 12 months and, if stable, again at 18 to 24 months.
  3. Nodule greater than 6 mm but less than or equal to 8 mm: reassessment CT at 3 to 6 months and, if stable, again at 9 to 12 months and at 24 months.
  4. Nodule greater than 8 mm: either reassessment CT at 3, 9, and 24 months to assess stability or perform contrast-enhanced CT, PET/CT, or biopsy or resection.

The Fleischner recommendations do not apply to patients with a history of malignancy, patients under 35 years with low risk of lung cancer, and in those patients with fever in which the nodules may be infectious.[79] For nodule reassessment, a noncontrast, thin-collimation, limited-coverage, low-dose CT scan is recommended by the Fleischner Society.[79] An example of a low-dose protoool io a 120-kilovolt (peak), 40–50-mAs algorithm reconstructed at 2.5 mm slice thickness with 2-mm intervals.

SUMMARY

With the increasing use of MDCT, more solitary pulmonary nodules are being detected. Although the majority of these lesions are benign, lung cancer constitutes an important consideration in the differential diagnosis of solitary pulmonary nodules. The goal of management is to correctly differentiate malignant from benign nodules to ensure appropriate treatment. Stratifying patients' risk factors for malignancy, including patient age, smoking history, and history of malignancy, is essential in the management of solitary pulmonary nodules. In terms of radiologic evaluation, obtaining prior films is important to assess for nodule growth. The detection of certain patterns of calcification and stability for 2 years or more have historically been the only useful findings for determining whether a nodule is or is not benign. However, recent technological advances in imaging, including MDCT and PET/CT, have improved nodule characterization and surveillance. For solid nodules, CT enhancement of less than 15 HU and hypometabolism on PET (SUV_{max} <2.5) favor a benign etiology. Potential pitfalls in nodule enhancement and PET evaluation of solitary pulmonary nodules include infectious and inflammatory conditions. Stratified according to patient risk factors for malignancy and nodule size, recent guidelines for the management of incidentally detected small pulmonary nodules have been useful in decision analysis. An important exception to these guidelines is the evaluation and management of the subsolid nodule. These lesions are not suitable for CT enhancement studies and may show low metabolic activity on PET imaging. Due to their association with bronchioloalveolar carcinoma and adenocarcinoma, subsolid nodules require a more aggressive approach in terms of reassessing serial imaging and/or obtaining tissue diagnosis. As data from the low-dose CT lung cancer screening trials are analyzed and further studies with new imaging techniques are performed, management strategies for the imaging evaluation of the solitary pulmonary nodule will continue to evolve.

REFERENCES

1. Austin JH, Muller NL, Friedman PJ, et al. Glossary of terms for CT of the lungs: recommendations of the Nomenclature Committee of the Fleischner Society. Radiology 1996;200(2):327–31.
2. Swensen SJ, Jett JR, Hartman TE, et al. CT screening for lung cancer: five-year prospective experience. Radiology 2005;235(1):259–65.
3. American Cancer Society. Cancer facts and figures 2006. Atlanta (GA): American Cancer Society; 2006.
4. Viggiano RW, Swensen SJ, Rosenow EC III. Evaluation and management of solitary and multiple pulmonary nodules. Clin Chest Med 1992;13:83–95.
5. Mountain CF. Revisions in the international system for staging lung cancer. Chest 1997;111:1710–7.
6. Coakley FV, Cohen MD, Johnson MS, et al. Maximum intensity projection images in the detection of simulated pulmonary nodules by spiral CT. Br J Radiol 1998;71(842):135–40.
7. Gruden JF, Ouanounou S, Tigges S, et al. Incremental benefit of maximum-intensity-projection images on observer detection of small pulmonary nodules revealed by MDCT. Am J Roentgenol 2002;179: 149–57.
8. Girvin F, Ko JP. Pulmonary nodules: detection, assessment, and CAD. Am J Roentgenol 2008;191: 1057–69.
9. Gurney JW, Lyddon DM, McKay JA. Determining the likelihood of malignancy in solitary pulmonary nodules with Bayesian analysis. Part II. Application. Radiology 1993;186:415–22.
10. Lee HJ, Im JG, Ahn JM, et al. Lung cancer in patients with idiopathic pulmonary fibrosis: CT findings. J Comput Assist Tomogr 1996;20(6): 979–82.
11. Bailey-Wilson JE, Amos CI, Pinney SM, et al. A major lung cancer susceptibility locus maps to chromosome 6q2325. Am J Hum Genet 2004;75:460–74.
12. Ginsberg MS, Griff SK, Go BD, et al. Pulmonary nodules resected at video-assisted thoracoscopic surgery: etiology in 426 patients. Radiology 1999; 213(1):277–82.
13. Herder GJ, van Tinteren H, Golding RP, et al. Clinical prediction model to characterize pulmonary nodules: validation and added value of 18F-fluorodeoxyglucose positron emission tomography. Chest 2005;128(4):2490–6.
14. Seltzer SE, Judy PF, Adams DF, et al. Spiral CT of the chest: comparison of cine and film-based viewing. Radiology 1995;197(1):73–8.
15. Henschke CI, McCauley DI, Yankelevitz DF, et al. Early lung cancer action project: overall design and findings from baseline screening. Lancet 1999;354:99–105.
16. Kaneko M, Eguchi K, Ohmatsu H, et al. Peripheral lung cancer: screening and detection with low-dose spiral CT versus radiography. Radiology 1996;201:798–802.
17. Sone S, Takashima S, Li F, et al. Mass screening for lung cancer with mobile spiral computed tomography scanner. Lancet 1998;351(9111):1242–5.
18. Zerhouni EA, Stitik FP, Siegelman SS, et al. CT of the pulmonary nodule: a cooperative study. Radiology 1986;160:319–27.
19. Zwirewich CV, Vedal S, Miller RR, et al. Solitary pulmonary nodule: high-resolution CT and radiologic-pathologic correlation. Radiology 1991;179:469–76.
20. Heitzman ER, Markarian B, Raasch BN, et al. Pathways of tumor spread through the lung: radiologic correlations with anatomy and pathology. Radiology 1982;144(1):3–14.
21. Winer-Muram HT. The solitary pulmonary nodule. Radiology 2006;239(1):34–49.
22. Lee YR, Choi YW, Lee KJ, et al. CT halo sign: the spectrum of pulmonary diseases. Br J Radiol 2005;78:862–5.
23. Kim SJ, Lee KS, Ryu YH, et al. Reversed halo sign on high-resolution CT of cryptogenic organizing pneumonia: diagnostic implications. Am J Roentgenol 2003;180:1251–4.
24. Wahba H, Truong MT, Lei X, et al. Reversed halo sign in invasive pulmonary fungal infections. Clin Infect Dis 2008;46(11):1733–7.
25. Siegelman SS, Khouri NF, Scott WW Jr, et al. Pulmonary hamartoma: CT findings. Radiology 1986;160: 313–7.

26. Muram TM, Aisen A. Fatty metastatic lesions in 2 patients with renal clear-cell carcinoma. J Comput Assist Tomogr 2003;27(6):869–70.

27. Siegelman SS, Khouri NF, Leo FP, et al. Solitary pulmonary nodules: CT assessment. Radiology 1986;160(2):307–12.

28. Siegelman SS, Zerhouni EA, Leo FP, et al. CT of the solitary pulmonary nodule. Am J Roentgenol 1980; 135:1–13.

29. Johnson TR, Krauss B, Sedlmair M, et al. Material differentiation by dual energy CT: initial experience. Eur Radiol 2007;17:1510–7.

30. Higashi Y, Nakamura H, Matsumoto T, et al. Dual-energy computed tomographic diagnosis of pulmonary nodules. J Thorac Imaging 1994;9(1):31–4.

31. Bhalla M, Shepard JA, Nakamura K, et al. Dual kV CT to detect calcification in solitary pulmonary nodule. J Comput Assist Tomogr 1995;19(1):44–7.

32. Swensen SJ, Yamashita K, McCollough CH, et al. Lung nodules: dual-kilovolt peak analysis with CT-multicenter study. Radiology 2000;214:81–5.

33. Seo JB, Im JG, Goo JM, et al. Atypical pulmonary metastases: spectrum of radiologic findings. Radiographics 2001;21(2):403–17.

34. O'Keefe ME, Good CA, McDonald JR. Calcification in solitary nodules of the lung. Am J Roentgenol 1957;77:1023–33.

35. Grewal RG, Austin JHM. CT demonstration of calcification in carcinoma of the lung. J Comput Assist Tomogr 1994;18:867–71.

36. Mahoney MC, Shipley RT, Corcoran HL, et al. CT demonstration of calcification in carcinoma of the lung. Am J Roentgenol 1990;154:255–8.

37. Henschke CI, Yankelevitz DF, Mirtcheva R, et al. CT screening for lung cancer: frequency and significance of part-solid and nonsolid nodules. Am J Roentgenol 2002;178:1053–7.

38. Noguchi M, Shimosato Y. The development and progression of adenocarcinoma of the lung. Cancer Treat Res 1995;72:131–42.

39. Colby TV, Wistuba II, Gazdar A. Precursors to pulmonary neoplasia. Adv Anat Pathol 1998;5: 205–15.

40. Yang ZG, Sone S, Takashima S, et al. High-resolution CT analysis of small peripheral lung adenocarcinomas revealed on screening helical CT. Am J Roentgenol 2001;176:1399–407.

41. Ohta Y, Shimizu Y, Kobayashi T, et al. Pathologic and biological assessment of lung tumors showing ground-glass opacity. Ann Thorac Surg 2006;81: 1194–7.

42. Woodring JH, Fried AM. Significance of wall thickness in solitary cavities of the lung: a follow-up study. Am J Roentgenol 1983;140:473–4.

43. Woodring JH, Fried AM, Chuang VP. Solitary cavities of the lung: diagnostic implications of cavity wall thickness. Am J Roentgenol 1980;135:1269–71.

44. Kui M, Templeton PA, White CS, et al. Evaluation of the air bronchogram sign on CT in solitary pulmonary lesions. J Comput Assist Tomogr 1996;20(6): 983–6.

45. Keogan MT, Tung KT, Kaplan DK, et al. The significance of pulmonary nodules detected on CT staging for lung cancer. Clin Radiol 1993;48(2):94–6.

46. Kunitoh H, Eguchi K, Yamada K, et al. Intrapulmonary sublesions detected before surgery in patients with lung cancer. Cancer 1992;70(7):1876–9.

47. Shimizu N, Ando A, Date H, et al. Prognosis of undetected intrapulmonary metastases in resected lung cancer. Cancer 1993;71(12):3868–72.

48. Lillington GA, Caskey CI. Evaluation and management of solitary multiple pulmonary nodules. Clin Chest Med 1993;14:111–9.

49. Good CA, Wilson TW. The solitary circumscribed pulmonary nodule. JAMA 1958;166:210–5.

50. Good CA. Management of patient with solitary mass in lung. Chic Med Soc Bull 1953;55:893–6.

51. Aoki T, Nakata H, Watanabe H, et al. Evolution of peripheral lung adenocarcinomas: CT findings correlated with histology and tumor doubling time. Am J Roentgenol 2000;174:763–8.

52. Hasegawa M, Sone S, Takashima S, et al. Growth rate of small lung cancers detected on mass CT screening. Br J Radiol 2000;73(876):1252–9.

53. Revel MP, Bissery A, Bienvenu M, et al. Are two-dimensional CT measurements of small noncalcified pulmonary nodules reliable? Radiology 2004;231(2): 453–8.

54. Erasmus JJ, Gladish GW, Broemeling L, et al. Interobserver and intraobserver variability in measurement of non-small-cell carcinoma lung lesions: implications for assessment of tumor response. J Clin Oncol 2003;21(13):2574–82.

55. Yankelevitz DF, Reeves AP, Kostis WJ, et al. Small pulmonary nodules: volumetrically determined growth rates based on CT evaluation. Radiology 2000;217(1):251–6.

56. Revel MP, Merlin A, Peyrard S, et al. Software volumetric evaluation of doubling times for differentiating benign versus malignant pulmonary nodules. Am J Roentgenol 2006;187(1):135–42.

57. Swensen SJ, Viggiano RW, Midthun DE, et al. Lung nodule enhancement at CT: multicenter study. Radiology 2000;214(1):73–80.

58. Yamashita K, Matsunobe S, Tsuda T, et al. Solitary pulmonary nodule: preliminary study of evaluation with incremental dynamic CT. Radiology 1995;194: 399–405.

59. Zhang M, Kono M. Solitary pulmonary nodules: evaluation of blood flow patterns with dynamic CT. Radiology 1997;205(2):471–8.

60. Shah SK, McNitt-Gray MF, Rogers SR, et al. Computer aided characterization of the solitary pulmonary nodule using volumetric and contrast

enhancement features. Acad Radiol 2005;12(10):1310–9.

61. Lowe VJ, Hoffman JM, DeLong DM, et al. Semiquantitative and visual analysis of FDG-PET images in pulmonary abnormalities. J Nucl Med 1994;35:1771–6.

62. Gould MK, Maclean CC, Kuschner WG, et al. Accuracy of positron emission tomography for diagnosis of pulmonary nodules and mass lesions: a meta-analysis. JAMA 2001;285(7):914–24.

63. Tan BB, Flaherty KR, Kazerooni EA, et al. American College of Chest Physicians. The solitary pulmonary nodule. Chest 2003;123(Suppl 1):89S–96S.

64. Gould MK, Ananth L, Barnett PG, et al. Veterans Affairs SNAP Cooperative Study Group. A clinical model to estimate the pretest probability of lung cancer in patients with solitary pulmonary nodules. Chest 2007;131(2):383–8.

65. Nomori H, Watanabe K, Ohtsuka T, et al. Evaluation of F-18 fluorodeoxyglucose (FDG) PET scanning for pulmonary nodules less than 3 cm in diameter, with special reference to the CT images. Lung Cancer 2004;45(1):19–27.

66. Lowe VJ, Fletcher JW, Gobar L, et al. Prospective investigation of PET in lung nodules (PIOPILN). J Clin Oncol 1998;16:1075–84.

67. Herder GJ, Golding RP, Hoekstra OS, et al. The performance of (18)F-fluorodeoxyglucose positron emission tomography in small solitary pulmonary nodules. Eur J Nucl Med Mol Imaging 2004;31:1231–6.

68. Erasmus JJ, McAdams HP, Patz EF Jr, et al. Evaluation of primary pulmonary carcinoid tumors using FDG PET. Am J Roentgenol 1998;170:1369–73.

69. Higashi K, Ueda Y, Seki H, et al. Fluorine-18-FDG PET imaging is negative in bronchioloalveolar lung carcinoma. J Nucl Med 1998;39(6):1016–20.

70. Sabloff BS, Truong MT, Wistuba II, et al. Bronchioalveolar cell carcinoma: radiologic appearance and dilemmas in the assessment of response. Clin Lung Cancer 2004;6(2):108–12.

71. Yi CA, Lee KS, Kim BT, et al. Tissue characterization of solitary pulmonary nodule: comparative study between helical dynamic CT and integrated PET/CT. J Nucl Med 2006;47(3):443–50.

72. Cook GJR, Wegner EA, Fogelman I. Pitfalls and artifacts in 18FDG PET and PET/CT oncologic imaging. Semin Nucl Med 2004;34(2):122–33.

73. Beyer T, Antoch G, Blodgett T, et al. Dual-modality PET/CT imaging: the effect of respiratory motion on combined image quality in clinical oncology. Eur J Nucl Med Mol Imaging 2003;30(4):588–96.

74. Osman MM, Cohade C, Nakamoto Y, et al. Respiratory motion artifacts on PET emission images obtained using CT attenuation correction on PET-CT. Eur J Nucl Med Mol Imaging 2003;30(4):603–6.

75. Goerres GW, Kamel E, Heidelberg TN, et al. PET-CT image co-registration in the thorax: influence of respiration. Eur J Nucl Med Mol Imaging 2002;29(3):351–60.

76. Goerres GW, Burger C, Kamel E, et al. Respiration-induced attenuation artifact at PET/CT: technical considerations. Radiology 2003;226(3):906–10.

77. Pan T, Mawlawi O, Nehmeh SA, et al. Attenuation correction of PET images with respiration-averaged CT images in PET/CT. J Nucl Med 2005;46(9):1481–7.

78. Truong MT, Pan T, Erasmus JJ. Pitfalls in integrated CT-PET of the thorax: implications in oncologic imaging. J Thorac Imaging 2006;21(2):111–22.

79. MacMahon H, Austin JH, Gamsu G, et al. Fleischner Society. Guidelines for management of small pulmonary nodules detected on CT scans: a statement from the Fleischner Society. Radiology 2005;237(2):395–400.

80. Gould MK, Fletcher J, Iannettoni MD, et al. American College of Chest Physicians. Evaluation of patients with pulmonary nodules: when is it lung cancer?: ACCP evidence-based clinical practice guidelines (2nd edition). Chest 2007;132(Suppl 3):108S–30S.

MDCT of Trachea and Main Bronchi

Cylen Javidan-Nejad, MD

KEYWORDS

• Tracheobronchial imaging • Trachea • Central airway
• Tracheomalacia

Diseases of the trachea and main bronchi are rare and present insidiously with nonspecific symptoms of dyspnea, cough, wheezing, and stridor. They commonly are misdiagnosed as asthma.[1]

Early recognition of tracheal disease is difficult, because the imaging findings are easily missed on imaging, such that the trachea has been regarded as the blind spot of the chest.[2] Timely diagnosis is further hampered, because symptoms of tracheal obstruction manifest only when the lesion occludes more than 75% of the tracheal lumen. At such point, the disease usually has advanced where similar therapeutic measures may not be feasible. If a tumor causes hemoptysis, it is discovered at an earlier stage.[3]

Once suspected, traditionally, many of these patients are evaluated by bronchoscopy, given its ability to directly visualize, biopsy, and sometimes treat lesions of the main airways. Bronchoscopy, however, is not well-tolerated by all patients, and it is associated with many complications, which can include minor ones, such as vasovagal reactions, nausea and vomiting, arrhythmias. More serious complications include sudden rise of intracranial pressure, pulmonary edema, laryngospasm, bronchospasm, and oxygen desaturation.[4] Furthermore, bronchoscopy is limited in evaluating the airway lumen beyond severe stenoses.[5] Therefore, for purposes of routine screening and treatment planning, a noninvasive method such as computed tomography (CT) is very helpful. With the advent and increased availability of multidetector CT, which allows fast volumetric image acquisition in a single breath hold and easy creation of two- and three-dimensional reformatted images of excellent quality, CT has become the imaging modality of choice for evaluating diseases of the trachea and main bronchi.[6,7]

MDCT TECHNIQUE

The inherent natural contrast of the lung parenchyma renders diagnostic imaging without use of intravenous contrast, at relatively lower radiation doses (110 to 140 kV and 50 to 80 mAs). The thinnest detector collimation is used when scanning. The newer multidetector scanners of 64 rows of detectors or more use detector collimators as thin as 0.625 mm. The images are reconstructed at a slice thickness of 1 mm, with 50% overlap, in the transaxial plane. A collimation of 0.625 mm creates a near-isometric resolution voxel of 0.4 mm.[8]

Imaging is performed twice, from the pharynx to the level of the first or second branching of the main bronchi, first at suspended end-inhalation, followed by scanning during active exhalation. The latter is performed only if there is a concern for tracheobronchomalacia. The advantage of active or forced exhalation is that it increases the sensitivity in diagnosis of subtle tracheobronchomalacia (**Fig. 1**).[9] Scanning should be performed only after coaching the patient with breathing instructions. For the dynamic exhalation portion of the examination, one should stress that the patient exhales without pursing his or her lips, because doing so artificially increases the intraluminal tracheal pressure, which may prevent manifestation of subtle tracheomalacia.[10]

To prevent scanning after the patient has finished active exhalation, it is imperative to know the fixed scan delay of the particular CT scanner being used. This is the time that lapses

Section of Cardiothoracic Imaging, Department of Radiology, Washington University School of Medicine, 510 South Kingshighway Blvd, Box 8131, St Louis, MO 63110, USA
E-mail address: javidanc@mir.wustl.edu

Radiol Clin N Am 48 (2010) 157–176
doi:10.1016/j.rcl.2009.10.003

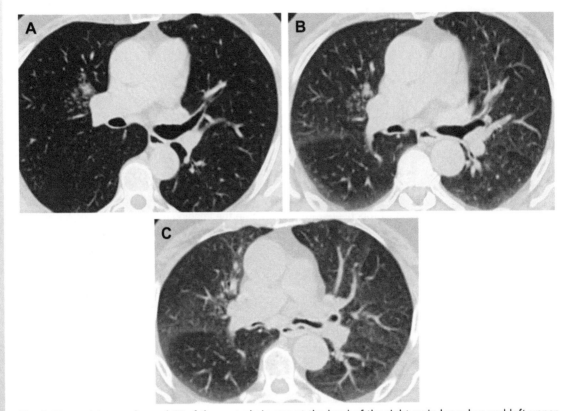

Fig. 1. Transaxial nonenhanced CT of the central airways at the level of the right main bronchus and left upper lobe bronchus in 49 year old man with chronic shortness of breath, not responding to treatment. The patient was imaged three times, per dynamic airway protocol, once at suspended end-inhalation (*A*), next at suspended end-expiration (*B*), and lastly during dynamic exhalation (*C*). The airways maintain normal caliber during suspended end-inhalation and end-expiration. However, when scanning was performed during active, forceful exhalation (*C*), marked narrowing of the lumina due to bronchial wall collapse is noted, diagnostic of bronchomalacia.

between when the technologist initiates the scan, and when the detectors rotate and imaging actually begins. Because forced exhalation only lasts 4 to 6 seconds, the scanning sequence should be as follows:

> The patient is told to take a deep breath
> The scanning is initiated
> Command to exhale is given only after that fixed time has transpired

The technologist must not use the automated patient instruction recording but should verbalize the command to exhale.[11]

The inherent motion artifact in the images of the lung parenchyma during active exhalation makes it difficult to use such images to diagnose coexisting small airway disease. For this reason, in the author's institution, the patient is scanned a third time, using a low-dose technique, from the thoracic inlet to the lung bases, at suspended end-exhalation to detect mosaic attenuation and air trapping.

Intravenous contrast is useful if tracheal stenosis is caused by a highly vascular mass such as a paraganglioma, or by extrinsic compression by a vessel, such as a pulmonary sling. Contrast use also improves visualization of segmental intraluminal bronchial masses, such as carcinoid tumors, which when arising in the segmental bronchi, cause postobstructive lung collapse and pneumonia, and may be obscured by the surrounding consolidated lung, unless intravenous contrast is used (**Fig. 2**).[8,11]

INTERPRETATION AND IMAGE AFTER PROCESSING

Interpretation should begin with viewing the transaxial images, with attention to the trachea and bronchial lumina and walls, and the surrounding mediastinal and hilar tissues. This initial screening allows a quick overview to identify disease, thereby directing the kind of postprocessed image to be created, to better display the abnormality.

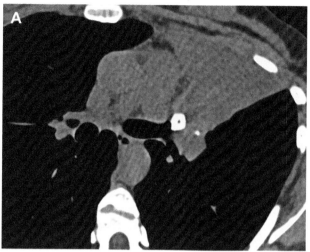
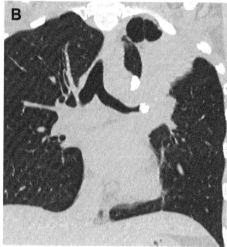

Fig. 2. Transaxial (*A*) and coronal (*B*) MPR images of nonenhanced CT of the chest in a 42-year old woman with chronic hemoptysis. A densely calcified broncholith, caused by erosion of calcified hilar lymph nodes into the airway lumina, obstructs the left upper lobe bronchus, causing complete collapse. The inherent dense calcification of this lesion makes it easily visible without use of intravenous contrast.

Multiplanar two- and three-dimensional reconstructed images not only provide a more anatomically meaningful portrayal of the airways, with use of such images, but also augment the identification of subtle and short segment airway stenosis. The relationship of mediastinal structures to the airways, depiction of the branching airways that have an oblique course relative to the transaxial plane, and understanding the craniocaudal extension of disease, are all understood better when employing such reformations.[11,12]

Two-dimensional multiplanar reformations (MPRs) in the coronal, sagittal, or oblique planes, can be created easily at the imaging PACS, or at a remote postprocessing station. These images display a section of single-voxel thickness, approximating 0.6 to 0.8 mm.[5,8] By creating an oblique coronal image aligned along the long axis of the trachea, to include the vocal cords and carina, one can create a single image of the trachea and main bronchi beyond what is visible with a laryngoscope (**Fig. 3**).[5]

Curved MPR is useful in measuring distances in a structure that has a nonlinear or curved axis. It involves straightening of that structure along its long axis and measuring distances between two points. It is also useful in obtaining a true cross-sectional diameter or area of that structure. It is crucial to create such images when stenosis or a lesion is measured in a bent or kinked trachea, which can be a normal tracheal alignment in older individuals. It also is used when a lesion or stenosis is located in a segmental bronchus or along a bronchial bifurcation, and accurate measurements of the lesion length, luminal narrowing, and distance from the carina need to be determined, for planning bronchoscopic stent placement or surgery.[7]

Three-dimensional multiplanar volume reformations display the combined information of a slab of chosen thickness in any given plane. If in such reformations, only the lowest attenuation pixels are projected in the chosen slab, a minimum intensity projection (MinIP) is created. This is useful for quickly displaying the distribution of air trapping and emphysema in the lung parenchyma. Its drawback in depicting airway disease is that it commonly underestimates the severity of asymmetric stenosis, to the extent that the intraluminal growth of a tumor can be missed. It is also very vulnerable to partial volume-averaging effects, leading to artificial decreased depiction of airway caliber, such that a severe stenosis can appear as airway total occlusion (**Fig. 4**).[7,8,12]

Creating volume-rendered reformatted images is based on isolating the surface of the luminal air column, by applying a segmentation threshold. If shading is applied to the other surface of these segmented data, a three-dimensional image of the entire tracheobronchial tree is generated. Such images are useful in providing an overview of pathology in the longitudinal plane. These images, similar to two- and three-dimensional MPRs, are subject to partial volume and stair step artifacts, and the degree of stenosis can be depicted inaccurately based on the threshold chosen for segmentation. CT bronchoscopy is a volume-rendered image where coloring similar to normal

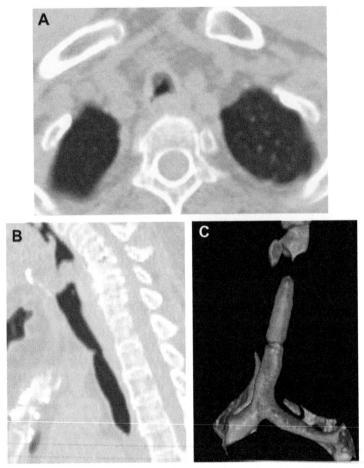

Fig. 3. Patient with history of prior intubation has stridor. Nonenhanced trachea CT shows a membrane-like soft-tissue extending into the tracheal lumen in the transaxial image (*A*). The sagittal reformatted image (*B*) best demonstrates that it has a shelf-like configuration and is located in the mid trachea, causing focal stenosis, due to prior intubation. Volume rendering (*C*) with arbitrary copper coloring, displays the waist-like short segment narrowing of the trachea. This technique involves post-processing where the surrounding lung parenchyma is segmented out to create an image only displaying the central airways. In this image the lung parenchyma posterior to the distal trachea and bilateral main bronchi have not been segmented out.

mucosa is applied to the segmented data as it is viewed from within. Many postprocessing engines allow navigating through the tracheal and bronchial lumina of these images, simulating a broncho-scopic experience (**Fig. 5**).[7,12]

It is of utmost importance that one should not overlook the transaxial CT images in favor of the postprocessed CT ones. The axial images are important to identify motion artifacts and various normal structures, which can easily simulate disease on postprocessed reformations. They are also valuable in evaluating the mediastinum and neighboring lung parenchyma.

CT OF NORMAL TRACHEA

The normal trachea measures approximately 10 to 12 cm in length, 2 to 4 cm of which are extrathoracic

and the remaining 6 to 8 cm in the thorax. The upper limits of normal for the trachea in the coronal and sagittal dimensions are 25 mm and 27 mm for men and 21 mm and 23 mm for women, respectively. The lower limit of normal in both coronal and sagittal planes is 13 mm for men and 11 mm for women. Pathologic widening or narrowing of the trachea refers to tracheal dimensions greater or less than these values, respectively.[13]

The tracheal wall gains its support through the horseshoe-shaped rings of hyaline cartilage, which uphold the anterior and lateral walls. A thin membrane comprises the posterior wall and is composed of smooth muscle and fibrous tissue.[14] The transaxial configuration of the trachea on CT is varied; it is usually round or oval in shape on inspiration, but it also can appear horseshoe-, triangular-, or pear-shaped.[15] On expiration, the

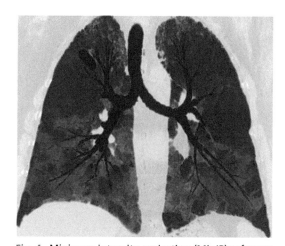

Fig. 4. Minimum intensity projection (MinIP) reformat of nonenhanced CT of a chest in a man who has undergone lung transplantation and suffers from chronic dyspnea. There are patchy areas of varying density. The low density areas represent air trapping and bronchiolitis obliterans (obliterative bronchiolitis), due to chronic rejection.

posterior membrane flattens or bows anteriorly, such that it decreases the sagittal diameter up to 30% in normal individuals.[14] Tracheal course in the chest can range from straight and vertical, to kinked and angled, where the trachea appears bent in more than one location, without focal narrowing.

The cartilaginous portion of the tracheal wall should not exceed 2 mm in thickness in normal individuals. Its posterior membrane is thinner and commonly imperceptible, detectable only because of the surrounding fat or obscured by the esophagus. Calcification of the tracheal cartilage is common in older individuals or patients receiving Coumadin (**Fig. 6**).[16]

TRACHEOBRONCHIAL DISEASES

Diseases of the central airways can be classified into two groups: those that cause luminal narrowing and those that cause luminal widening. Such grouping can be subdivided further, based on their extent of involvement, into localized or focal

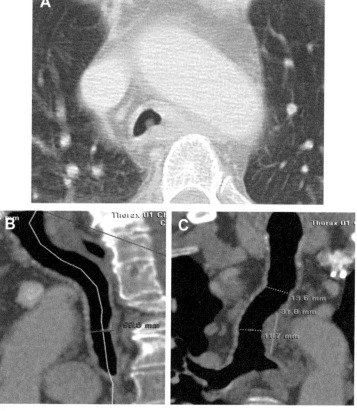

Fig. 5. Transaxial (A), curved MPR (B) and coronal reformatted images of CT of the airway shows a small lesion arising from that posterior wall of the trachea (A). Curved MPR helps measure the distance of this lesion from the carina (B) and creates a straightened image of the trachea, allowing the entire trachea to be seen on the coronal reformatted image (C). Biopsy revealed squamous cell carcinoma.

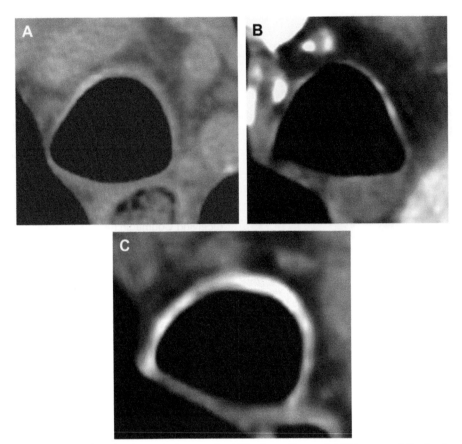

Fig. 6. Normal variation of tracheal morphology and calcification – Transaxial CT images of the trachea of three different people taken at suspended end-inhalation. Trachea can have an oval shape on cross-sectional imaging, where the cartilaginous portion of the wall is non-calcified (A). A triangular configuration with minimal calcification of the left lateral wall is also a normal appearance (B). Dense uniform calicification in a horse-shoe shaped trachea of an older woman, also a normal variation (C).

and long-segment or diffuse diseases. It is important to recognize that such grouping is arbitrary, as certain diseases can involve the airways in both focal and diffuse forms. Because most central airway diseases fall in the two categories of focal narrowing and diffuse narrowing, in this article, the discussion is limited to these two groupings.

FOCAL NARROWING

Short-segment luminal narrowing most commonly is caused by malignant or benign neoplasms arising from the airway, or by stenoses in the setting of prior trauma and medical intervention such as tracheostomy or endotracheal intubation. In daily practice, the most common intraluminal mass seen is mucus. Identifying air bubbles in this pseudolesion can help distinguish it from a polyp. Sometimes it is necessary to repeat the scan after the patient coughs to assess for

a change in morphology, to differentiate mucus from a mass (Fig. 7).[17]

Neoplasms

Primary malignant neoplasms
Primary tumors of the trachea and main bronchi are rare and represent only 1% of tracheobronchial neoplasms. Ninety percent of such tumors are malignant, and of those, 86% are caused by squamous cell carcinoma (SCC) and adenoid cystic carcinoma (ACC). Carcinoid and mucoepidermoid tumors occur with less frequency in the central airways.[3]

SCC is the most common primary malignancy of the central airways. It arises from the surface epithelium and is strongly associated with smoking. Forty percent of patients with airway SCC develop head and neck or lung cancers at a point in their lives. SCC affects men two to four times more often than women, and it frequently presents between the ages of 50 and 60. It is

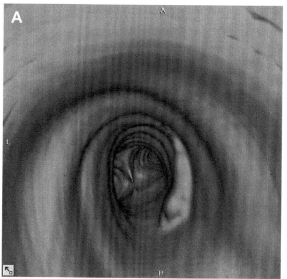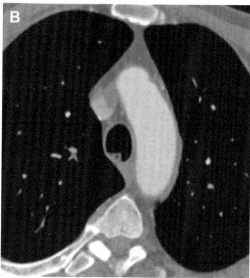

Fig. 7. Virtual bronchoscopy volume rendering of non-enhanced CT of the trachea (*A*) demonstrates a focal polyp-like lesion arising from the right inferolateral wall of the trachea. When the original transaxial CT image of the trachea (*B*) is viewed at that same level, the lesion appears to have bubbles of air within it. It is not a neoplasm, it is mucus.

commonly infiltrative, with a large exophytic component at the time of diagnosis. Mediastinal lymphadenopathy and pulmonary metastases are common. These lesions have high uptake on FDG-positron emission tomography (PET) imaging (**Fig. 8**).[18,19]

ACC is the most common lung cancer that arises from the salivary glands in the airway, and it is the second most common primary malignancy of the trachea. It is not associated with smoking and occurs with equal frequency among men

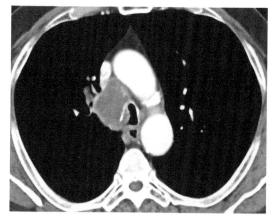

Fig. 8. Fifty six year old man with long history of smoking has hemoptysis. Non-enhanced transaxial CT of chest reveals a mass arising from the right tracheal wall, growing both into the lumen and exo-phytically, infiltrating the mediastinum.

and women. Its age of occurrence is at a younger age than SCC, most commonly in the fourth decade of life. It occurs mostly in the trachea and proximal bronchi. ACC appears as an intraluminal focal mass on bronchoscopy and even CT, but because it grows along the submucosa of the airway, there is circumferential wall thickening of the airway with infiltrative growth along a long craniocaudal segment, best appreciated on coronal and sagittal MPR images. ACC grows slowly and rarely is associated with regional lymphadenopathy or distant metastases. It shows variable FRG uptake on PET imaging, where the higher the grade of the tumor, the more avid the FDG uptake (**Fig. 9**).[18,19]

Mucoepidermoid carcinoma (MEC) and carcinoid tumors are other primary malignancies of the airways and relative to SCC and ACC, they arise in the more distal airways, most commonly in the lobar and segmental bronchi. MEC is a tumor arising from the minor salivary glands, but it is more rare than ACC. Carcinoid tumors are neuroendocrine neoplasms that can excrete hormones and neuroamines, such as corticotropin (ACTH), serotonin, somatostatin, and bradykinin. Based on the mitotic activity of the tumor cells, its grading ranges from low-grade typical tumors, to intermediate-grade atypical locally aggressive tumors, to high-grade small cell carcinoma.[18,19]

MEC and carcinoid tumors have many common features. Both present with hemoptysis and symptoms of lung collapse and repeated infections, and

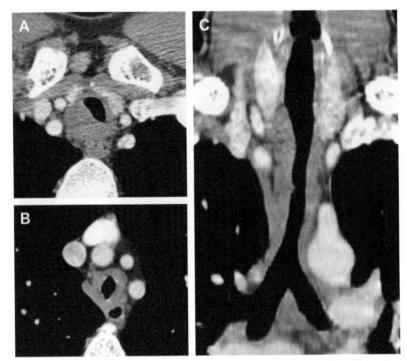

Fig. 9. Thirty five year old man with several months of stridor has a contrast-enhanced CT of the chest to further evaluate the cause. Transaxial image of the trachea at the level of the thoracic inlet (*A*) shows a large mass arising from the right posterolateral tracheal wall, obstructing more than half the luminal area. There is circumferential tracheal wall thickening, seen both at the level of the mass and on the transaxial image of trachea lower in the chest (*B*), at the level of the great vessels of the superior mediastinum. Coronal reformation (*C*) best demonstrates the craniocaudal growth of this tumor along the tracheal wall, which upon biopsy was proven to be adenoidcystic carcinoma.

neither is associated with smoking or shows gender predilection. On CT and bronchoscopy, they appear as smooth-margined or lobulated, oval or round endoluminal masses (Fig. 10). Both can have internal calcifications. CT shows that these masses arise from the airway wall, causing focal wall thickening, which helps differentiate such lesions from benign airway tumors, which lack wall invasion. Postobstructive atelectasis, mucus plugging, and repeated pneumonia are frequent features. Because both lesions are vascular, they demonstrate enhancement with contrast. The degree of enhancement is variable (Fig. 11).[18,19]

Metastases

Metastases to the trachea and main bronchi are commonly caused by local invasion, such as thyroid, laryngeal, esophageal, and lung cancers. More rarely endoluminal metastases are caused by hematogenous spread from primary malignancies such as colorectal, breast, and renal cell carcinoma, sarcomas, melanoma, and hematogenous malignancies such plasmacytoma and granulocytic carcinoma or chloroma. Such metastases are diagnosed, on average, 4 years after the

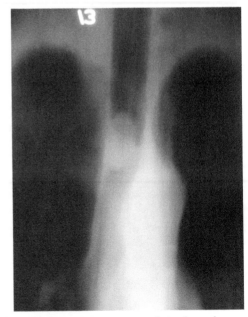

Fig. 10. Coronal tomogram of trachea shows an oblong-shaped mass growing endoluminally in the lower trachea, which was a mucoepidermoid carcinoma. Before the widespread availability of CT, such tomograms were routinely used in evaluating the trachea.

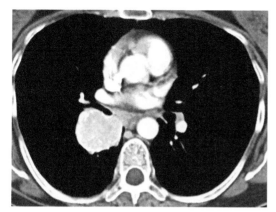

Fig. 11. Forty one year old woman with hemoptysis and chronic cough is further evaluated by contrast-enhanced CT of the chest. Transaxial image at the level of the lower lobe bronchi shows a large enhancing mass arising from the left lower lobe bronchus.

primary malignancy has been discovered. Hemoptysis and coughing are the most common presenting symptoms. CT can detect such metastases and direct bronchoscopy for biopsy.[20]

Metastatic lesions are usually solitary, but they may be multiple. They could have imaging features simulating primary tracheal malignancies such as squamous cell and adenoidcystic carcinoma. If they occur in the main bronchi, they can present with lobar collapse. A prior history of extratracheal malignancy is most helpful in determining the etiology of such lesions (**Fig. 12**).[1,19]

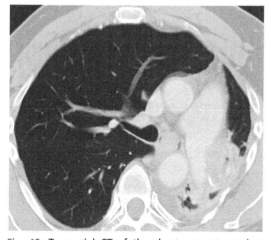

Fig. 12. Transaxial CT of the chest reconstructed at lung window settings in a patient with known history of melanoma shows a mass occupying the entire lumen of the left main bronchus, causing near-complete collapse of the left lung with marked shift of the mediastinum into the left hemithorax.

Benign neoplasm

Benign neoplasms of the trachea are much less common than malignant ones, and they have the common appearance of focal, well-defined intraluminal lesions that do not invade the tracheal wall or adjacent mediastinum. Of these, squamous cell papillomas and polyps are the most common.[21]

Squamous cell papillomas are benign neoplasms, and they have two forms: multiple or juvenile laryngotracheal papillomatosis, and solitary, which is less frequent and occurs in adults. The multiple form, or laryngotracheal papillomatosis, is caused by infection with human papillomavirus types 6 and 11, acquired by birth or by sexual transmission. It most commonly presents in children younger than 4 years of age, and it begins as a laryngeal mass. In a fraction of such children, especially if incompletely treated, multiple trachea and bronchial polyps develop later in adolescence or young adulthood, as a result of endobronchial dissemination. When the distal airways are involved, these lesions manifest as pulmonary nodules that usually cavitate. Such patients can present with repeated infections and symptoms of airway obstruction. Medical management and surgical management are aimed at slowing the rate of papilloma growth using antiviral and cytotoxic agents, and excision of endoluminal lesions using electrocautery, cryotherapy, and CO_2 laser. The high risk of malignant transformation of such lesions warrants continued surveillance by CT and bronchoscopy, especially when pulmonary nodules have developed.[21,22]

The term polyp is attributed to the solitary form of squamous cell papillomas. They are also called inflammatory, or fibroepithelial polyps and are more common in middle-aged smokers. They are believed to be caused by chronic mucosal irritation, either by hot or corrosive gases, endobronchial foreign bodies, or by broncholiths. These lesions usually regress after removal of the caustic agent and do not have a high tendency for malignant transformation (**Fig. 13**).[21]

Non-neoplastic Etiologies

Iatrogenic and post-traumatic stenoses
Strictures most commonly are caused by iatrogenic means, where the inflated cuff of an endotracheal or tracheostomy tube inserts local pressure on the tracheal mucosa and cartilage of the subglottic trachea and impedes blood flow. This leads to ischemic necrosis and eccentric or circumferential intimal hyperplasia and luminal stenosis. Less commonly, similar stenosis is located several centimeters above the carina, caused by the tip of the endotracheal tube or tracheostomy tube

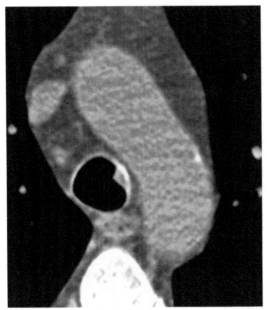

Fig. 13. Transaxial image of nonenhanced CT of the airway of a smoker reveals a solitary polyp arising from the left lateral wall of the lower trachea. Benign lesions have the common feature of being well-circumscribed and do not cause tracheal wall thickening or extend into the mediastinum.

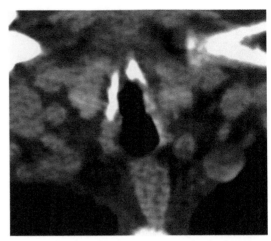

Fig. 14. Nonenhanced transaxial CT of the trachea of a patient with history of prior tracheostomy and stridor, shows narrowing of the tracheal lumen a few centimeter below the vocalcords. The lateral walls of the trachea have collapsed inward and there is a defect along the anterior midline of the tracheal arc-like cartilage.

damaging the tracheal wall, causing focal mucosal and cartilage ischemia and damage. Tracheostomy tubes, at the site of the stoma, permanently damage the anterior arc-like cartilaginous ring along the midline, resulting in inward collapse of the lateral walls of the trachea with associated focal scarring and irregular wall thickening. Regardless of the cause, the stenosis can develop/or manifest much later than the traumatic event. The location of stenosis, history of endotracheal intubation or tracheostomy, and in stomal injury, the typical morphology of the cartilaginous ring deformity, help one correctly identify the iatrogenic etiology of the stenosis (**Fig. 14**).[23]

Traumatic injury of the airway is caused, either by perforation of the tracheal wall at the time of intubation, by blunt trauma to the trachea, or by shearing injury to the main stem bronchi located where the bronchi are anchored to the hilar pleura. These injuries heal with strictures, commonly creating an hourglass configuration of the airway lumen.[1,23,24]

CT imaging depicts the site, morphology, length, and location of the tracheal narrowing. Because the wall thickening is sometimes thin and web-like, coronal, sagittal, and curved MPRs are needed to detect it, given the increased sensitivity of such techniques in revealing subtle stenoses. They are also necessary to accurately measure luminal dimensions, length of stenosis, and distance from the vocal chords or carina; all information needed for treatment planning. The narrowing is typically less than 3 cm in length and is either symmetric or eccentric, causing an hourglass-shaped stenosis.[24]

DIFFUSE NARROWING

Narrowing of the airway beyond a length of 3 cm is considered long-segment narrowing.[24] There are many causes of diffuse tracheobronchial luminal narrowing. For ease of discussion, they can be categorized into two groups, based on the absence or presence of airway wall thickening. It is important to note that many of the inflammatory, infiltrative, and infectious diseases of the airway that cause narrowing associated with diffuse smooth or nodular wall thickening become fibrotic in their later stages, causing cicatricial stenosis without much wall thickening.

DIFFUSE NARROWING WITHOUT WALL THICKENING
Saber Sheath Trachea

Saber sheath trachea occurs in the setting of chronic obstructive lung disease. Luminal narrowing affects only the coronal diameter of the intrathoracic trachea, sparing the extrathoracic portion. It is usually asymptomatic and an incidental finding on chest radiographs and CT. Sometimes mild tracheomalacia on expiratory images is discovered (see **Fig. 13**).[14]

Tracheobronchomalacia

Tracheobronchomalacia is another cause of diffuse narrowing without associated airway wall thickening. The diffuse pattern, best diagnosed with dynamic expiratory imaging, can manifest as either inward collapse of the tracheal cartilage or exaggerated anterior collapse of the posterior membrane, and it can be associated with abnormal cross-sectional morphology of trachea, where the coronal diameter exceeds that of the sagittal diameter, creating a flattened, frown-shaped appearance of the trachea on CT.[15,25] Commonly, a decrease of 50% of the cross-sectional area is used as the criteria for diagnosis; however, Boiselle and colleagues[26] have demonstrated a wide range of airway collapsibility in normal individuals. They therefore suggested applying a threshold of 75% of decreased cross-sectional luminal area for more specificity (Fig. 15).

Tracheobronchomalacia can be seen in chronic obstructive pulmonary disease. In such situations, the luminal narrowing is caused by exaggerated anterior bowing of the posterior membrane, rather than collapse of the cartilaginous wall.[27] If focal, malacia is more likely caused by focal congenital partial or complete absence of a cartilaginous ring, or as the sequelae of trauma or focal infection. Vascular rings are associated with focal tracheobronchomalacia, possibly because of chronic airway compression.[28]

Mounier-Kuhn disease, or congenital tracheobronchomegaly, is associated with diffuse tracheomalacia in its moderate and severe forms. It is caused by congenital abnormality of the connective tissue of the airway cartilage and membranes between the cartilaginous rings, which manifests relatively later in life, especially if the individual is a smoker. Although this entity is usually discussed as a cause of diffuse luminal widening, it is mentioned here in cases where the tracheomalacia is severe and CT imaging is performed at end-expiration; the airway collapses, and it appears diffusely narrowed. CT taken on inspiration is diagnostic in displaying that abnormally enlarged caliber of the central airways (Fig. 16).[29,30]

DIFFUSE NARROWING WITH WALL THICKENING
Acute Inflammation

Airway wall thickening causing long-segment luminal narrowing can be seen with acute tracheal inflammation. This can be caused by inhalation of noxious fumes but is more commonly caused by an acute or subacute infection. In children, such tracheal swelling most commonly is caused by parainfluenza virus, resulting in layngotracheobronchitis (croup).[31] Ventilator-associated tracheobronchitis is a common nosocomial infection of adults hospitalized in the intensive care unit. It predominantly is caused by gram-negative bacteria, and it is

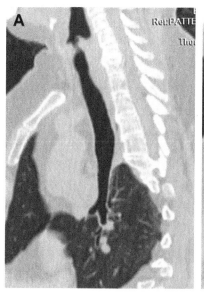
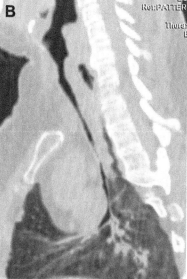

Fig. 15. Fifty one year old woman with chronic cough and wheezing. Coronal multiplanar reformats of CT of chest performed at suspended end inhalation (*A*) and during forced exhalation (*B*), according to the dynamic trachea protocol, shows marked exaggerated relaxation of the posterior membrane of the entire intrathoracic trachea, causing severe diffuse narrowing, with areas of complete luminal obliteration.

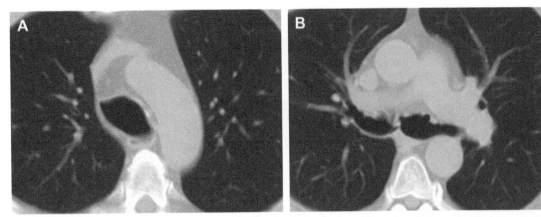

Fig. 16. Transaxial CT images of the chest, at the levels of the trachea (*A*) and main bronch (*B*) demonstrate marked enlargement of the lumina of the trachea and main bronchi in patient with Mounier-Kuhn syndrome. The configuration of the trachea on cross sectional is such that the coronal diameter exceeds the sagittal diameter, a morphology indicative of tracheomalacia.

associated with fever, cough, increased sputum production, and associated lower respiratory tract inflammation, in the absence of pneumonia. CT and bronchoalveolar lavage with cultures are most helpful in diagnosis.[32]

Invasive tracheal aspergillosis is a rare and highly fatal cause of progressive airway obstruction in immunocompromised patients. Ulcerative tracheobronchitis after lung transplantation initially is limited to the anastomosis sites of the main bronchi, due to the relative ischemia, but it can spread to involve the trachea also. Ulceration, necrosis, and pseudomembrane formation are pathologic features. On CT, nonspecific diffuse wall thickening of the central airways is noted; however, generally diagnosis is made by bronchoscopy. Treatment is debridement of the affected mucosa, in addition to oral antifungal therapy (**Fig. 17**).[33–35]

Chronic Infection

Rhinoscleroma is a chronic granulomatous infection caused by *Klebsiella rhinoscleromatis*. It is an endemic disease in Guatemala, El Salvador, Egypt, India, Indonesia, Poland, Hungary, and Russia. It usually affects the nasal mucosa, but can involve the larynx, and much less commonly, the tracheobronchial tree. It progresses slowly if untreated, with periods of remissions and relapse, eventually causing extensive airway destruction. CT findings are subglottic stricture and nodular

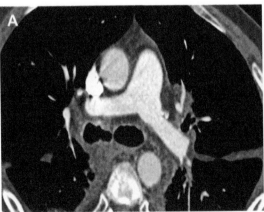
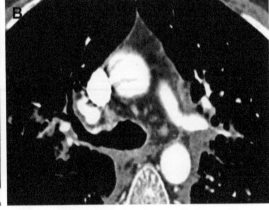

Fig. 17. Thirty nine year old man hospitalized after bilateral lung transplantation has low grade fevers. No pneumonia was identified, however on transaxial images of contrast-enhanced CT of the chest at the levels of the main bronchi (*A*) and right upper lobe bronchus (*B*) diffuse wall thickening of the airway is noted, causing luminal narrowing, especially of the right main bronchus. The surround fat planes are indistinct due to inflammatory changes. Biopsy revealed aspergillus in the airway wall, with mucosal ulceration, consistent with invasive tracheobronchial aspergillosis.

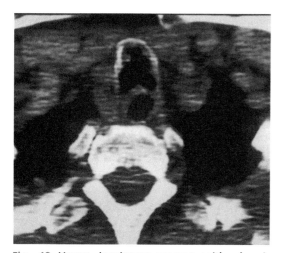

Fig. 18. Young immigrant woman with chronic cough. Transaxial image of CT of chest shows multiple noncalcified nodules arising from the tracheal wall. Biopsy revealed Klebsiella rhinoscleroma infection of the airways.

wall thickening of the trachea and central bronchi, leading to concentric narrowing of their lumens. There is no associated calcification. The involvement can be localized or diffuse. The mainstay of treatment is surgical debridement and prolonged antibiotic therapy (Fig. 18).[24,36,37]

Tuberculosis (TB) of the tracheobronchial tree is seen much less frequently with current improved antibiotic treatment regimens. The stenosis caused by TB can manifest in the setting of acute infection or several years later. It typically involves the distal trachea and main bronchi. It spreads to the central airways by peribronchial lymphatic pathways and by local extension from adjacent TB lymphadenitis.[23] The disease begins as edema and lymphocytic infiltration of the airway submucosa and tubercle formation. The granulation tissue destroys and replaces the mucosa, leading to fibrosis and airway stenosis. In the acute phase, the disease involves the main bronchi symmetrically; however, late, fibrotic TB is more common in the left mainstem bronchus. Mediastinal lymphadenopathy is common. On CT, there is diffuse circumferential

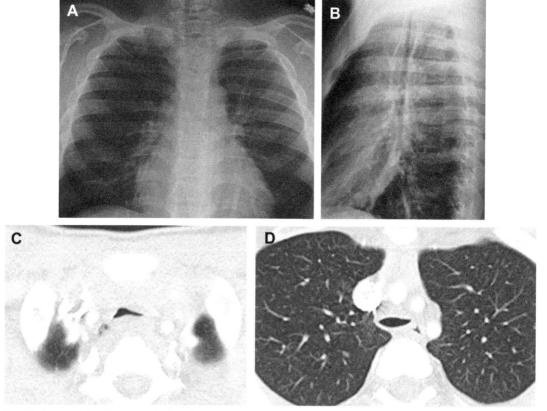

Fig. 19. Transaxial CT images of the chest at the levels of extrathoracic (A) and intrathoracic trachea (B) of a 21 year old man with chronic cough and repeated pneumonia shows diffuse tracheomalacia where the trachea appears flattened (C, D).

thickening of distal tracheal and bronchial walls, with irregular luminal narrowing and peribronchial soft tissue thickening, involving a long segment of the airway.[38,39]

Diffuse laryngeotracheobronchial papillomatosis can have numerous polypoid lesions involving the airway mucosa, causing nodular wall thickening and luminal narrowing. The lesions are not calcified. Parenchymal cavitary nodules are common when there is extensive disease.[24]

Relapsing Polychondritis

Relapsing polychondritis (RP) is a rare multisystem disorder characterized by recurrent inflammation and destruction of cartilage. Fifty percent of patients with RP develop respiratory tract involvement at some point of their disease. Airway involvement is a poor prognostic sign and is the leading cause of death. Its cause is unknown; however, an immune-mediated mechanism is postulated. It can develop at any age, but most commonly is diagnosed in the fourth and fifth decades of life. It is more frequent in whites and shows no gender predilection.[40]

The most common findings on inspiratory CT are smooth and diffuse airway wall thickening, sparing the posterior membrane, and increased airway wall attenuation, which ranges from a subtle increase to frank calcification. Progressive

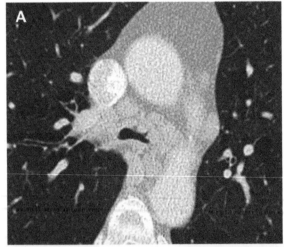

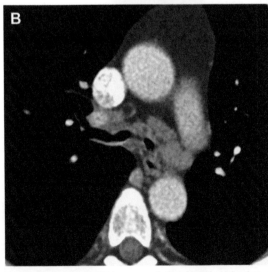
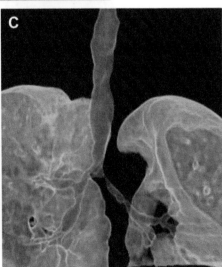

Fig. 20. Nonenhanced CT images of a woman with chronic cough and known diagnosis of C-ANCA positive granulomatosis of the lungs, shows nodular non-calcified soft tissue thickening around the airways at the level of the carina (A), causing luminal narrowing as evidenced on the transaxial image of the trachea (B). Volume rendered post-processed image (C) in the coronal plane shows marked nodular wall narrowing of the distal trachea, bilateral main and lobar bronchi.

cartilage calcification frequently is seen over serial imaging. Both the trachea and main bronchi are involved equally. Luminal narrowing is diffuse, but not always the predominant feature. Although the wall thickening is most commonly smooth, nodular thickening can sometimes occur. Tracheobronchomalacia is considered a key feature of this disease, and may be the only airway abnormality detected on CT, early in the process. If appropriate dynamic expiratory CT is performed, tracheomalacia and air trapping are detected in over 90% of such patients. Fixed airway narrowing occurs when fibrosis sets in after chronic inflammation (**Fig. 19**).[41,42]

Wegener Granulomatosis

Wegener or C-ANCA positive granulomatosis is characterized by necrotizing granulomatous inflammation and necrotizing vascultis affecting the small arteries, veins and capillaries. It has a predilection for the upper respiratory tract, such as the sinuses and nasal mucosa, the kidneys, and the lungs. Tracheobronchial involvement occurs in 50% of patients, usually in conjunction with disease manifestation elsewhere. Subglottic stenosis is the most frequent airway manifestation. Sometimes the airway involvement is isolated, leading to delayed diagnosis. Occasionally after successful remission with immunosuppressive therapy of other manifestations of disease elsewhere, the airway involvement either

is diagnosed for the first time or continues to progress to scarring and stenosis (**Fig. 20**).[24,43]

Patients younger than 30 years old are more prone to having airway involvement. Common symptoms are dyspnea, wheezing, and hemoptysis, usually from concomitant pulmonary disease with alveolar hemorrhage. CT shows focal or long segments of circumferential mass-like wall thickening of the trachea and bronchi, associated with thickening and calcification of the cartilaginous rings. Mucosal ulceration noted on bronchoscopy may be hard to identify on CT. Bronchiectasis and peribronchial thickening of small airways are common. Airway lesions demonstrate partial or complete improvement with treatment. Tracheomalacia or bronchomalacia can occur as a result of the chronic inflammation.[43]

Amyloidosis

Tracheobronchial amyloidosis (TBA) is a rare disease that results from abnormal extracellular deposition of amyloid and autologous fibrillar proteins in a beta-pleated sheet configuration, which leads to formation of submucosal plaques or nodules. It can be associated with systemic disease, or isolated to the trachea. Patients present with nonspecific symptoms of chronic cough or wheezing, and diagnosis is based on biopsy, which shows green birefringence of Congo-red stained deposits when viewed under polarized light. TBA is more common in men,

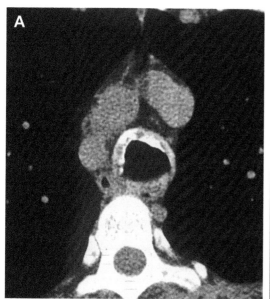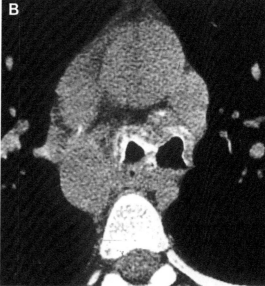

Fig. 21. Amyloidosis of the airway causing diffuse calcification and wall thickening of the trachea (*A*) and bilateral main bronchi (*B*) on transaxial images of nonenhanced CT of the chest.

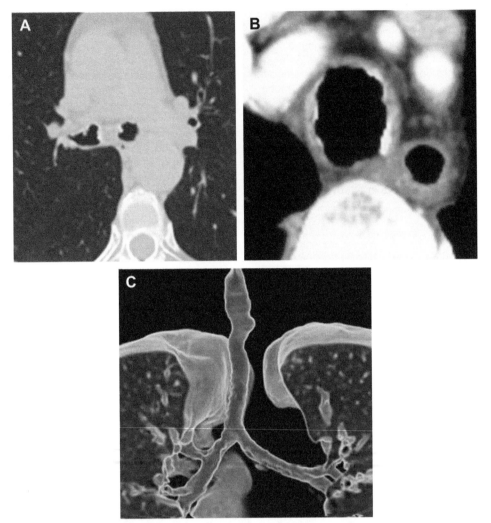

Fig. 22. Tracheobronchopathia osteochondroplastica causing calcified nodules protruding into the tracheal lumen (*A*) and causing luminal narrowing of the main bronchi (*B*) on transaxial CT images of the chest. Volume-rendered post-processed image (*C*) shows the distribution of disease.

most commonly first presenting in the fifth and sixth decades of life.[24,44,45]

CT findings include focal or diffuse irregular and asymmetric wall thickening, with mural calcifications, causing luminal narrowing. Concentric or eccentric structuring is a possible associated finding. It can involve anywhere from the trachea to the segmental bronchi in contiguous segments.[24] Nodular thickening can occlude the airway lumen, causing atelectasis, postobstructive pneumonia, or air trapping. Magnetic resonance imaging (MRI) can be helpful, where the amyloid deposits show intermediate T1-signal intensity and low T2-signal intensity (**Fig. 21**).[44]

There is no established treatment for TBA. Resection is not curative, and lesions recur 6 to 12 months after surgery.[24] External-beam radiation therapy has been shown to improve pulmonary function, with visible improvement on CT and bronchoscopy.[45]

Sarcoidosis

Tracheal and bronchial stenosis in association with sarcoidosis is unusual. Airway involvement can occur in the absence of lung parenchymal manifestations of sarcoidosis. The larynx and lobar bronchi are affected more commonly than the trachea. When it occurs, tracheal stenosis is a late manifestation of disease. The progressive luminal stenosis with smooth or nodular wall thickening may be treated with prolonged courses of corticosteroids and repeated tracheal dilations.[24,31,46]

Tracheobronchopathia Osteochondroplastica

Tracheobronchopathia osteochondroplastica (tracheopathia osteoplastica TPOP) is a disease of the distal trachea and mainstem and lobar bronchi, causing nodular narrowing of the airway lumina. It is caused by benign proliferation of bone and cartilage, creating numerous 1 to 3 mm nodules in the submucosa of the cartilaginous portion of the airway wall. It spares the posterior membranous wall of the trachea. On pathologic specimens in the submucosa, cartilaginous and osseous islands of tissue with close association to the perichondrium are found. Foci of bone marrow with active hematopoiesis also are identified. One theory of its histogenesis is that the nodules are ecchondroses and exosostoses of the cartilaginous rings.[47]

It usually is discovered incidentally in adults in their fourth and fifth decades of life. Women and men are affected equally, and there is no association with smoking. The presence or lack of symptoms depends on the degree of luminal narrowing. Symptoms range from none to coughing, hoarseness, wheezing, and hemoptysis. A superimposed infection may spur on the onset of symptoms. The disease sometimes is discovered because of difficult intubation.[48]

On chest radiography, nodular, long-segment narrowing of the trachea is noted on the frontal radiograph only. CT best demonstrates the dense or calcified nodules protruding into the airway lumen, narrowing it along the coronal diameter. The presence of nodules in TPOP differentiates it from saber-sheath trachea, which also narrows

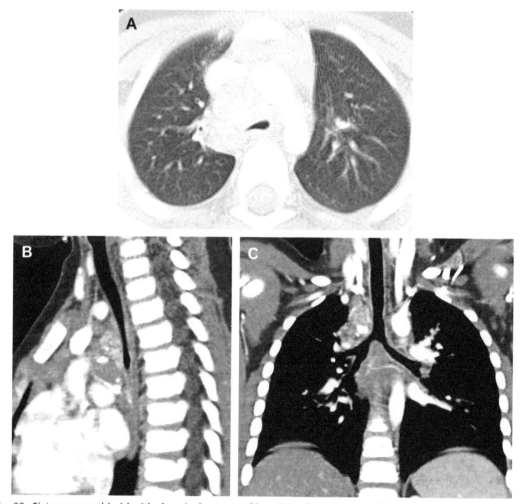

Fig. 23. Sixteen-year-old girl with chronic shortness of breath and past history of histoplasmosis causing mediastinal lymphadenopathy several years ago, has a CT of chest to evaluate the cause. Transaxial image at the level of the trachea (*A*) shows luminal narrowing by external compression of the anterior wall. Sagittal (*B*) and coronal (*C*) double-oblique reformatted images show a long segment of tracheal narrowing by a large calcified mediastinal mass due to fibrosing mediastinitis.

the coronal diameter, but has no wall thickening (Fig. 22).[47,48]

The main differential diagnosis consists of amyloidosis, Wegener granulomatosis, and lymphoma, which also can have submucosal nodules. These entities do not spare the posterior wall of the trachea. Occasionally pathology is necessary to confirm the diagnosis.

TPOP is easily differentiated from tracheobronchial papillomatosis, as the latter lacks calcification of the submucosal nodules and is associated with parenchymal nodules. In TPOP, the mediastinal fat is intact, thereby differentiating it from mediastinal fibrosis, which also can calcify. Nodular wall thickening in RP is rare. Another entity easily confused with TPOP is diffuse tracheobronchial chondrocalcification, which is normal in older individuals, but can be seen prematurely with warfarin use. This form of chondral calcification can be discontinuous, simulating nodules. The calcifications, however, never protrude into the lumen to cause narrowing (Fig. 23).[47,48]

The goal of treatment is to provide symptomatic relief and varies from patient to patient.

Severe conditions that are complicated by bleeding, severe obstructive symptoms, or recurrent infections require more aggressive intervention. Bronchoscopic therapeutic methods can be used, which include endobronchial Nd:YAG laser photoevaporation, coring through rigid bronchoscopy, and stenting.[47,48]

Fibrosing Mediastinitis

Fibrosing mediastinitis (FM) or sclerosing mediastinitis is rare condition where there is excessive fibrous tissue deposition in the mediastinum. Its exact cause is unknown, and it has been postulated that it is caused by an immunologic reaction to an infection or other allergens. CT demonstrates localized or diffuse and confluent soft tissue, commonly calcified, in the mediastinum and hila, which obliterate the normal fat planes and compress the neighboring vessels and airways. If associated with histoplasmosis and other granulomatous diseases, calcified mediastinal lymph nodes also are seen. Tracheobronchial narrowing occurs in severe cases, where vascular involvement is already present. The cicatricial and infiltrative nature of the disease process causes localized or long-segment airway narrowing with irregular wall thickening.[49,50]

Other Non-neoplastic Causes

Inflammatory bowel disease, such as Crohn and ulcerative colitis, and other inflammatory diseases such as Behcet syndrome rarely can cause tracheobronchitis.[14,24] Ulcerative colitis is the most common frequent of these to involve the airways. Almost always the airway involvement is discovered after the gastrointestinal manifestations have developed. The mechanism of wall thickening is mucosal ulceration, diffuse and chronic submucosal inflammation, leading to fibrosis and irregular wall thickening and luminal stenosis.[51]

SUMMARY

Tracheobronchial imaging has undergone a major revolution since the advent of MDCT. The improved spatial and temporal resolution not only allows reformatting images that enhance the comprehension of disease before bronchoscopy or surgery, it has introduced newer techniques such as dynamic expiratory imaging to evaluate for tracheomalacia, which can be a subtle, but a confounding entity for patients and clinician alike. Tracheobronchial diseases can be arbitrarily divided into those that cause focal and diffuse narrowing and widening. Such groupings can help develop a practical approach in evaluating diseases of the central airways.

REFERENCES

1. Kwong JS, Muller NL, Miller RR. Diseases of the trachea and main-stem bronchi: correlation of CT with pathologic findings. Radiographics 1992;12:645–57.
2. Berkmen YM. The trachea: the blind spot in the chest. Radiol Clin North Am 1984;22:539–62.
3. Naidich DP, Webb WR, Grenier PA, et al. Imaging of the airways—functional and radiologic correlations. Philadelphia: Lippincott Williams Wilkins; 2005. p. 70–105.
4. British Thoracic Society Bronchoscopy Guidelines Committee. British Thoracic Society guidelines on diagnostic flexible bronchoscopy. Thorax 2001; 56(Suppl 1):1–21.
5. Koletsis EN, Kalogeropoulou C, Prodromaki E, et al. Tumoral and nontumoral trachea stenoses: evaluation with three-dimensional CT and virtual bronchoscopy. J Cardiothorac Surg 2007;2:18.
6. Prokop M. General principles of MDCT. Eur J Radiol 2003;45:S4–10.
7. Boiselle PM, Ernst A. Recent advances in central airway imaging. Chest 2002;121(5):1651–60.
8. Beigelman-Aubry C, Brillet PY, Grenier PA. MDCT of the airways: technique and normal results. Radiol Clin North Am 2009;47:185–201.
9. Baroni RH, Feller-Kopman D, Nishino M, et al. Tracheobronchomalacia: comparison between end-expiratory and dynamic expiratory CT for evaluation of central airway collapse. Radiology 2005;235(2):635–41.
10. Bankier AA, O'Donnell CR, Boiselle PM. Quality initiatives—respiratory instructions for CT examinations of

the lungs: a hands-on guide. Radiographics 2008;28: 919–31.

11. Boiselle PM, Lee KS, Ernst A. Multidetector CT of the central airways. J Thorac Imaging 2005;20(3):186–95.

12. Grenier PA, Beigelman-Aubry C, Fetita C, et al. New frontiers in CT imaging of airway disease. Eur Radiol 2002;12:1022–44.

13. Breatnach E, Abbott GC, Fraser AG. Dimensions of the normal human trachea. AJR Am J Roentgenol 1984;142:903–6.

14. Webb EM, Elicker BM, Webb WR. Pictorial essay-using CT to diagnose non-neoplastic tracheal abnormalities: appearance of the tracheal wall. AJR Am J Roentgenol 2000;174:1315–21.

15. Boiselle PM, Ernst A. Tracheal morphology in patients with tracheomalacia: prevalence of inspiratory lunate and expiratory "frown" shapes. J Thorac Imaging 2006;21(3):190–6.

16. Joshi A, Berdon WE, Ruzal-Shapiro C, et al. CT detection of tracheobronchial calcification in an 18-year-old on maintenance warfarin sodium therapy: cause and effect? AJR Am J Roentgenol 2000;175(3):921–2.

17. Westra D, Verbeeten B Jr. Some anatomical variants and pitfalls in computed tomography of the trachea and mainstem bronchi. I. Mucoid pseudotumors. Diagn Imaging Clin Med 1985;54(5):229–39.

18. Park CM, Goo JM, Lee HJ, et al. Tumors in the tracheobronchial tree: CT and FDG PET features. Radiographics 2009;29:55–71.

19. Ferretti GR, Bithigoffer C, Righini CA, et al. Imaging of tumors of the trachea and central bronchi. Radiol Clin North Am 2009;47:227–41.

20. Durdun AB, Demirag F, Sokak ME, et al. Endobronchial metastases: a clinicopathological analysis. Respirology 2005;10(4):510–4.

21. Ko JM, Jung JI, Park SH, et al. Benign tumors of the tracheobronchial tree: CT–pathologic correlation. AJR Am J Roentgenol 2006;186:1304–13.

22. Bondaryev A, Makris D, Breen DP, et al. Airway stenting for severe endobronchial papillomatosis. Respiration 2009;77:455–8.

23. Grenier PA, Beigelman-Aubry C, Brillet PY. Nonneoplatic tracheal and bronchial stenosis. Radiol Clin North Am 2009;47:243–60.

24. Prince JS, Duhamel DR, Levin DL, et al. Nonneoplastic lesions of the tracheobronchial wall: radiologic findings with bronchoscopic correlation. Radiographics 2002;22:S215–30.

25. Carden KA, Boiselle PM, Waltz DA, et al. Tracheomalacia and tracheobronchomalacia in children and adults. Chest 2005;127:984–1005.

26. Boiselle PM, O'Donnell CR, Bankier AA, et al. Tracheal collapsibility in healthy volunteers during forced expiration: assessment with multidetector CT. Radiology 2009;252(1):255–62.

27. Sverzellati N, Rastelli A, Chetta A, et al. Airway malacia in chronic obstructive pulmonary disease: prevalence, morphology and relationship with emphysema, bronchiectasis and bronchial wall thickening. Eur Radiol 2009;19(7):1669–78.

28. Lee EY, Boiselle PM. Tracheobronchomalacia in infants and children: multidetector CT evaluation. Radiology 2009;252(1):7–22.

29. Giannoni S, Benassai C, Allori O, et al. Tracheomalacia associated with Mounier-Kuhn syndrome in the Intensive Care Unit: treatment with Freitag stent. A case report. Minerva Anestesiol 2004;70(9):651–9.

30. Menon B, Aggarwal B, Iqbal A. Mounier-Kuhn syndrome: report of 8 cases of Tracheobronchomegaly with associated complications. South Med J 2008;101(1):83–7.

31. Muller NL, Miller RR, Ostrow DN, et al. Clinico-radiologic-pathologic conference diffuse thickening of the tracheal wall. J Can Assoc Radiol 1989;40:213–5.

32. Nseir S, Ader F, Marquette CH. Nosocomial tracheobronchitis. Curr Opin Infect Dis 2009;22:148–53.

33. Kramer MR, Denning DW, Marshall SE, et al. Ulcerative tracheobronchitis after lung transplantation. A new form of invasive aspergillosis. Am Rev Respir Dis 1991;144:552–6.

34. Warman M, Lahav J, Feldberg E, et al. Invasive tracheal aspergillosis treated successfully with voriconazole: clinical report and review of the literature. Ann Otol Rhinol Laryngol 2007;116(10):713–6.

35. Franquet T, Muller NL, Oikonomou A, et al. Aspergillus infection of the airways: computed tomography and pathologic findings. J Comput Assist Tomogr 2004;28(1):10–6.

36. Verma G, Kanawaty D, Hyland R. Rhinoscleroma causing upper airway obstruction. Can Respir J 2005;12(1):43–5.

37. Simons ME, Granato L, Oliveira RCB, et al. Rhinoscleroma: case report. Braz J Otorhinolaryngol 2006;72(4):568–71.

38. Smati B, Boudaya MS, Ayadi A, et al. Tuberculosis of the trachea. Ann Thorac Surg 2006;82:1900–1.

39. Kim Y, Lee KS, Yoon JH, et al. Tuberculosis of the trachea and main bronchi: CT findings in 17 patients. AJR Am J Roentgenol 1997;168:1051–6.

40. Faix LE, Branstetter BF. Uncommon CT findings in relapsing polychondritis. AJNR Am J Neuroradiol 2005;26:2134–6.

41. Behar JV, Choi YW, Hartman TA, et al. Relapsing polychondritis affecting the lower respiratory tract. AJR Am J Roentgenol 2002;178:173–7.

42. Lee KS, Ernst A, trentham DE, et al. Relapsing polychondritis: prevalence of expiratory CT airway abnormalities. Radiology 2006;240(2):565–73.

43. Prakash UB, Golbin JM, Edell ES, et al. Airway involvement in Wegener's granulomatosis. Rheum Dis Clin North Am 2007;33:755–75.

44. Gilad R, Milillo P, Som PM. Severe diffuse systemic amyloidosis with involvement of the pharynx, larynx,

and trachea. CT and MR findings. AJNR Am J Neuroradiol 2007;28:1557–8.

45. Poovaneswaran S, Abdul Razak AR, Lockman H, et al. Tracheobronchial amyloidosis: utilization of radiotherapy as a treatment modality. Medscape J Med 2008;10(2):42.

46. Brandstetter RD, Messina MS, Sprince NL, et al. Tracheal stenosis due to sarcoidosis. Chest 1981; 80:656.

47. Restrepo S, Pandit M, Villamil MA, et al. Tracheobronchopathia osteochondroplastica—helical CT findings in 4 cases. J Thorac Imaging 2004;19(2):112–6.

48. Jabbardarjani HR, Radpey B, Kharabian S, et al. Tracheobronchopathia osteochondroplastica: presentation of ten cases and review of literature. Lung 2008; 186:293–7.

49. Devaraj A, Griffin N, Nicholson AG, et al. Computed tomography findings in fibrosing mediastinitis. Clin Radiol 2007;62:781–6.

50. Rossi SE, McAdams HP, Rosado-de-Christenson ML, et al. From the archives of the AFIP- fibrosing mediastinitis. Radiographics 2001;21:737–57.

51. Wilcox P, Miller R, Miller G, et al. Airway involvement in ulcerative colitis. Chest 1987;92(1):18–22.

Volumetric Expiratory HRCT of the Lung: Clinical Applications

Mizuki Nishino, MD[a],*, George R. Washko, MD[b,c], Hiroto Hatabu, MD, PhD[d,e]

KEYWORDS

- Computed tomography (CT) • Lung • High-resolution CT
- Expiratory high-resolution CT • Volumetric

Expiratory high-resolution CT scan (HRCT) of the chest offers a powerful adjunct to inspiratory HRCT in the detection of lung diseases involving the small airways by reflecting the interplay of air in the alveoli, the pulmonary interstitium, and pulmonary blood volume.[1–5] The hallmark of expiratory airflow obstruction has been the radiographic finding of air trapping where lung regions with a lesser degree of increase in expiratory attenuation than normal are thought to be indicative of retained gas in the secondary pulmonary lobule.[1,3] This process can be found in a variety of lung diseases with obstructive physiology, including asthma, bronchiectasis, and emphysema.

A major limitation to acquiring expiratory CT scans on all patients is the associated radiation exposure. Because of this, in 2003, two of the authors (Nishino and Hatabu) and their colleagues[6,7] developed a clinical volumetric expiratory HRCT protocol with the decreased tube current that provides volumetric data sets of the entire thorax at end-inspiration and at end-expiration without increasing radiation dose and examination time. These volumetric data sets of expiratory HRCT images allow for full visualization of the airway and lung parenchyma, with the added value of the three-dimensional and multiplanar capability (**Fig.** 1).[6,7] Volumetric expiratory HRCT has since been used for evaluation of diffuse lung disease with suspected airway abnormalities. More recently, the Chronic Obstructive Pulmonary Disease Gene (COPDGene) Study, a multicenter investigation of the genetic epidemiology of subjects with chronic obstructive pulmonary disease (COPD) supported by National Institute of Health, adopted volumetric inspiratory and expiratory HRCT for its protocol.

COPD

COPD is defined as incompletely reversible expiratory airflow obstruction.[8] It is typically related to tobacco smoke exposure and is the result of remodeling of the small airways with obliteration of their lumen and loss of lung elastic recoil due to emphysematous destruction of the parenchyma.[9] Standard objective measures of both of these processes, airway disease and emphysema have been well established using inspiratory CT scanning.[10] Less well recognized are the potential contributions that expiratory CT scanning can be made to further understanding of these processes using quantitative measures of gas trapping and CT attenuation gravitational gradients.

[a] Department of Radiology, Dana-Farber Cancer Institute, Harvard Medical School, 44 Binney Street, Boston, MA 02215, USA
[b] Division of Pulmonary and Critical Care Medicine, Brigham and Women's Hospital, 75 Francis Street, Boston, MA 02215, USA
[c] Harvard Medical School, Boston, MA, USA
[d] MRI Program, Center for Pulmonary Functional Imaging, Brigham and Women's Hospital, 75 Francis Street, Boston, MA 02215, USA
[e] Department of Radiology, Center for Pulmonary Functional Imaging, Brigham and Women's Hospital, Harvard Medical School, 75 Francis Street, Boston, MA 02215, USA
* Corresponding author.
E-mail address: Mizuki_Nishino@dfci.harvard.edu (M. Nishino).

Radiol Clin N Am 48 (2010) 177–183
doi:10.1016/j.rcl.2009.09.003
0033-8389/09/$ – see front matter © 2010 Published by Elsevier Inc.

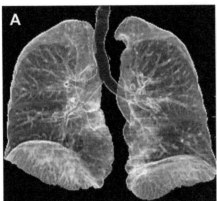
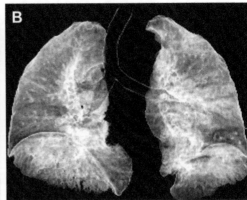

Fig. 1. A 70-year-old woman with a history of bronchial asthma. (*A, B*) The reconstructed images with volume rendering of the posterior two-thirds of the lungs at end-inspiration and end-expiration using an ADW workstation. Volume and attenuation changes after expiration are visually displayed in a 3-dimensional fashion, providing easy recognition of air trapping. There are marked changes in the configuration of the airway conducting to the areas of air trapping. (*From* Nishino M, Boiselle PM, Copeland JF, et al. Value of volumetric data acquisition in expiratory high-resolution CT of the lung. J Comput Assist Tomogr 2004;28:209–14; with permission.) ADW, Advanced Development Workstation.

Densitometric assessments of the lung parenchyma have been accepted methods for quantitatively examining CT scan burdens of emphysema since the 1980s.[10] These methods have been benchmarked against histopathologic examination and have been integral to most CT scan-based epidemiologic studies of subjects with COPD.[10–13] With the advent of volumetric expiratory CT scan imaging protocols came the recognition that similar densitometric methods can be applied to these images. Recently, Akira and colleagues[14] found that such objective analysis of the expiratory images of subjects with COPD may offer stronger correlates to lung function than inspiratory scans in subjects with severe disease. Additional studies in larger cohorts will likely support such observations and further argue for the phenotypic information available in expiratory CT scans.

It has been known that CT demonstrates an attenuation gradient in the normal lung, with the greatest density in dependent lung regions and the least density in nondependent lung regions. In 1993, Webb and colleagues[2] reported that the anteroposterior attenuation gradient is discontinuous at the major fissure, and that the posterior aspect of the upper lobe has greater attenuation than the anterior aspect of the lower lobe. It was also noted that the anteroposterior intralobar attenuation gradient was accentuated during expiration. Departure from these gradients could imply local abnormalities in lung compliance, distribution of mechanical stress, or distensibility of vessels.[2,15] However, the significance of the loss of this intralobar attenuation gradient has not been determined in detail.

The authors investigated 21 consecutive patients with emphysema studied with volumetric expiratory HRCT, and 6 patients with normal HRCT. The anterior-posterior intralobar attenuation gradients were quantified on end-inspiratory and end-expiratory sagittal reformations using a lung analysis software program.[16] The quantitative values of the intralobar attenuation gradients were correlated with pulmonary function test results (**Figs. 2** and **3**). The intralobar attenuation gradients in the patients with forced expiratory volume in 1 second (FEV_1), by percent, of less than 70% were significantly smaller compared with those in patients with $FEV_1(\%)$ greater than 70% in right lower lobe at end-inspiration, and right and left lower lobes at end-expiration. There was a significant positive correlation between the intralobar attenuation gradient and pulmonary function test results in bilateral lower lobes, when the cutoff values of 70% for $FEV_1(\%)$ and 0.002 for attenuation gradient were used. The intralobar attenuation gradients in bilateral lower lobes at end-expiration were significantly correlated with FEV_1 and FEV_1 per forced vital capacity (FVC). These results indicated that the quantitatively measured intralobar attenuation gradients correlate with obstructive changes on pulmonary function tests in patients with emphysema, especially at end-expiration in the lower lobes, suggesting a potential utility of these gradients as a functional indicator of emphysema.[16]

BRONCHIECTASIS

Bronchiectasis is an airway disease associated with chronic progressive inflammatory changes

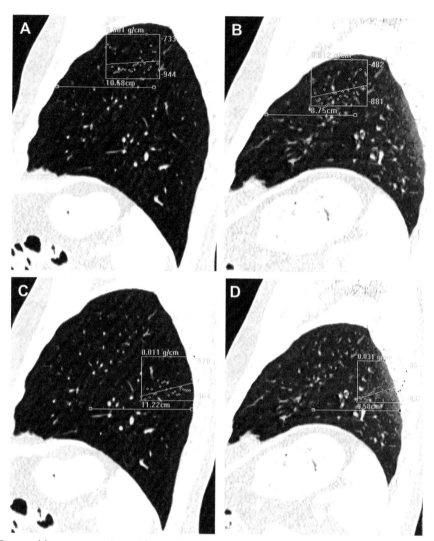

Fig. 2. A 38-year-old man presenting with cough and wheezing, with normal pulmonary function test results of FEV_1 (% predicted): 84, FVC (% predicted): 84, FEV_1/FVC (% predicted): 100. Quantitative measurement of the intralobar anteroposterior attenuation gradient in the left upper lobe shows attenuation gradient of 0.001 g/cm at (A) end-inspiration, which increased to 0.012 g/cm at (B) end-expiration, demonstrating the presence of normal attenuation gradient accentuated at end-expiration. Quantitative measurement of the intralobar anteroposterior attenuation gradient in the left lower lobe shows attenuation gradient of 0.011 g/cm at (C) end-inspiration, which increased to 0.031 g/cm at (D) end-expiration, also demonstrating the presence of normal attenuation gradient accentuated at end-expiration. (From Nishino M, Roberts DH, Sitek A, et al. Loss of anteroposterior intralobar attenuation gradient of the lung: Correlation with pulmonary function. Acad Radiol 2006;13(5):589–97; with permission.)

of the bronchial wall, which leads to irreversible abnormal bronchial dilatation and airflow obstruction.[17,18] The pathophysiologic mechanism is generally considered as multifactorial. Air trapping is often seen in patients with bronchiectasis on expiratory CT scan, and is considered one of the major determinants of airflow obstruction in bronchiectasis.[19,20] In addition to bronchial dilatation, the chronic airway inflammation in bronchiectasis may cause bronchial wall weakness and loss of

dynamic integrity, resulting in excessive collapsibility of the airway, namely bronchomalacia. In mid 1960s, Fraser and colleagues[21] reported the prominent collapse of the large airways on expiration in bronchiectasis based on the evaluation using cinefluorography evaluation. However, the frequency and severity of bronchomalacia in association with the resultant air trapping remained to be determined in patients with bronchiectasis. The authors studied 46 patients with

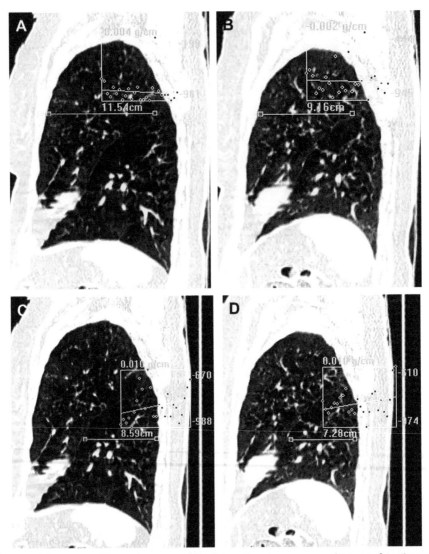

Fig. 3. A 70-year-old woman with emphysema, with obstructive changes on pulmonary function test; FEV$_1$ (% predicted): 35, FVC (% predicted): 78, FEV$_1$/FVC (% predicted): 45. Quantitative measurement of the intralobar anteroposterior attenuation gradient in the left upper lobe shows attenuation gradient of −0.004 g/cm at (A) end-inspiration, and −0.002 g/cm at (B) end-expiration, demonstrating loss of intralobar attenuation gradient on both images. Quantitative measurement of the intralobar anteroposterior attenuation gradient in the left lower lobe shows attenuation gradient of 0.010 g/cm both at (C) end-inspiration, and at (D) end-expiration, demonstrating loss of normal attenuation gradient. (*From* Nishino M, Roberts DH, Sitek A, et al. Loss of antero-posterior intralobar attenuation gradient of the lung: correlation with pulmonary function. Acad Radiol 2006;13(5):589–97; with permission.)

bronchiectasis evaluated by volumetric expiratory high-resolution CT scan and pulmonary function tests to evaluate the frequency and severity of bronchomalacia in bronchiectasis, to compare the extent of air trapping in bronchiectasis patients with or without bronchomalacia, and to correlate the severity of bronchomalacia and the extent of air trapping versus pulmonary function. Of 46 patients with bronchiectasis, 32 patients (70%) were noted to have bronchomalacia. Air trapping was observed in 43 patients (93%). The extent of air trapping in patients with bronchomalacia was significantly greater compared with the patients without bronchomalacia (*P* = .0308, chi-squared test) (**Fig. 4**).[22]

SARCOIDOSIS

Sarcoidosis is a multisystemic disease of unknown cause characterized by the presence of

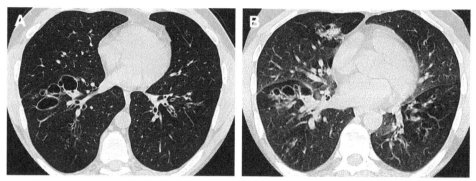

Fig. 4. A 47-year-old woman with bronchiectasis. Pair of (A) end-inspiratory and (B) end-expiratory scans obtained at the level of inferior pulmonary veins show cystic bronchiectasis in right lower lobe and (A) cylindrical bronchiectasis in lower lobes at end-inspiration, which demonstrate excessive collapsibility at end-expiration, indicating bronchomalacia (grade 2). (B) Note multiple radiolucent areas compared with adjacent lung at end-expiration in the bilateral lower lobes, indicating air trapping (grade 3). (From Nishino M, Siewert B, Roberts DH, et al. Excessive collapsibility of bronchi in bronchiectasis: evaluation on volumetric expiratory high-resolution CT. J Comput Assist Tomogr 2006;30(3):474–8; with permission.)

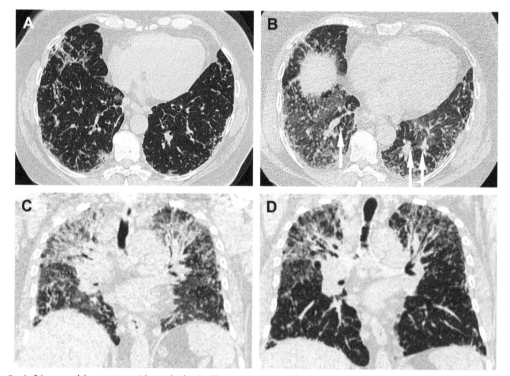

Fig. 5. A 64-year-old woman with pathologically proven sarcoidosis. A pair of (A) end-inspiratory and (B) end-expiratory scans obtained at the lung base showing nodular thickening of the interlobular septum and fissures. At end-expiration, multiple areas of air trapping in both lower lobes are noted. (B) The segmental and subsegmental bronchi conducting to the areas of air trapping are severely collapsed, indicating bronchomalacia (arrows). Reformatted coronal images on (C) end-inspiration and (D) end-expiration at the level of the carina showing marked peribronchovascular interstitial thickening, ground-glass opacities, and small nodules, predominantly in the upper lobes. (D) Note the severely narrowed bronchi at end-expiration. (From Nishino M, Kuroki M, Roberts DH, et al. Bronchomalacia in sarcoidosis: evaluation on volumetric expiratory high-resolution CT of the lung. Acad Radiol 2005;12(5):596–601; with permission.)

noncaseating granulomatous inflammation that may involve all parts of the lung, including the airways. Characteristic HRCT findings of pulmonary sarcoidosis include nodular thickening of bronchovascular bundles, small nodules, and ground-glass opacities.[23] The presence of air trapping on expiratory CT scan in sarcoidosis was described by Gleeson and colleagues[24] in 1996. Since then, air trapping on expiratory CT scan is considered as evidence of small-airway obstruction and has been reported in sarcoidosis in association with incomplete lung emptying at end-expiration.[25–27]

In the authors' preliminary review of cases of sarcoidosis evaluated with volumetric expiratory HRCT, bronchomalacia was unexpectedly but frequently observed on the end-expiratory images. The authors examined the CT scans of 18 subjects with pathologically proven sarcoidosis who underwent clinical volumetric expiratory high-resolution computed tomography. Bronchomalacia was noted in 11 of 18 patients (61%) with sarcoidosis (mild, n = 6; moderate, n = 4; and severe, n = 1). Air trapping was observed in 17 of 18 patients (94%; grade 1 [1%–25%], n = 8; grade 2 [26%–50%], n = 9) (Fig. 5). The extent of air trapping in patients with bronchomalacia was significantly greater than that in patients without bronchomalacia (P = .027, chi-squared test).[28] Given the propensity of sarcoidosis to involve the central and peripheral airways, sarcoidosis may cause increased airway collapsibility resulting in bronchomalacia. These results demonstrated that bronchomalacia may be frequently associated with sarcoidosis. Further investigation is required to determine the clinical sequela of bronchomalacia in this population.

SUMMARY AND FUTURE DIRECTIONS

Volumetric HRCT is useful in the evaluation of a variety of diffuse lung diseases with suspected airway abnormalities, including emphysema, bronchiectasis, and sarcoidosis. It also provides volumetric assessment of the entire thorax at end-inspiration and at end-expiration and allowing for detailed analysis of the airway and parenchyma. Obviously, this field of volumetric expiratory HRCT is work-in-progress. While the HRCT provides a static view of lung morphology, volumetric expiratory HRCT provides complementary dynamic and functional information of the pulmonary airway and parenchyma. Without question, quantified data analysis of volumetric expiratory HRCT is crucial for further use and application of volumetric expiratory HRCT. Standardization of image acquisition and postprocessing in CT examinations will be necessary for the real application of such quantified

data derived from volumetric expiratory HRCT to daily clinical medical practice.[29] The authors are confident that more advanced works in this field will be published, and this technique will come into practice in the next 3 to 5 years.

REFERENCES

1. Stern EJ, Webb WR, Warnock ML, et al. Bronchopulmonary sequestration: dynamic, ultrafast, high-resolution CT evidence of air trapping. AJR Am J Roentgenol 1991;157:947–9.
2. Webb WR, Stern EJ, Kanth N, et al. Dynamic pulmonary CT: findings in healthy adult men. Radiology 1993;186:117–24.
3. Stern EJ, Webb WR, Gamsu G. Dynamic quantitative computed tomography. A predictor of pulmonary function in obstructive lung diseases. Invest Radiol 1994;29:564–9.
4. Arakawa H, Webb WR. Air trapping on expiratory high-resolution CT scans in the absence of inspiratory scan abnormalities: correlation with pulmonary function tests and differential diagnosis. AJR Am J Roentgenol 1998;170:1349–53.
5. Arakawa H, Webb WR, McCowin M, et al. Inhomogeneous lung attenuation at thin-section CT: diagnostic value of expiratory scans. Radiology 1998;206:89–94.
6. Nishino M, Hatabu H. Volumetric expiratory high-resolution CT of the lung. Eur J Radiol 2004;52:180–4.
7. Nishino M, Boiselle PM, Copeland JF, et al. Value of volumetric data acquisition in expiratory high-resolution CT of the lung. J Comput Assist Tomogr 2004; 28:209–14.
8. Pauwels RA, Buist AS, Calverley PM, et al. GOLD Scientific Committee. Global strategy for the diagnosis, management, and prevention of chronic obstructive pulmonary disease. NHLBI/WHO Global Initiative for Chronic Obstructive Lung Disease (GOLD) Workshop summary. Am J Respir Crit Care Med 2001;163:1256–76.
9. Hogg JC, Macklem PT, Thurlbeck WM. Site and nature of airway obstruction in chronic obstructive lung disease. N Engl J Med 1968;278:1355–60.
10. Müller NL, Staples CA, Miller RR, et al. "Density mask". An objective method to quantitate emphysema using computed tomography. Chest 1988;94:782–7.
11. Gevenois PA, de Maertelaer V, De Vuyst P, et al. Comparison of computed density and macroscopic morphometry in pulmonary emphysema. Am J Respir Crit Care Med 1995;152:653–7.
12. Gevenois PA, De Vuyst P, de Maertelaer V, et al. Comparison of computed density and microscopic morphometry in pulmonary emphysema. Am J Respir Crit Care Med 1996;154:187–92.
13. Patel BD, Coxson HO, Pillai SG, et al. Airway wall thickening and emphysema show independent familial

aggregation in chronic obstructive pulmonary disease. Am J Respir Crit Care Med 2008;178:500–5.

14. Akira M, Toyokawa K, Inoue Y, et al. Quantitative CT in chronic obstructive pulmonary disease: inspiratory and expiratory assessment. AJR Am J Roentgenol 2009;192:267–72.

15. Millar AB, Denison DM. Vertical gradients of lung density in supine subjects with fibrosing alveolitis or pulmonary emphysema. Thorax 1990;45:602–5.

16. Nishino M, Roberts DH, Sitek A, et al. Loss of anteroposterior intralobar attenuation gradient of the lung: correlation with pulmonary function. Acad Radiol 2006;13(5):589–97.

17. Reid LM. Reduction in bronchial subdivision in bronchiectasis. Thorax 1950;5:233–47.

18. Ip M, Lauder IJ, Wong WY, et al. Multivariate analysis of factors affecting pulmonary function in bronchiectasis. Respiration 1993;60:45–50.

19. Roberts HR, Wells AU, Milne DG, et al. Airways obstruction in bronchiectasis: correlation between computed tomography features and pulmonary function tests. Thorax 2000;55:198–204.

20. Hansell DM, Wells AU, Rubens MB, et al. Bronchiectasis: functional significanceof areas of decreased attenuation at expiratory CT. Radiology 1994;193: 369–74.

21. Fraser RG, Macklem PT, Brown WG. Airway dynamics in bronchiectasis: a combined cinefluorographic-manometric study. AJR Am J Roentgenol 1965;93:821–35.

22. Nishino M, Siewert B, Roberts DH, et al. Excessive collapsibility of bronchi in bronchiectasis: evaluation on volumetric expiratory high-resolution CT. J Comput Assist Tomogr 2006;30(3):474–8.

23. Muller NL, Kullnig P, Miller RR. The CT findings of pulmonary sarcoidosis: analysis of 25 patients. AJR Am J Roentgenol 1989;152:1179–82.

24. Gleeson FV, Traill ZC, Hansell DM. Evidence of expiratory CT scans of small-airway obstruction in sarcoidosis. AJR Am J Roentgenol 1996;166: 1052–4.

25. Hansell DM, Milne DG, Wilsher ML, et al. Pulmonary sarcoidosis: morphologic associations of airflow obstruction at thin-section CT. Radiology 1998;209: 697–704.

26. Davies CW, Tasker AD, Padley SP, et al. Air trapping in sarcoidosis on computed tomography: correlation with lung function. Clin Radiol 2000;55:217–21.

27. Magkanas E, Voloudaki A, Bouros D, et al. Pulmonary sarcoidosis. Correlation of expiratory high-resolution CT findings with inspiratory patterns and pulmonary function tests. Acta Radiol 2001;42:494–501.

28. Nishino M, Kuroki M, Roberts DH, et al. Bronchomalacia in sarcoidosis: evaluation on volumetric expiratory high-resolution CT of the lung. Acad Radiol 2005;12(5):596–601.

29. Hatabu H. Are we ready? A time for measurement of physiological parameters of the lung using multidetector row CT scans. Acad Radiol 2009;16:249.

Multidetector CT Scan in the Evaluation of Chest Pain of Nontraumatic Musculoskeletal Origin

Travis J. Hillen, MD, MS, Daniel E. Wessell, MD, PhD*

KEYWORDS

• Multidetector CT • Chest pain • Musculoskeletal

Chest pain is a very common symptom resulting in emergency department visits and admissions to the hospital.[1,2] There are many potential causes of acute nontraumatic chest pain ranging from relatively benign causes, such as gastroesophageal reflux, to life-threatening causes, such as myocardial infarction. While history and physical examination, along with targeted basic diagnostic testing, remain the mainstay in the evaluation of chest pain, advanced imaging with a thin-collimation multidetector computed tomography scan (MDCT) plays an increasing role. In the emergency setting, MDCT is obtained routinely to evaluate acute chest pain in suspected cases of pulmonary embolism (PE) and aortic dissection. Additionally, at many sites the MDCT triple rule-out is being used for suspected coronary artery disease.

The MDCT-imaging protocols for PE and aortic dissection studies use relatively high kilovolts peak and mAs with thin collimation. These parameters are typically set to values that are very similar to those used in dedicated musculoskeletal imaging protocols. These imaging techniques, along with dedicated reconstructions using high-resolution reconstruction kernels and multiplanar reformatting, allow for superb imaging of the thoracic musculoskeletal structures. Thus, the images obtained with thin-collimation MDCT are excellent for evaluating PE and aortic dissection,[3] plus other causes of chest pain, including chest pain of musculoskeletal origin.

Musculoskeletal diseases are very common causes of chest pain in the general population (approximately 10%–15% adults and 24% children).[4–6] One of the most common causes of musculoskeletal chest pain, costochondritis, is routinely diagnosed by physical examination and not by chest CT scan.[7,8] However, many other causes of musculoskeletal chest pain can be visualized on thin-collimation MDCT examinations. These include (1) infectious causes, such as discitis/osteomyelitis and sternoclavicular septic arthritis; (2) rheumatic causes, such as ankylosing spondylitis (AS), with and without fracture; and synovitis, acne, palmoplantar pustulosis, hyperostosis, and osteitis (SAPHO); and (3) systemic diseases resulting in bone findings, such as osteoporosis with insufficiency fractures, neoplasm (with or without pathologic fracture), and sickle cell disease with bone infarcts or avascular necrosis. These entities are not the most common causes of acute nontraumatic chest pain and may

Division of Diagnostic Radiology, Section of Musculoskeletal Radiology, Mallinckrodt Institute of Radiology, Washington University School of Medicine, 660 South Euclid Avenue, Campus Box 8131, St Louis, MO 63110, USA
* Corresponding author.
E-mail address: wesselld@mir.wustl.edu (D.E. Wessell).

Radiol Clin N Am 48 (2010) 185–191
doi:10.1016/j.rcl.2009.09.007
0033-8389/09/$ – see front matter © 2010 Elsevier Inc. All rights reserved.

not even be in the initial differential diagnosis when a thin-collimation MDCT chest CT scan is ordered. However, in total they do account for a significant minority of the causes of acute chest pain. Given the excellent capability of thin-section MDCT with coronal and sagittal reformatting to depict these musculoskeletal disease entities, the cardio-thoracic imager must have a basic familiarity with their imaging appearances.

INFECTIOUS CAUSES OF CHEST PAIN
Discitis/Osteomyelitis

Discitis/osteomyelitis is an uncommon cause of chest pain but is important to diagnose given the consequences of recognition failure. In adults, dis-citis can have a slow insidious onset and the classic signs of infection, fever and chills, may not be present. A common presentation is back pain. In adults, the infection is thought to most often arise via hematogenous spread of infection at another site (eg, upper respiratory tract infec-tion, urinary tract infection). The most common infectious organism is *Staphylococcus aureus*, which accounts for greater than 50% of infections. Infection begins in the disk with loss of disk space and subsequent invasion or destruction of the adjacent vertebral body. The CT scan findings of early discitis/osteomyelitis are subtle and difficult to visualize in the axial plane.[9] MDCT with sagittal and coronal reformatations improves identification of early disk-height loss and endplate destruc-tion.[10] On the sagittal and coronal reformatted images, all of the disk spaces can be viewed simultaneously and thus even subtle changes at

a single level are readily seen as being different from the adjacent levels. As the disease prog-resses the vertebral body involvement may become more advanced and potentially result in vertebral body collapse.

In some cases, there may be concomitant development of adjacent soft tissue infection or epidural abscess. While the disk and vertebral body involvement is often best seen on sagittal or coronal reformatted images with bone window-ing, the adjacent soft tissue involvement is often best seen on the transverse (axial) images with soft tissue windowing. The exact extent and char-acter of the soft tissue component may be better evaluated with magnetic resonance imaging.

Discitis/osteomyelitis may present with acute chest pain (**Fig. 1**). Sagittally reformatted images clearly demonstrate the disk-centered process with adjacent vertebral body destruction and provide a useful adjunct to transverse images. Windowing for bone and soft tissue allows for eval-uation of both the involvement of the vertebral bodies and the adjacent soft tissues.

Disk space narrowing is very common owing to degenerative disk disease. The main diagnostic dilemma with dicsitis/osteomyelitis is differenti-ating it from degenerative disk disease. Degenera-tive disk disease results in disk-space narrowing, but is differentiated from discitis/osteomyelitis by the absence of endplate destruction at the adja-cent vertebral bodies. In degenerative disk disease, the endplates can appear quite irregular because of remodeling, but are usually between normal and increased in density, without any destruction of the endplates. Additionally, discitis

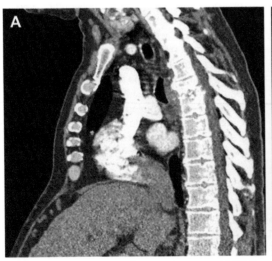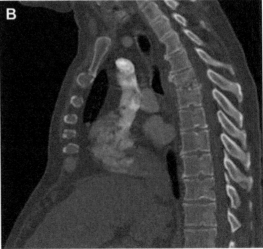

Fig. 1. Mid-sagittal image from a PE protocol MDCT examination for acute chest pain with soft-tissue (*A*) and bone (*B*) windowing demonstrating disk-centered destruction of midthoracicvertebral bodies with associated phlegmon consistent with discitis/osteomyelitis.

usually involves a single disk space while degenerative disk disease often, but not always, involves multiple levels. One important exception is discitis/osteomyelitis due to atypical organisms such as mycobacteria and fungi, which can involve multiple contiguous levels. Additionally, the indolent nature of these atypical infections can result in increased density of the vertebral bodies. The presence of an adjacent soft tissue mass or paraspinal fluid collection favors a diagnosis of discitis/osteomyelitis, be it of pyogenic or atypical origin.

Sternoclavicular Septic Arthritis

Sternoclavicular joint septic arthritis accounts for less than 1% of septic arthritis in the general population.[11] The most common organism is *Staphylococcus aureus*. The risk factors include intravenous drug abuse, diabetes mellitus, central line infection, immunosuppression, and distant infection. As with any suspected septic arthritis, in the vast majority of cases synovial fluid analysis is crucial and joint aspiration is often the best initial diagnostic and potentially therapeutic procedure. Therefore, it should not be delayed by advanced imaging. However, as in the case of discitis/osteomyelitis, septic arthritis may not be in the initial differential diagnosis and, thus, advanced imaging of this entity with CT scan may be obtained. CT scan findings include erosions of the manubrium and clavicle at the sternoclavicular joint with fluid and adjacent soft tissue swelling (**Fig. 2**) that, depending on the severity of the infection, can extend into the mediastinum.[12] The sternoclavicular joints can be evaluated on either the straight transverse images or on oblique coronal reformatted images set up off a midline sagittal image along the body of the sternum.

RHEUMATIC CAUSES OF CHEST PAIN
AS

AS is an inflammatory disorder that typically begins as inflammation at the tendinous and ligamentous insertions on the bones. The disorder typically waxes and wanes with new reactive bone formation occurring with each flare of the disease. AS classically affects the axial joints with findings of sacroiliitis and progressive ossification of the spinal ligaments, disks, and facet joints. Approximately one-half million people in the United States have AS, with a 3 to 1 ratio of men to women. A common early presenting feature of the disease includes the presence of chest pain,[13] which often worsens with expansion of the thoracic cavity. Because of this, the chest pain in AS can easily be mistaken for pleuritic chest pain. Thus, it is common for patients with

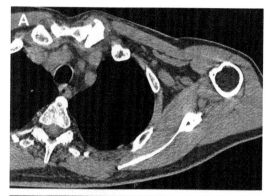
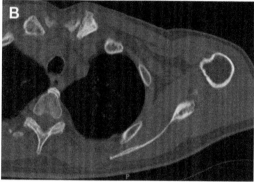

Fig. 2. Transverse (axial) image with soft tissue (*A*) and bone (*B*) windowing from a MDCT examination of the chest in a patient with suspected sternoclavicular osteomyelitis. There is joint-centered destruction of the left sternoclavicular joint with associated abscess. As should be the case with any case of suspected septic arthritis, the left sternoclavicular joint was aspirated and the patient underwent subsequent irrigation and debridement of the left sternoclavicular joint.

AS to undergo thin-section MDCT of the chest as part of the evaluation of their chest pain.

While they are easily recognizable on conventional lateral radiographs of the thoracic spine, the gracile syndesmophytes, which are characteristic of AS, are not as easily recognizable on direct transverse (axial) CT scan images. Sagittal reformats readily depict the syndesmophytes and coronal reformats satisfactorily demonstrate the ossification that can be seen within the costal cartilages. In suspected cases, correlation with any available pelvic imaging may be helpful to evaluate for the classic changes of sacroiliitis or ankylosis of the sacroiliac joints.

With increasing ossification of the spine, there is less mobility and increasing risk for fracture. Patients with AS may develop spinal fractures with even minor trauma (**Fig. 3**). Spinal fracture in a patient with AS can have serious consequences, including spinal instability with neurologic defects

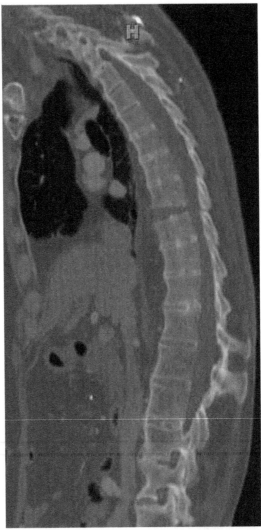

Fig. 3. Sagittal reformatted image obtained from a thin-section MDCT examination performed for aortic dissection. This patient's acute upper back pain was thought to be due to aortic dissection given his relatively minor trauma. Note the findings of AS, including ossification of the spinal ligaments and disks. There is a fracture of the ossified anterior and posterior longitudinal ligaments with associated widening of the disk space between T9 and T10. Fractures through the syndesmophytes at the T9-T10 level with widening of the disk space at this level suggest disruption of the anterior and posterior longitudinal ligaments. Although not seen on this midline sagittal image, the fracture extended to involve the posterior elements. The patient also underwent MR imaging, which confirmed disruption of the anterior and posterior longitudinal ligaments without signal abnormality in the cord. The patient subsequently underwent surgical stabilization via an instrumented posterior spinal fusion from T7 to T12.

secondary to central canal stenosis or hematoma.[14,15]

SAPHO Syndrome

SAPHO syndrome is a rare disease of unknown cause with findings including synovitis, acne, palmoplantar pustulosis, hyperostosis, and osteitis. Approximately 28% of patients with palmoplantar pustulosis have anterior chest wall pain and 18%

of these patients have radiographic anterior chest wall changes.[16] Usually, SAPHO involves the anterior chest wall followed by the spine.[17,18] MDCT evaluation of the anterior chest wall demonstrates hyperostotic and erosive changes (Fig. 4) with joint space narrowing most commonly at the sterno-costoclavicular joint and hyperostosis and anky-losis at the costochondral junctions.[17] The use of reformatted images in the coronal oblique plane oriented parallel to the sternum effectively demonstrates these findings. Patients with SA-PHO also commonly have findings in the spine, including erosions of the vertebral body corners, osteosclerosis, paravertebral ossifications, and discovertebral junction lesions.[17–19] The differential diagnosis for the lesions of the anterior chest wall and spine includes inflammatory and crystalline arthropathies. However, the physical examination findings described above should help lead to the diagnosis.

SYSTEMIC DISEASES WITH MUSCULOSKELETAL FINDINGS
Osteoporosis with Insufficiency Fracture

Osteoporosis is a common disorder associated with aging, characterized by decreased bone mineral density affecting more women than men. With decreasing bone mineral density, there is resultant increased risk for fracture. Common locations for osteoporotic fractures include the femur, spine, pelvis, and sacrum. In 1995 alone, the estimated expense for the treatment of osteoporotic fractures was $13.8 billion.[20] Osteoporotic compression fractures in the thoracic spine commonly result in both back and chest pain.[21] Another cause of chest pain related to osteoporotic fractures includes sternal insufficiency fractures, which are often, but not always, associated with increasing thoracic kyphosis (**Fig. 5**).[22,23] Sternal insufficiency fractures have been shown to cause chest pain similar to the chest pain of myocardial infarction and PE.[24–26] MDCT evaluation of both vertebral compression fractures and sternal insufficiency fractures is best performed in the sagittal plane. Compression fractures of the spine are characterized by anterior loss of vertebral body height. If severe enough, they can extend into the posterior aspect of the vertebral body and be associated with retropulsion of bone fragments resulting in central canal narrowing. Sternal insufficiency fractures are characterized as either buckling (displaced) or nondisplaced.[22,23]

Neoplasm with or Without Pathologic Fracture

Metastatic disease to the skeleton is the third most common location of metastases and is much more common than primary malignancy of the skeleton.[27] Metastases or primary skeletal neoplasms of the bones in the chest can involve the spine, ribs, sternum, scapulae, and clavicles. Metastases are often painful with or without associated

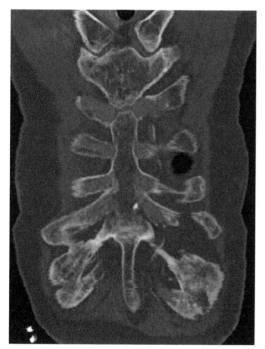

Fig. 4. Oblique coronal reformatted image along the plane of the sternal body from a MDCT examination originally ordered as a PE protocol to evaluate the patient's chest pain and shortness of breath. Examination demonstrates hyperostosis of the costochondral junctions with associated sternoclavicular erosions or inflammatory arthritis in a patient with SAPHO. While this can be an age-related change, the extensive ossification along with ankylosis, and the erosions at the right sternoclavicular joint, suggest SAPHO syndrome. Given the imaging findings, the clinical examination can be directed to evaluate for typical skin changes.

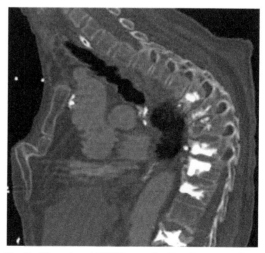

Fig. 5. PE protocol MDCT examination for acute chest pain in a patient with osteoporosis from chronic steroid treatment post-lung transplantation shows a marked thoracic kyphosis secondary to multiple vertebral insufficiency fractures and associated sternal insufficiency fractures.

pathologic fracture.[28] Fractures of metastases to bones in the chest often occur with no trauma or only minimal trauma and may result in chest pain.[29] MDCT is more sensitive than conventional radiographs at detecting metastases and is able to detect metastases in bone marrow before cortical destruction has occurred.[28,30] Imaging features are varied depending on the primary malignancy and the extent of involvement of the bones. Typically, the lesions are lytic, blastic (sclerotic), or a combination of both (Fig. 6). In addition to the detection of metastases, MDCT is often used as imaging guidance for skeletal biopsy if the primary cancer is not known.

Sickle Cell Disease with Bone Infarcts

Sickle cell anemia is the most common single gene disorder affecting black Americans. Acute chest pain in sickle cell disease is most often the result of either pain crisis or acute chest syndrome. Pain crisis is the most common cause of hospitalization in patients with sickle cell disease and is the result of acute bone ischemia or infarct.[31] Acute chest syndrome is defined as an acute illness associated with an infiltrate on chest radiography.[32] It is thought to represent a common clinical manifestation of several different pathologic processes, including fat embolism secondary to bone infarct, infection, or vascular occlusion.[33] MDCT is sometimes used in the evaluation of sickle cell disease associated acute chest pain to evaluate for causes of the chest pain including

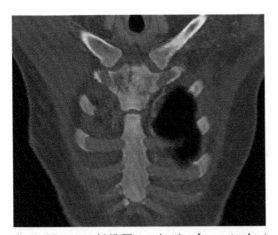

Fig. 6. PE protocol MDCT examination for acute chest pain in a patient with lung cancer metastatic to the manubrium with a pathologic fracture. The patient had a known history of lung cancer and the MDCT examination was obtained to evaluate for suspected PE. While the presence of the lesion was evident on the straight transverse (axial) images, the extent of the lesion and the associated pathologic fracture is better elucidated on the coronal reformats.

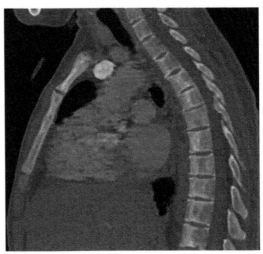

Fig. 7. Mid-line sagittal reformatted image from a PE protocol MDCT examination of the chest. Bone findings of sickle cell disease, including sternal and vertebral body bone infarcts and multiple H-shaped vertebral bodies. The extensive areas of patchy increased bone density seen in the vertebral bodies and sternum are classic for old bone infarcts. In the acute setting, these infarcts can be extremely painful. While infarcts are typically not visible on MDCT in the acute setting, the presence of old bone infarcts on an otherwise normal MDCT examination of the chest should raise suspicion that an acute bone infarct may be the cause of the patient's pain.

PE. The bone infarcts associated with acute chest pain are not readily identified by MDCT in the acute setting. However, manifestations of chronic bone infarction (Fig. 7) and avascular necrosis are often seen on MDCT examinations in patients with sickle cell disease as H-shaped vertebral bodies, humeral head avascular necrosis, and as chronic infarcts in ribs, scapula, or vertebral bodies.[34]

SUMMARY

Acute nontraumatic chest pain is a common presenting symptom to the emergency department. Often, it is evaluated by MDCT with PE, aortic dissection, or coronary artery protocols. The parameters used for these MDCT protocols are very similar to those used in protocols for dedicated imaging of the musculoskeletal system. Thus, these studies are not only effective in evaluating for these traditional vascular causes of chest pain, but also in evaluating musculoskeletal causes of chest pain, including those of infectious, rheumatologic, and systemic causes. In essence, every MDCT of the chest is also a musculoskeletal examination of the chest and anyone interpreting these images must be familiar with the MDCT-imaging appearance of common musculoskeletal causes of acute nontraumatic chest pain.

REFERENCES

1. Clinical policy for the initial approach to adults presenting with a chief complaint of chest pain, with no history of trauma. American College of Emergency Physicians. Ann Emerg Med 1995;25:274.
2. Graff LG, Dallara J, Ross MA, et al. Impact on the care of the emergency department chest pain patient from the Chest Pain Evaluation Registry (CHEPER) study. Am J Cardiol 1997;80:563.
3. Johnson TRC, Nikolaou K, Wintersperger BJ, et al. ECG-gated 64-MDCT angiography in the differential diagnosis of acute chest pain. AJR Am J Roentgenol 2007;188:76.
4. Karlson BW, Herlitz J, Pettersson P, et al. Patients admitted to the emergency room with symptoms indicative of acute myocardial infarction. J Intern Med 1991;230:251.
5. Selbst SM, Ruddy RM, Clark BJ, et al. Pediatric chest pain: a prospective study. Pediatrics 1988;82:319.
6. Kocis KC. Chest pain in pediatrics. Pediatr Clin North Am 1999;46:189.
7. Disla E, Rhim HR, Reddy A, et al. Costochondritis. A prospective analysis in an emergency department setting. Arch Intern Med 1994;154:2466.
8. Habib PA, Huang GS, Mendiola JA, et al. Anterior chest pain: musculoskeletal considerations. Emerg Radiol 2004;11:37.
9. Stabler A, Reiser MF. Imaging of spinal infection. Radiol Clin North Am 2001;39:115.
10. Tali ET. Spinal infections. Eur J Radiol 2004;50:120.
11. Ross JJ, Shamsuddin H. Sternoclavicular septic arthritis: review of 180 cases. Medicine (Baltimore) 2004;83:139.
12. Pollack MS. Staphylococcal mediastinitis due to sternoclavicular pyoarthrosis: CT appearance. J Comput Assist Tomogr 1990;14:924.
13. Dawes PT, Sheeran TP, Hothersall TE. Chest pain—a common feature of ankylosing spondylitis. Postgrad Med J 1998;64:27.
14. Wang YF, Teng MMH, Chang CY, et al. Imaging manifestations of spinal fractures in ankylosing spondylitis. AJNR Am J Neuroradiol 2005;26:2067.
15. Hitchon PW, From AM, Brenton MD, et al. Fractures of the thoracolumbar spine complicating ankylosing spondylitis. J Neurosurg 2002;97(2 Suppl):218.
16. Jurik AG. Anterior chest wall involvement in patients with pustulosis palmoplantaris. Skeletal Radiol 1990;19:271.
17. Cotton A, Flipo RM, Mentre A, et al. SAPHO syndrome. Radiographics 1995;15:1147.
18. Boutin RD, Resnick D. The SAPHO syndrome: an evolving concept for unifying several idiopathic disorders of bone and skin. AJR Am J Roentgenol 1998;170:585.
19. Laredo JD, Vuillemin-Bodaghi V, Boutry N, et al. SAPHO syndrome: MR appearance of vertebral involvement. Radiology 2007;242:825.
20. Ray NF, Chan JK, Thamer M, et al. Medical expenditures for the treatment of osteoporotic fractures in the United States in 1995: report from the National Osteoporosis Foundation. J Bone Miner Res 1997;12:24.
21. Patel U, Skingle S, Campbell GA, et al. Clinical profile of acute vertebral compression fractures in osteoporosis. Rheumatology 1991;30:418.
22. Cooper K. Insufficiency fractures of the sternum: a consequence of thoracic kyphosis? Radiology 1988;167:471.
23. Chen C, Chandnani V, Kang HS, et al. Insufficiency fracture of the sternum caused by osteopenia: plain film findings in seven patients. AJR Am J Roentgenol 1990;154:1025.
24. Rutledge DI. Spontaneous fracture of the sternum simulating myocardial infarction. Postgrad Med 1962;32:502.
25. Vassalo L. Spontaneous fracture of the sternum simulating pulmonary embolism. Br J Clin Pract 1969;23:288.
26. Schapira D, Nachtigal A, Scharf Y. Spontaneous fracture of the sternum simulating myocardial infarction. Clin Rheumatol 1995;14:478.
27. Berretoni BA, Carter JR. Current concepts: review mechanisms of cancer metastasis to bone. J Bone Joint Surg 1986;68:308.
28. Rosenthal DI. Radiologic diagnosis of bone metastases. Cancer 1997;80:1595.
29. Rubens RD. Bone metastases—the clinical problem. Eur J Cancer 1998;34:210.
30. Helms CA, Cann CE, Brunelle FO, et al. Detection of bone-marrow metastases using quantitative computed tomography. Radiology 1981;140:745.
31. Kumar DS, Yadavali RP, Concepcion LA, et al. Acute chest pain in a young woman with a chronic illness. Br J Radiol 2008;81:261.
32. Lane P. Sickle cell disease. Pediatr Clin North Am 1996;43:639.
33. Lonergan GF, Cline DB, Abbondanzo SL. From the archives of the AFIP: sickle cell anemia. Radiographics 2001;21:971.
34. Keeley K, Buchanan GR. Acute infarction of long bones in children with sickle cell anemia. J Pediatr 1982;101:170.

Thoracic Applications of Dual Energy

Martine Remy-Jardin, MD, PhD*, Jean-Baptiste Faivre, MD,
Francois Pontana, MD, Anne-Lise Hachulla, MD,
Nunzia Tacelli, MD, Teresa Santangelo, MD,
Jacques Remy, MD

KEYWORDS

- Multidetector computed tomography • Dual energy
- Thoracic applications • Imaging

Recent technological advances in multidetector computed tomography (MDCT) have led to the introduction of dual-source CT, which allows acquisition of CT data at the same energy, so called dual-source scanning, or at 2 distinct tube voltage settings during a single acquisition, termed dual-energy (DE) imaging. Although the advantage of the former scanning mode is the improvement of temporal resolution, the latter offers new options for CT imaging, because it allows tissue characterization and functional analysis with morphologic evaluation. Over the last 3 years, these new diagnostic approaches in the management of respiratory disorders have attracted much interest. It is definitely too early to draw definitive conclusions on dual-energy CT applications; however, the objective of this article is to review the results already reported with the first generation of dual-source CT systems. Alternative approaches, although not yet evaluated in the conditions of routine clinical practice, have been developed by other manufacturers, such as rapid kV switching and sandwich detectors to generate multiple kV data-sets using a single system.

TECHNICAL CONSIDERATIONS
DE on a Dual-source CT System

The dual-source MDCT system consists of 2 acquisition systems mounted onto the rotating gantry of the scanner, with an angular offset of about 90°. In the first generation of dual-source CT systems, one tube detector (tube A) covered the entire 50-cm diameter scan field of view (FOV), whereas the second tube detector (tube B) was restricted to a central 26-cm diameter FOV. On the second generation of dual-source CT scanners, this configuration has been modified with a tube B detector now covering a 33-cm diameter FOV, thus avoiding the previously encountered limitations of DE postprocessing for large patients. The acquisition parameters most commonly selected include 140 kilovolt (peak) (kV[p]) and 50 to 70 milliampere-second (mAs) for tube A and 80 kV(p) and 330 mAs for tube B. The tube B current is adjusted to compensate for the lower photon output at the lower voltage. The gantry rotation time is 0.33 seconds with a pitch of 0.5 to 0.8. A collimation of 0.6 to 1.2 mm can be chosen, enabling reconstructions of 1- and 1.5-mm thick sections, respectively. The adaptation of the z-flying focal spot for 64 detectors allows coverage of 19.2 mm, with a collimation of 0.6 mm (0.6 mm × 32) or 16.8 mm, with a collimation of 1.2 mm (1.2 mm × 14). With the aforementioned scanning parameters, the average scan duration for an adult chest examination is 13 seconds; with the adjunct of automatic angular (x, y) modulation of the milliamperage, the average dose-length product (DLP) of such a scanning protocol is 280 milligray (mGy).cm.[1,2] This average DLP value is higher than the average DLP of 150 mGy.cm of standard single-energy CT angiographic examinations but much lower compared with the legally required levels (European reference values of 650 mGy.cm).

Department of Thoracic Imaging, Hospital Calmette, University Lille Nord de France, Boulevard Jules Leclercq, F-59000 Lille, France
* Corresponding author.
E-mail address: mremy-jardin@chru-lille.fr (M. Remy-Jardin).

Radiol Clin N Am 48 (2010) 193–205
doi:10.1016/j.rcl.2009.08.013

Apart from the larger tube B-detector FOV previously mentioned, several additional technical modifications have been introduced in the second generation of dual-source CT systems, which have an impact on the feasibility and overall quality of DECT scans. Because of the shorter rotation time, increased pitch, and higher coverage, the average scanning time is reduced by more than 50%, which allows scanning of all categories of respiratory patients, even if dyspneic. The increase in the angular offset of the 2 acquisitions systems, from 90° to 95°, reduces cross-scatter radiation from the second tube-detector system, and an improved filtration of high energy allows improved spectral decomposition. Lastly, the average temporal dissociation between the 2 acquisitions in the z axis is around 0.08 second, which excludes major patient movement between the acquisitions.

Principles of DE Imaging

X-ray matter interactions in the diagnostic imaging range are dominated by the photoelectric and the Compton effects. The predominance of these 2 effects varies with the energy of the X-ray beam and the physical composition of the organs or lesions to be imaged. For example, iodine, calcium, or any other element with a high atomic number has a predominant photoelectric interaction at high tube voltages. As opposed to single-energy imaging, which results in an anatomic depiction of the imaged area based on the spatial distribution of object attenuation, DECT is sensitive to the object's chemical composition.[3] Consequently, DECT will be able to separate materials with different atomic numbers, despite similar attenuation coefficients. Whereas air, tissues, liquids, and fat have almost similar coefficient attenuation values at 80 and 140 kV(p) and thus, no possibility of specific recognition with DE, it is possible to distinguish between iodine and calcium by their different absorptiometric characteristics at low and high kilovoltages.

Similarly, the injection or inhalation of substances with high atomic numbers, such as iodine ($Z = 53$), xenon ($Z = 54$), or krypton ($Z = 36$), that are not always detectable with single-energy because of suboptimal levels of enhancement, can allow depiction and quantification of perfusion or ventilation abnormalities by means of the contrast agent absorptiometric characteristics at DECT. The clinical relevance of this scanning mode is the possibility of detecting functional alterations in the absence of morphologic or densitometric abnormalities on single-energy CT scans. Besides this technical approach based on

the "three-material decomposition" principle, there are other techniques available, such as the ρZ-projection that converts DE data to mass density and effective atomic number information. In an experimental study, Mahnken and colleagues[4] have demonstrated that this technique was suited to quantitatively assessing these parameters of ex-vivo body fluid samples and suggested that, in clinical routine, it might be useful for characterizing fluid collections even in enhanced CT.

RECONSTRUCTIONS OF DE DATA SETS

Three series of reconstructions can be generated from a DE data set. Firstly, the data delivered by detector A and detector B is reconstructed separately and analyzed independently. Secondly, the separate 80- and 140-kV(p) images can be fused and weighted images calculated. Both categories of reconstructions are made without the benefit of DE processing for material decomposition. Thirdly, it is possible to generate images based on the so-called three-material decomposition principle, which can be considered in specific clinical situations.

Fusion of Tube A and Tube B Images

To avoid separate analysis of 80-kV(p) and 140-kV(p) images, it is possible to fuse CT data sets of different tube energies into a unique blended data set with desirable properties. Important properties include high contrast and low noise, optimal lesion conspicuity, and artifact suppression.[5] According to the nomenclature used by Behrendt and colleagues,[6] a weighting factor of 0.0 results in 100% image information derived from the 140-kV(p) image and 0% information taken from the 80-kV(p) image. A weighting factor of 1.0 leads to the opposite, namely 100% image information from the 80-kV(p) image and 0% information from the 140-kV(p) image. The other weighting factors generate fused images between these 2 extremes; the weighting factor used for image fusion can be freely chosen. Because the enhancement of iodine is stronger at lower tube voltage settings, the consequence of using different weighting factors is a variable contrast enhancement of the fused images.[4,7,8] However, one should consider that high enhancement values are accompanied by streak artifacts caused by beam-hardening at the border of high-contrast areas, resulting in deficient detail accuracy and image quality. Such artifacts can, for example, mask small but clinically relevant calcifications or endoluminal defects in small vessels. For DECT angiographic examinations, the usual weighting factor is 0.4 which leads to creation of images resembling 120-kV(p) images with a reduction in noise compared with a single-source scan. They are obtained with a dedicated DE convolution kernel that draws 60% of the fused image from the 140-kV(p) image and 40% from the 80-kV(p) image (**Fig. 1**). Because the optimal weighting between image contrast and noise varies according to the amount, concentration, and rate of injection of contrast medium and with vessel diameters, further research is needed to optimize this parameter in the various categories of CT angiographic examinations obtained in routine clinical practice.

In the aforementioned fusion process, also called linear blending, there is a uniform application of a fixed weighting function for all pixels that reduces both noise and high signal. Nonlinear blending can be used to refine the process. The use of a modified sigmoid blending function strongly weighs the low Hounsfield unit (HU) values toward the 140-kV(p) image and the high HU values toward the 80–kV(p) image, with subsequent potential for improved contrast-to-noise ratio.[5] As underlined by physicists, one of the primary challenges is optimizing the selection of nonlinear blending parameters that may be organ-specific. From a practical standpoint, it should be emphasized that the "weighted average image" data set that results from combining the information from both tubes is reconstructed in real time at the CT-acquisition workstation and is subsequently available for clinical interpretation.

Material-Specific Imaging

Using material decomposition algorithms, it is possible to create separate material-specific images depicting the constituent materials of interest in the image volume.[3] From a practical standpoint, the user has to determine the idealized material triplet within the voxels of the examined anatomic region. If the substance of interest is iodine within lung parenchyma, it is assumed that the idealized material triplet necessary to apply to three-material decomposition is composed of iodine, air, and soft tissues. To generate images demonstrating the distribution of iodine alone, often called perfusion imaging, the images are created after selecting voxels of lung parenchyma by thresholding, subsequently excluding mediastinal structures and central pulmonary vessels in the lung parenchyma. If the user wants to analyze lung perfusion in normal lung parenchyma, that is, lung parenchyma devoid of any infiltrative process, the attenuation values of the final image range between −600 HU and −1000 HU (**Fig. 2**). However, the upper value of this HU selection has to be increased to −200 HU if the lung parenchyma shows features of mild infiltration, such as areas of ground glass attenuation. Vendor-supplied default parameters are used for low- and high-kV soft tissue densities, whereas air attenuation does not vary with the kilovoltage. If the substance of interest is iodine within mediastinal vessels, the new idealized material triplet is now composed of iodine, fat, and soft tissues. Similarly, the material decomposition algorithm allows creation of an iodine map of mediastinal structures that can be subtracted from the original contrast-enhanced images, thus creating a "virtual" unenhanced image, often called a "virtual noncontrast scan" (**Fig. 3**). Although mostly described for cervical[9,10] and cranial[11] CT angiographic examinations, it is also possible to exclude bone from a DE chest CT scan, a process called "virtual bone subtraction" or "dual-energy bone removal." In summary, the parameters that can be adjusted by the user are (a) the CT values of the input materials at low and high energies; (b) the threshold values for the evaluation (minimum and maximum HU values); and (c) the range which refers to the number of adjacent voxels used by the system for interpolation during

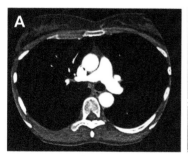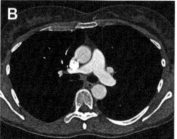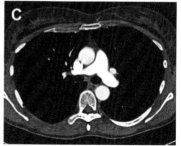

Fig. 1. Normal dual-energy CT angiogram obtained in a 35-year-old woman suspected of acute PE, illustrating the image quality of the diagnostic scans. (*A*) 80 kV(p) image. (*B*) 140 kV(p) image. (*C*) Weighted average image (0.4 weighting factor). Note the higher iodine conspicuity in (*A*) and decreased noise in (*C*).

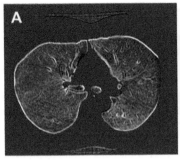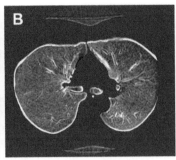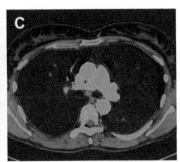

Fig. 2. Same patient as in **Fig. 1**, illustrating the 3 series of lung perfusion scans which can be generated from a given data set. (*A*) Native perfusion scan, 2-mm thick, obtained at the level of the upper lung zones. (*B*) Maximum intensity projection, 4-mm thick, obtained at the same level as (*A*). Note the more homogeneous appearance of lung perfusion compared with (*A*). Thin peripheral rim devoid of perfusion information in the left axillary region due to the small size of the tube B FOV on (*A*, *B*). (*C*) Fusion of the native perfusion scan and the mediastinal diagnostic scan, reconstructed with the same section thickness (2-mm thick) at the same anatomic level.

the calculation of the three-material decomposition.[12] All the aforementioned selections are defined once for each application and subsequently automatically provided by the workstation to allow simple clinical use. The material-specific data sets are volumetric and therefore can be evaluated as reconstructed axial images or processed by conventional 3-dimensional applications, such as multiplanar reconstruction, maximum intensity projection, and volume-rendered reformation.

CLINICAL APPLICATIONS

Thoracic applications of DE rely on the possibility of identifying contrast medium or specific tissue infiltration characterized by a high atomic number, which cannot be precisely detected with single energy CT.

Perfusion Imaging

On the basis of single-source CT, 2 approaches have been investigated for the detection of perfusion abnormalities, one using color-coded maps

of lung density in humans,[13–15] whereas other authors have investigated a subtraction technique using precontrast and postcontrast conventional CT images in experimental animal studies.[16,17] Although both approaches demonstrated the detectability of perfusion defects by CT, the feasibility of this approach in clinical practice has substantial limitations pertaining to scanning times and levels of radiation exposure. The availability of dual-source CT and the subsequent possibility of scanning patients with DE has offered another alternative for lung perfusion imaging.[18]

Technical approach of lung perfusion with DECT

Perfusion imaging is based on quantification of the enhancement in tissue and blood at certain time points following intravenous administration of contrast medium.[19] Consequently, lung perfusion with DECT does not correspond to blood flow analysis as such, because it represents a measurement at one time point only, but it provides an iodine map of the lung microcirculation. Within normal lung parenchyma, the iodine content of the

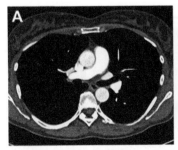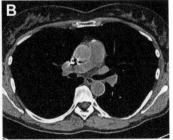

Fig. 3. Same patient as in **Fig. 1**, illustrating the possibility of creating a virtual noncontrast scan from a CT angiographic acquisition. (*A*) Weighted average image (0.4 weighting factor), obtained at the level of the right pulmonary artery. (*B*) After identification of iodine within mediastinal vessels, it is removed from the image, creating a virtual noncontrast image at the same anatomic level. Note the presence of streak artifacts within the superior vena cava that cannot be subtracted.

capillary bed can be assimilated into the "parenchymographic" phase of a conventional or digital angiogram. There are numerous parameters known to influence the iodine distribution within pulmonary capillaries. Some are technically related, whereas others are linked to the anatomic or physiologic circumstances of data acquisition. The enhancement within lung microvessels depends on the volume and flow rate of the contrast agent administered and on the contrast medium administration site: a peripheral vein, a central venous catheter with its extremity positioned at the level of the superior vena cava, or a right-sided cardiac cavity. Moreover, all the anatomic structures through which the iodinated contrast agent courses above and below the pulmonary capillary level, involving the systemic venous return, the right side of the heart, the large pulmonary arteries and veins, the left side of the heart, the aorta, and peripheral arteries, will affect the iodine distribution within lung microcirculation.[20] One should not underestimate the influence of the systemic arterial circulation in the analysis of the iodine content of pulmonary microvessels. Because of its role in collateral supply and the numerous anastomoses within the pulmonary circulation, the systemic circulation can compensate for, or create functional obstacles to, the pulmonary blood flow and thus, modify the iodine content within pulmonary capillaries. The anatomic status of the lung parenchyma needs to be integrated; for example, an atelectatic lung zone remains perfused, but less than within normally ventilated areas. Lastly, there are also some physiologic changes in lung perfusion to integrate into its final interpretation, such as the considerable reduction in the pulmonary capillary bed beyond the age of 60.

The authors' experience in lung perfusion is mainly derived from DECT angiographic examinations indicated in the clinical setting of acute pulmonary embolism (PE).[2] The tube voltages are set at 140 kV (tube A) and 80, (tube B), with the 80-kV tube current adjusted to 6 times the 140-kV tube, that is, 330 as compared with 50 mAs to compensate for the lower photon output at the lower voltage. Collimation is 32 × 0.6 mm with the z-flying focal spot, enabling reconstruction of 64 slices per rotation; the gantry rotation time is 0.33 seconds, with a pitch of 0.5. Because analysis of small-sized vessels is more accurately obtained on 1-mm thick scans, the 0.6 mm collimation is routinely chosen over the 1.2 mm. The acquisitions are done from top to bottom of the chest with an injection protocol similar to that of a standard CT angiogram obtained with single energy on a similar 64-slice CT scanner (120 mL of a 35% contrast

agent; flow rate: 4 mL/s). The scan is initiated by bolus tracking within the ascending aorta, with a threshold of 100 HU to trigger data acquisition. The examinations are systematically obtained with an automatic angular (x, y) modulation of the milliamperage. Two categories of images are routinely reconstructed: "diagnostic scans" and "lung perfusion scans." Diagnostic scans correspond to contiguous 1-mm thick transverse CT scans, generated from the raw spiral projection data of tube A and tube B, with a weighting factor of 0.4, viewed at lung and mediastinal window settings. Lung perfusion scans are generated after determination of the iodine content of every voxel of the lung parenchyma on the separate 80- and 140-kV(p) images. Three series of images can be created, including native perfusion scans, maximum intensity projections (MIPs) of lung perfusion, and fused images of native perfusion scans and diagnostic scans. Native perfusion scans and MIP images of lung perfusion can be generated as grayscale or color-coded images. All generated images can be displayed as transverse scans, completed, whenever necessary, by coronal and sagittal reformations. Each data set can also be used to generate virtual noncontrast images, useful for extracting iodine when searching for intramural or endoluminal calcifications of pulmonary arteries.

Indications

Even if DE acquisition does not correspond to true perfusion imaging, because it visualizes only blood volume and not blood flow, several advantages of this imaging technique can be highlighted. Compared to scintigraphy and magnetic resonance imaging (MRI), it is the only imaging modality able to provide high-quality morphologic analysis and functional information on the pulmonary circulation from the same data set, justifying the moderate increase in the overall radiation dose compared with single-source CT. It is the only technique allowing comparison of CT angiograms acquired at different energies in the same patient, at the same time point after contrast medium injection, and within strictly similar hemodynamic conditions. The possibility of reconstruction at intermediate energies (90 kV[p], 100 kV[p], 110 kV[p], 120 kV[p], and 130 kV[p]) enables one to obtain the best adapted spectral optimization. In cases of suboptimal arterial concentration of contrast medium, the low-energy acquisition enables one to generate images with increased vascular enhancement. Although this technique needs further validation, several applications of pulmonary micro-CT angiography can be suggested in the present conditions of DECT use.

Acute PE The first advantage of DECT is the ability to use the diagnostic information available from the tube B, set at 80 kV. As this tube voltage optimizes the contrast-to-noise ratio within pulmonary vessels,[21] it can help detect peripheral endoluminal clots, known to be better visualized than on images acquired at 120 or 140 kV. The diagnosis of acute PE can also benefit from perfusion scans on which it is possible to identify perfusion defects beyond obstructive clots.[2,22,23] Perfusion defects in the adjacent lung parenchyma have the typical triangular shape well known from pulmonary angiographic, scintigraphic, and MRI perfusion studies (Fig. 4). The usefulness of diagnostic and perfusion scans in acute PE has recently been investigated by Nunes and colleagues[24] In a study group of 30 consecutive patients with no underlying cardiorespiratory disease and in whom acute PE was diagnosed on dual-energy MDCT angiograms, these investigators have compared the diagnostic information of both series of images. Diagnostic scans identified peripheral endoluminal clots in 25.5% of segments, whereas 74.5% of segments showed no endoluminal abnormalities. Perfusion scans identified perfusion defects in 57% of the segments with endoluminal clots, beyond obstructive and nonobstructive clots, and normal results in the remaining 43% with endoluminal clots, although they identified embolic-type perfusion defects in 4% of the segments without endovascular abnormalities. These results demonstrate an obvious diagnostic complementarity between the 2 series of images,

in agreement with the results recently reported by Thieme and colleagues.[22]

Regarding pulmonary emboli in general, including obstructive and nonobstructive clots, the diagnostic accuracy of perfusion scans was limited, having only 58% sensitivity and 92% specificity. A homogeneous contrast distribution had a negative predictive value for PE of 93.9%. Depiction of PE-type defects on perfusion scans could help improve the depiction of peripheral acute PE, reported as an unsuspected finding in 6% of unselected inpatients referred for CT angiographic examinations.[25] DECT can also help differentiate lung infarction from nonspecific peripheral lung consolidation, sometimes mimicking a Hampton bump. The iodine map can also be used as an additional parameter in the assessment of pulmonary artery obstruction score in the clinical context of acute PE.[24]

Chronic PE Similar to what is achievable for acute PE, DECT angiography can allow depiction of perfusion defects beyond chronic clots (Fig. 5). Four vascular characteristics of chronic PE can benefit from DECT. Firstly, chronic PE is responsible for a mosaic pattern of lung attenuation, characterized by areas of ground glass attenuation with enlarged vascular sections, intermingled with areas of normal lung attenuation and smaller vascular sections. When present, these findings are highly suggestive of redistribution of blood flow; however, they are not systematically observed in chronic PE. In such circumstances,

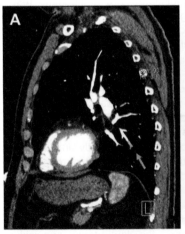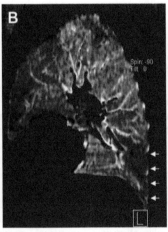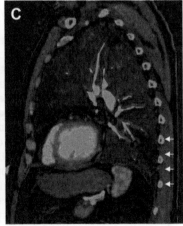

Fig. 4. Referral of 53-year-old man for clinical suspicion of acute PE. (A) Sagittal diagnostic image at the level of the left hemithorax, showing an obstructive endoluminal clot within the posterior segmental artery of the left lower lobe (arrow). (B) Maximum intensity projection. (C) Fused image of native perfusion and diagnostic scans, obtained at the same level as (A), showing a triangular, peripheral perfusion defect beyond the obstructive clot in the left lower lobe (arrows). Note the additional presence of hypoperfused areas in the anterior and apical regions, secondary to the presence of multiple endoluminal clots.

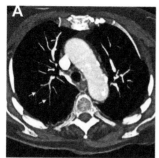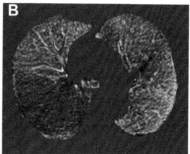

Fig. 5. Referral of 85-year-old woman for worsening of dyspnea in the context of chronic thromboembolic disease. (A) Maximum intensity projection generated from the weighted average data set at the level of the upper lung zones. Note the presence of severely stenosed pulmonary arterial branches in the posterior segment of the right upper lobe (arrows). (B) Native perfusion scan at the same anatomic level showing a perfusion defect in the posterior segment of the right upper lobe.

DECT has the potential to recognize ground glass attenuation of vascular origin by means of the high iodine content within the areas of ground glass attenuation, thus allowing it to be distinguished from ground glass attenuation secondary to abnormal filling of the airspaces as observed in various infiltrative lung diseases.[26] Secondly, chronic PE can lead to the development of calcifications within partially or completely occlusive chronic clots and within pulmonary artery walls, when chronic PE is complicated by longstanding or severe pulmonary hypertension. Such calcifications can be detected by means of virtual noncontrast imaging, always accessible from DECT data sets. Thirdly, the images generated at 80 kV can be used to improve the visualization of the systemic collateral supply present in chronic PE, originating from bronchial and nonbronchial systemic arteries. Lastly, it is possible to demonstrate links between the severity of pulmonary arterial obstruction, development of systemic collateral supply, and perfusion impairment in chronic PE.[27]

Other pulmonary vascular disorders When a patient is referred for pulmonary hypertension of unknown origin, CT plays an important role owing to its ability to evaluate noninvasively central and peripheral pulmonary arteries. Three conditions share a heterogeneous spatial distribution of the underlying vascular lesions: chronic PE, pulmonary veno-occlusive disease, and pulmonary capillary hemangiomatosis. Pathologic reports indicate dilated alveolar capillaries in pulmonary veno-occlusive disease and proliferation of capillaries within alveolar walls in pulmonary capillary hemangiomatosis. Such capillary proliferation can lead to ground glass opacity in diffuse, geographic, mosaic, perihilar, patchy, or centrilobular patterns.[28] Reports from pulmonary arteriographic and perfusion scintigraphic findings have already documented these peripheral vascular lesions,[29,30] which are likely to be detectable using DECT angiography.

Pretherapeutic and follow-up studies of pulmonary arteriovenous malformations can also be obtained with DECT. One objective is to improve the detection of small-sized pulmonary arterial branches that may supply the malformation, which, once recognized, may lead to consideration of the malformation with a complex rather than simple angioarchitecture. Depending on the complexity of the malformation, this finding may be a strong argument for reconsidering the therapeutic option and choosing surgery instead of embolotherapy. The second objective is to obtain an optimized depiction of small-sized systemic arteries that can supply the aneurysm before treatment or that may develop after occlusion of the pulmonary artery or arteries feeding the malformation. Because of the small diameter of the aforementioned arteries, reconstruction of images with various weighing factors can be useful, especially those considering a high percentage of 80 kV. In the long-term follow-up of successful embolization procedures, the organized thrombus around deposited coils and its potential recanalization could also benefit from DECT acquisitions.

Obstructive airway diseases Chronic obstructive pulmonary disease (COPD) is defined by irreversible airflow limitation, with variable contributions of airway obstruction and parenchymal destruction. High-resolution CT (HRCT) is currently the method of choice for the noninvasive assessment of emphysema and has been shown to correlate well with the pathology.[31,32] Because the severity of lung destruction and the distribution of lung perfusion determine the functional consequences of emphysematous changes, much attention has been given to the analysis of lung perfusion alterations in COPD patients. To date, this functional information in COPD patients has been approached noninvasively by perfusion scintigraphy, single photon emission CT (SPECT), and MR. Lung perfusion scintigraphy has been specifically used to evaluate patients with severe emphysema who were candidates for lung volume reduction surgery.[33–36] Although this technique can provide information on the perfusion pattern in patients with severe emphysema, it suffers from low spatial resolution. SPECT has the potential for superior evaluation but it is rarely used because it is time consuming and not widely available.[37,38] MRI seem to be a more promising technique because of its high diagnostic accuracy in the detection of perfusion abnormalities and the ability to provide lobar and segmental analysis of perfusion defects.[39–41] However, none of these techniques can assess lung morphologic changes that remain based on HRCT images. Therefore, matching lung destruction and impaired pulmonary perfusion requires a combination of morphologic and functional information or creation of fusion images with an additional modality.

The advent of DECT technology offers the possibility of a simultaneous approach of structure and function in respiratory patients, which has been recently applied to the evaluation of pulmonary perfusion in smokers. Investigating 47 smokers with differing severity of airway obstruction, Pansini and colleagues[42] have shown that regional alterations of lung perfusion can be depicted by DECT in patients with predominant emphysema matching parenchymal destruction (Fig. 6). Apart from destructive changes, perfusion alterations in smokers can also be linked to pulmonary vascular remodeling caused by cigarette smoke products, which has been identified at an early stage of the disease.[43] This functional evaluation of emphysema is achievable at a lobar level,[42] similar to that reported for morphologic analysis on 3-dimensional HRCT.[44] Further evaluation of DECT is required after implementation of the most recent technological advances expected to allow reduction of artifacts, better temporal resolution, and improved spectral characterization for quantifying the amount of iodine within the pulmonary microcirculation. In such technical conditions, it is likely that DECT will be superior to the association of HRCT and MR perfusion aimed at reaching similar objectives.[40]

Ventilation Imaging

In clinical practice, pulmonary function tests are routinely used to assess lung function, providing global measurements of airflow, lung volumes, and gas exchange from which are inferred primary structural and functional alterations. However, they cannot approach regional changes, which has engendered much interest in the combined structural and functional approach accessible to DECT. The high atomic number of xenon has raised immediate interest in this contrast agent for regional assessment of lung function, otherwise and previously used to generate ventilation studies in animals and healthy human volunteers with single-energy CT.[45–54]

The first clinical experience with xenon ventilation at DECT has recently been reported by Chae and colleagues[55] (Fig. 7). Investigating 8 healthy volunteers and 4 patients with chronic obstructive lung diseases, these investigators were able

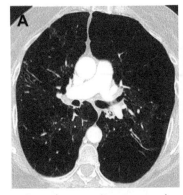 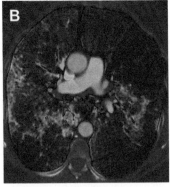

Fig. 6. Chronic obstructive pulmonary disease secondary to cigarette consumption in 68-year-old man. (A) 1-mm thick, weighted average image (0.4 weighting factor) of the lung parenchyma showing extensive emphysematous destruction in the upper lobes, more pronounced on the left side. (B) Fused image of the native perfusion scan and the mediastinal diagnostic scan at the same level as (A), illustrating the matching of areas of marked hypoattenuation on the perfusion image and areas of severe emphysematous changes on the diagnostic image on both sides.

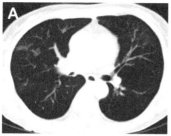 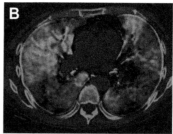

Fig. 7. Severe dyspnea in the context of bronchiolitis obliterans secondary to bone marrow transplantation in 51-year-old woman (A) 3-mm thick, weighted average image of the lung parenchyma, showing a mosaic pattern of lung attenuation on both sides. (B) On color-coded xenon map, there are multifocal areas showing decreased xenon enhancement (ventilation defects) in both lungs. Most of ventilation defects are matched with low attenuation areas on the diagnostic scan. (Courtesy of Joon Beom Seo, MD, PhD, Seoul, South Korea.)

to directly visualize the degree of enhancement caused by xenon in the lung parenchyma, by performing material differentiation without additional unenhanced acquisitions. From a practical standpoint, the subjects were asked to inhale a high concentration (66%) of oxygen for 3 minutes before inhaling a mixture of 30% xenon and 70% oxygen for 1.5 minutes. The CT protocol included 1 unenhanced and 9 xenon-enhanced scans over the carina, which were obtained during the wash-in and washout phases, completed by a single acquisition over the entire thorax at the end of xenon inhalation. Healthy volunteers showed homogeneous enhancement throughout the lung with an average maximum degree of xenon enhancement of 23.78 HU, whereas multiple ventilation defects were seen in the 4 patients.

Although the investigators demonstrated the feasibility of such approaches, their approach suffers from several limitations. The first deals with the high radiation exposure of this protocol. The mean of total DLP of dynamic scanning was 540.7 mGy.cm for adult subjects and 123.5 mGy.cm for pediatric subjects, whereas the acquisition of the entire thorax was 233.3 mGy.cm and 60.5 mGy.cm for adult and pediatric subjects, respectively. Moreover, they experienced side effects of xenon which is soluble in blood and tissue. The evaluation failed in two of the 12 subjects included in this study who reported having an uncomfortable feeling at the end of the wash-in period, namely abnormal resistance in respiration. This is not surprising because one of the major adverse effects of xenon is respiratory depression. To avoid these complications, one could consider the mixture of xenon and krypton already proposed for ventilation studies with single-energy CT[56] or the replacement of xenon by stable krypton, which has none of the unwanted side effects. Moreover, single-breath techniques should also be reconsidered for ventilation studies, because they minimize radiation dose and are applicable to high-speed volumetric DE scanning. As opposed to multibreath washout or wash-in studies that provide information regarding the regional distribution of pulmonary ventilation under dynamic or tidal breathing conditions, the single-breath approach can only provide information of ventilation under static conditions.[53] Despite obvious interest in this new method, ethical considerations on the patient's radiation exposure should temper the use of DECT in children for investigating well-known pathophysiological conditions, such as collateral ventilation in bronchial atresia.[57]

DE in the Evaluation of Pulmonary Nodules

Before the advent of the current DECT technology, the utility of DE in the recognition of calcified lung nodules had been investigated by comparing the information of 2 successive single-source CT acquisitions, obtained at 80 kV and 140 kV, respectively.[58] This dual-kV(p) analysis did not appear to be helpful in the identification of benign lung nodules in the studied population, partly because the median increase in mean CT nodule attenuation measurement from 140 to 80 kV(p) images was very low and because nearly 10% of malignant nodules also contain calcifications. Despite these mitigated preliminary results, further investigations have been undertaken with dual-source CT, aimed at taking advantage of this technology in the diagnostic approach of solitary lung nodules.

One application is providing a virtual nonenhanced and an iodine-enhanced image from a single scanning after iodine contrast material injection, by material differentiation of iodine. If one is able to detect calcification on a virtual nonenhanced image and directly measure the iodine component on an iodine-enhanced image, this technique may prevent additional nonenhanced scanning and the patient's radiation exposure will be reduced. This objective was recently evaluated by Chae and colleagues[59] who demon-strated that the iodine component could be successfully differentiated from the enhanced soft tissue. With regard to the detection of calcifi-cations, the investigators reported that most of the calcifications in nodules and lymph nodes were detected on virtual nonenhanced image. However, a limited proportion of calcifications (6.2%) were not depicted because, during material decomposition, the signal is lowered because part of the calcium is moved to the iodine image. Obscured calcifications on enhanced weighted average image were detected on virtual nonen-hanced image, suggesting that this image could be helpful when high attenuation is equivocal on an enhanced CT image. The investigators compared the CT numbers between virtual and real images and showed reliable concurrence between CT numbers on nonenhanced weighted average image and virtual nonenhanced image and between CT numbers on iodine-enhanced image and degree of enhancement (the latter being calculated as the difference in CT numbers on enhanced weighted average image and nonen-hanced weighted average image). These results suggest that DECT can provide information on the degree of enhancement from a single data set whereas 2 successive scans are necessary with single-energy CT.

In addition to the reduction in radiation expo-sure, this approach may also reduce measurement errors because of different positioning of the region of interest on the serial images of dynamic scanning, thus providing more precise information on the degree of vascularization within the nodule. However, this technique can only be applied to lung nodules covered by the 2-detector systems, namely nodules located inside the FOV of the smaller detector. Although each tube has 24 rows of 1.2 mm, the investigators recommend using only some of them (14 × 1.2 mm) to allow for an improved scatter-correction by using the outer rows. In summary, the diagnostic benefits of DE as applied to lung nodules do not seem as spectacular as those encountered with perfusion imaging. However, one might expect a potential role of this technique in monitoring the transit of iodinated contrast material to improve evaluation of tumoral angiogenesis.

Diffuse and Focal Hyperdense Thoracic Diseases

Lung parenchymal hyperdense disorders
Attenuation higher than muscle seen as dense diffuse pulmonary opacities can be due to calcium deposits in pulmonary metastatic calcification and

pulmonary alveolar microlithiasis,[60] iodine accu-mulation in amiodarone lung toxicity, or inhalation or intravenous administration of materials with high atomic numbers, such as talcum powder deposition in talcosis.[61] When the underlying disease is known, the nature of the hyperdense material can be deduced. Conversely, the cause of the hyperdense infiltration has to be investi-gated, and this can be done with DECT. Because of the smaller tube-B FOV, switching the kV(p) of the 2 tubes and obtaining the 80 kV(p) examination at low energy with the largest FOV is recommen-ded for evaluating all hyperdense parenchymal lesions, including the most peripheral ones.

Hilar hyperdense lesions
Imaging of occupational or environmental respira-tory diseases must include depiction of lung parenchymal changes and careful analysis of mediastinal and hilar lymph nodes. When they reach the bronchioloalveolar level, inhaled particles are phagocytosed by bronchoalveolar macrophages. Most bronchoalveolar macro-phages migrate up the ciliary elevator, whereas some of them migrate into lymphatics to flow to hilar lymph nodes.[62] They can then remain confined within lymph nodes or migrate toward the systemic venous return. The concentration of particles can be higher within lymph nodes than within the lung parenchyma,[63] explaining why CT can depict them as hyperattenuating structures simulating calcifications within normal-sized or enlarged lymph nodes.[64,65] In case of inhaled particles of high atomic numbers, DECT could provide structural information on the mineral content of hyperattenuating lymph nodes. Among professional exposures to agents with high atomic numbers, one should think of dental laboratory technicians potentially exposed to inhalation of chromium, molybdenum, cobalt, and tungsten; aluminium workers; and mica- and talc-exposed workers. The difficulty of DE imaging of hyperatte-nuating lymph nodes in exposed workers is mainly linked to the differences in mineralogic composi-tion of the inhaled dust, varying according to their geographic origin. Were this difficulty to be over-come, DECT could attempt to define relationships between lymph node characteristics and paren-chymal lung alterations secondary to specific occupational exposures.[66,67]

SUMMARY

The introduction of DECT is changing the noninva-sive approach to management of chest disorders by adding functional assessment to high-spatial and high-resolution diagnostic imaging. To date, the most investigated application has been iodine mapping at pulmonary CT angiography, often called lung perfusion imaging. The material decomposition achievable with this technology opens up new options for recognizing substances poorly characterized with single-energy CT. Radiologists should also be aware of the opportunities and challenges of developing new functional imaging biomarkers and contrast agents applicable to this new imaging modality. The experience reported in the literature over the last 3 years has been exclusively limited to DE imaging using dual-source CT technology. However, radiologists should follow alternative technological approaches currently under development.

REFERENCES

1. Johnson TR, Krauss B, Sedlmair M, et al. Material differentiation by dual energy CT: initial experience. Eur Radiol 2007;17:1510–7.

2. Pontana F, Faivre JB, Remy-Jardin M, et al. Lung perfusion with dual-energy multidetector-row CT (MDCT): feasibility for the evaluation of acute pulmonary embolism in 117 consecutive patients. Acad Radiol 2008;15:1494–504.

3. Petersilka M, Bruder H, Krauss B, et al. Technical principles of dual source CT. Eur J Radiol 2008;68: 362–8.

4. Mahnken AH, Stanzel S, Hiesmann B. Spectral ρZ-projection method for characterization of body fluids in computed tomography: ex-vivo experiments. Acad Radiol 2009;16:763–9.

5. Holmes DR III, Fletcher JG, Apel A, et al. Evaluation of non-linear blending in dual-energy computed tomography. Eur J Radiol 2008;68:409–13.

6. Behrendt FF, Schmidt B, Plumhans C, et al. Image fusion in dual energy computed tomography. Effect on contrast enhancement, signal-to-noise ratio and image quality in computed tomography angiography. Invest Radiol 2009;44:1–6.

7. Nakayama Y, Awai K, Funama Y, et al. Abdominal CT with low tube voltage: preliminary observations about radiation dose, contrast enhancement, image quality and noise. Radiology 2005;237: 945–51.

8. Szucks-Farkas Z, Verdun FR, von Allmen G, et al. Effect of X-ray tube parameters, iodine concentration, and patient size on image quality in pulmonary computed tomography angiography: a chest-phantom-study. Invest Radiol 2008;43:374–81.

9. Watanabe Y, Uotani K, Nakazawa T, et al. Dual-energy direct bone removal CT angiography for evaluation of intracranial aneurysm or stenosis: comparison with conventional digital substraction angiography. Eur Radiol 2009;19:1019–24.

10. Lell MM, Kramer M, Klotz E, et al. Carotid computed tomography angiography with automated bone suppression. A comparative study between dual energy and bone subtraction techniques. Invest Radiol 2009;44:322–7.

11. Morhard D, Fink C, Graser A, et al. Cervical and cranial computed tomographic angiography with automated bone removal. Dual energy computed tomography versus standard computed tomography. Invest Radiol 2009;44:293–7.

12. Godoy MC, Naidich DP, Marchiori E, et al. Basic principles and postprocessing techniques of dual-energy CT: illustrated by selected congenital abnormalities of the thorax. J Thorac Imaging 2009;24: 152–9.

13. Wildberger JE, Niethammer MU, Klotz E, et al. Multislice CT for visualization of pulmonary embolism using perfusion weighted color maps. Röfo 2001; 173:289–94.

14. Herzog P, Wildberger JE, Niethammer MU, et al. CT perfusion imaging of the lung in pulmonary embolism. Acad Radiol 2003;10:1132–46.

15. Coulden RA, Brown SJ, Clements L, et al. Mosaic perfusion in pulmonary hypertension: how does multislice CT compare with perfusion scintigraphy? Radiology 2000;217:S384–5.

16. Screaton NJ, Coxson HO, Kalloger SE, et al. Detection of lung perfusion abnormalities using computed tomography in a porcine model of pulmonary embolism. J Thorac Imaging 2003;18:14–20.

17. Wildberger JE, Klotz E, Ditt H, et al. Multislice computed tomography perfusion imaging for visualization of acute pulmonary embolism: animal experience. Eur Radiol 2005;15:1378–86.

18. Klotz E, Remy J, Pontana F, et al. Lung perfusion. In: Remy-Jardin M, Remy J, editors. Integrated cardiothoracic imaging with MDCT. 1st edition. Berlin: Springer; 2009. p. 363–78.

19. Miles KA. Perfusion imaging with computed tomography: brain and beyond. Eur Radiol 2006; 16(Suppl 7):M37–43.

20. Gil J, Ciurea D. Functional structure of the pulmonary circulation. In: Peacock AJ, editor. Pulmonary circulation. A handbook for clinicians. London: Chapman and Hall Medical; 1996. p. 1–11.

21. Gorgos A, Remy-Jardin M, Tacelli N, et al. Evaluation of peripheral pulmonary arteries at 80 kV and at 140 kV: dual-energy CT assessment in 40 patients. J Comput Assist Tomogr 2009, in press.

22. Thieme SF, Johnson TR, Lee C, et al. Dual-energy CT for assessment of contrast material distribution in the pulmonary parenchyma. AJR Am J Roentgenol 2009;193:144–9.

23. Zhang LJ, Zhao YE, Wu SY, et al. Pulmonary embolism detection with dual-energy CT. Experimental study of dual-source CT in rabbits. Radiology 2009;52:61–70.

24. Nunes G, Remy-Jardin M, Faivre JB, et al. Evaluation of acute pulmonary embolism with dual-energy

CT: respective usefulness of morphologic and functional information [abstract]. French Society of Radiology, Paris, October 2009.

25. Ritchie G, McGurk S, McCreath C, et al. Prospective evaluation of unsuspected pulmonary embolism on contrast enhanced multidetector CT (MDCT) scanning. Thorax 2007;62:536–40.

26. Pontana F, Faivre JB, Remy-Jardin M, et al. Lung perfusion with dual-energy multidetector-row CT (MDCT): can it help recognize ground-glass opacities (GCO) of vascular origin? Radiology SSC 06-05. [abstract]. 2008;337–8.

27. Renard B, Faivre JB, Remy-Jardin M, et al. Dual-energy CT angiography of chronic thromboembolic disease: can it help recognize links between the severity of pulmonary arterial obstruction and perfusion defects? [abstract no. SSQ04–03] Radiological Society of North America, Chicago November 2009.

28. Ito K, Tchiki T, Ohi K, et al. Pulmonary capillary hemangiomatosis with severe pulmonary hypertension. Circ J 2003;67:793–5.

29. Frazier AA, Franks TJ, Mohammed TLH, et al. Pulmonary veno-occlusive disease and pulmonary capillary hemangiomatosis. Radiographics 2007;27:867–82.

30. Lippert JL, White CS, Cameron EW, et al. Pulmonary capillary hemangiomatosis: radiographic appearance. J Thorac Imaging 1998;13:49–51.

31. Gevenois PA, De Vuyst P, de Martelaere V, et al. Comparison of computed density and microscopic morphometry in pulmonary emphysema. Am J Respir Crit Care Med 1996;154:187–92.

32. Newell JD Jr, Hogg JC, Snider GL. Report of a workshop: quantitative computed tomography scanning in longitudinal studies of emphysema. Eur Respir J 2004;23:769–75.

33. Thurnheer R, Engel H, Weder W, et al. Role of perfusion scintigraphy in relation to chest computed tomography and pulmonary function in the evaluation of candidates for lung volume reduction surgery. Am J Respir Crit Care Med 1999;159:301–10.

34. Claverley JR, Desai SR, Wells AU, et al. Evaluation of patients undergoing lung volume reduction surgery: ancillary information available from computed tomography. Clin Radiol 2000;55:45–50.

35. Cerderlund K, Höberg S, Jorfeldt L, et al. Lung perfusion scintigraphy prior to lung volume reduction surgery. Acta Radiol 2003;44:246–51.

36. Washko GR, Reilly JJ. Radiographic evaluation of the potential lung volume reduction surgery candidate. Proc Am Thorac Soc 2008;5:421–6.

37. Fujita E, Nagasaka Y, Kozuka T, et al. Correlation among the indices of high-resolution computed tomography, pulmonary function tests, pulmonary perfusion scans and exercise tolerance in cases of chronic pulmonary emphysema. Respiration 2002; 69:30–7.

38. Suga K, Kawakami Y, Iwanaga H, et al. Assessment of anatomic relation between pulmonary perfusion and morphology in pulmonary emphysema with breath-hold SPECT-CT fusion images. Ann Nucl Med 2008;22:339–47.

39. Fink C, Puderbach M, Bock M, et al. Regional lung perfusion: assessment with partially parallel three-dimensional MR imaging. Radiology 2004;231: 175–84.

40. Ley-Zaporozhan J, Ley S, Eberhardt R, et al. Assessment of the relationship between lung parenchymal destruction and impaired pulmonary perfusion on a lobar level with emphysema. Eur J Radiol 2007;63:76–83.

41. Jang YM, Oh YM, Seo JB, et al. Quantitatively assessed dynamic contrast-enhanced magnetic resonance imaging in patients with chronic obstructive pulmonary disease: correlation of perfusion parameters with pulmonary function test and quantitative computed tomography. Invest Radiol 2008;43: 403–10.

42. Pansini V, Remy-Jardin M, Faivre JB, et al. Assessment of lobar perfusion in smokers according to the presence and severity of emphysema: preliminary experience with dual-energy CT angiography. Eur Radiol 2009 [Epub ahead of print].

43. Peinado VI, Pizarro S, Barbera JA. Pulmonary vascular involvement in COPD. Chest 2008;134:808–14.

44. Revel MP, Faivre JB, Remy-Jardin M, et al. Automated lobar quantification of emphysema in patients with severe COPD. Eur Radiol 2008;18:2723–30.

45. Gur D, Drayer BP, Borovetz HS, et al. Dynamic computed tomography of the lung: regional ventilation measurements. J Comput Assist Tomogr 1979; 3:749–53.

46. Chon D, Simon BA, Beck KC, et al. Differences in regional wash-in and wash-out time constants for xenon-ventilation studies. Respir Physiol Neurobiol 2005;148:65–83.

47. Gur D, Shabason L, Borovetz HS, et al. Regional pulmonary ventilation measurements by xenon enhanced dynamic computed tomography: an update. J Comput Assist Tomogr 1981;5:678–83.

48. Herbert DL, Gur D, Shabason L, et al. Mapping of human local pulmonary ventilation by xenon enhanced computed tomography. J Comput Assist Tomogr 1982;6:1088–93.

49. Kreck TC, Krueger MA, Altemeier WA, et al. Determination of regional ventilation and perfusion in the lung using xenon and computed tomography. J Appl Physiol 2001;91:1741–9.

50. Marcucci C, Nyhan D, Simon BA. Distribution of pulmonary ventilation using Xe-enhanced computed tomography in prone and supine dogs. J Appl Physiol 2001;90:421–30.

51. Murphy DM, Niecewicz JT, Zabbatino SM, et al. Local pulmonary ventilation using nonradioactive

xenon-enhanced ultrafast computed tomography. Chest 1989;96:799–804.

52. Robertson HT, Kreck TC, Krueger MA. The spatial and temporal heterogeneity of regional ventilation: comparison of measurements by two high-resolution methods. Respir Physiol Neurobiol 2005;148:85–95.

53. Tajik JK, Chon D, Won C, et al. Subsecond multisection CT of regional pulmonary ventilation. Acad Radiol 2002;9:130–46.

54. Simon BA. Regional ventilation and lung mechanics using x-ray CT. Acad Radiol 2005;12:1414–22.

55. Chae E, Seo J, Goo H, et al. Xenon ventilation CT using a dual-energy technique of dual-source CT: initial experience. Radiology 2008;248:615–24.

56. Chon D, Beck KC, Simon BA, et al. Effect of low-xenon and krypton supplementation on signal/noise of regional CT-based ventilation measurements. J Appl Physiol 2007;102:1535–44.

57. Goo HW, Chae EJ, Seo JB, et al. Xenon ventilation CT using a dual-source dual-energy technique: dynamic ventilation abnormality in a child with bronchial atresia. Pediatr Radiol 2008;38:1113–6.

58. Swensen SJ, Yamashita K, McCollough CH, et al. Lung nodules: dual-kilovolt peak analysis with CT-multicenter study. Radiology 2000;214:81–5.

59. Chae EJ, Song JW, Seo JB, et al. Clinical utility of dual-energy CT in the evaluation of solitary pulmonary nodules: initial experience. Radiology 2008;249: 671–81.

60. Marchiori E, Franquet T, Davaus Gasparetto T, et al. Consolidation with diffuse or focal high attenuation. J Thorac Imaging 2008;23:298–304.

61. Yoon HK, Moon HS, Park SH, et al. Dendriform pulmonary ossification in patient with rare earth pneumoconiosis. Thorax 2005;60:701–3.

62. Corry D, Kulkarni P, Lipscomb AF. The migration of bronchoalveolar macrophages into hilar lymph nodes. Am J Pathol 1984;115:321–8.

63. Sherson D, Maltbaek N, Heydorn K. A dental technician with pulmonary fibrosis: a case of chromium-cobalt alloy pneumoconiosis? Eur Respir J 1990;3: 1227–9.

64. Vahlensieck M, Overlack A, Müller KM. Computed tomographic high-attenuation mediastinal lymph nodes after aluminium exposition. Eur Radiol 2000;10: 1945–6.

65. Akira M, Kozuka T, Yamamoto S, et al. Inhalational talc pneumoconiosis: radiographic and CT findings in 14 patients. AJR Am J Roentgenol 2007;188: 326–33.

66. Ooi CG, Khong PL, Cheng RS, et al. The relationship between mediastinal lymph node attenuation with parenchymal lung parameters in silicosis. Int J Tuberc Lung Dis 2003;7: 1199–206.

67. Boroto K, Remy-Jardin M, Flohr T, et al. Thoracic applications of dual-source CT technology. Eur J Radiol 2008;68:375–84.

Index

Note: Page numbers of article titles are in **boldface** type.

Radiol Clin N Am 48 (2010) 207–212
doi:10.1016/S0033-8389(09)00206-1

Moving?

Make sure your subscription moves with you!

To notify us of your new address, find your **Clinics Account Number** (located on your mailing label above your name), and contact customer service at:

Email: journalscustomerservice-usa@elsevier.com

800-654-2452 (subscribers in the U.S. & Canada)
314-447-8871 (subscribers outside of the U.S. & Canada)

Fax number: 314-447-8029

Elsevier Health Sciences Division
Subscription Customer Service
3251 Riverport Lane
Maryland Heights, MO 63043

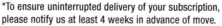

Printed and bound by CPI Group (UK) Ltd, Croydon, CR0 4YY

08/06/2025

01896875-0013